Advances in Neurosurgery 20

K. Piscol, M. Klinger, M. Brock (Eds.)

Neurosurgical Standards

Cerebral Aneurysms

Malignant Gliomas

With 164 Figures

Springer-Verlag
Berlin Heidelberg New York London Paris
Tokyo Hong Kong Barcelona Budapest

Proceedings of the 42th Annual Meeting
of the Deutsche Gesellschaft für Neurochirurgie
Bremen, May 5-8, 1991

Prof. Dr. Kurt Piscol
Neurochirurgische Klinik
Zentralkrankenhaus St.-Jürgen-Str.
W-2800 Bremen 1, FRG

Prof. Dr. Margareta Klinger
Neurochirurgische Klinik der Universität Erlangen-Nürnberg
Schwabachanlage 6 (Kopfklinikum), W-8520 Erlangen, FRG

Prof. Dr. Mario Brock
Neurochirurgische Klinik und Poliklinik
Universitätsklinikum Steglitz, Freie Universität Berlin
Hindenburgdamm 30, W-1000 Berlin 45, FRG

ISBN 3-540-54838-6 Springer-Verlag Berlin Heidelberg New York
ISBN 0-387-54838-6 Springer-Verlag New York Berlin Heidelberg

Library of Congress Cataloging-in-Publication Data. Neurosurgical standards, cerebral aneurysms, malignant gliomas / K. Piscol, M. Klinger, M. Brock (eds.). p. cm. – (Advances in neurosurgery; 20) "Proceedings of the 42th Annual Meeting of the Deutsche Gesellschaft für Neurochirurgie, Bremen, May 5-8, 1991" – T.p. verso. Includes bibliographical references and index.
ISBN 3-540-54838-6 (alk. paper). – ISBN 0-387-54838-6 (alk. paper)
1. Intracranial aneurysms–Surgery-Standards–Congresses. 2. Gliomas–Surgery–Standards-Congresses. I. Piscol, Kurt. II. Klinger, M. (Margareta), 1943– . III. Brock, M. (Mario), 1938– . IV. Deutsche Gesellschaft für Neurochirurgie. Tagung 42th: 1991 : Bremen, Germany. V. Series. [DNLM: 1. Cerebral Aneurysm–surgery–congresses. 2. Glioma–therapy–congresses. 3. Cerebral Aneruysm–surgery–congresses. 4. Glioma–therapy–congresses. 5. Neurosurgery–standards–congresses. W1 AD684N v.20] RD594.2.N48 1992 617.4'81–dc20 DNLM/DLC for Library of Congress 92-2145 CIP

Typesetting: Springer $\TeX$ in-house system

11/3130 - 5 4 3 2 1 0 – Printed on acid-free paper

Contents

Malignant Gliomas

Winning Poster and Lecture Presentations

List of Contributors

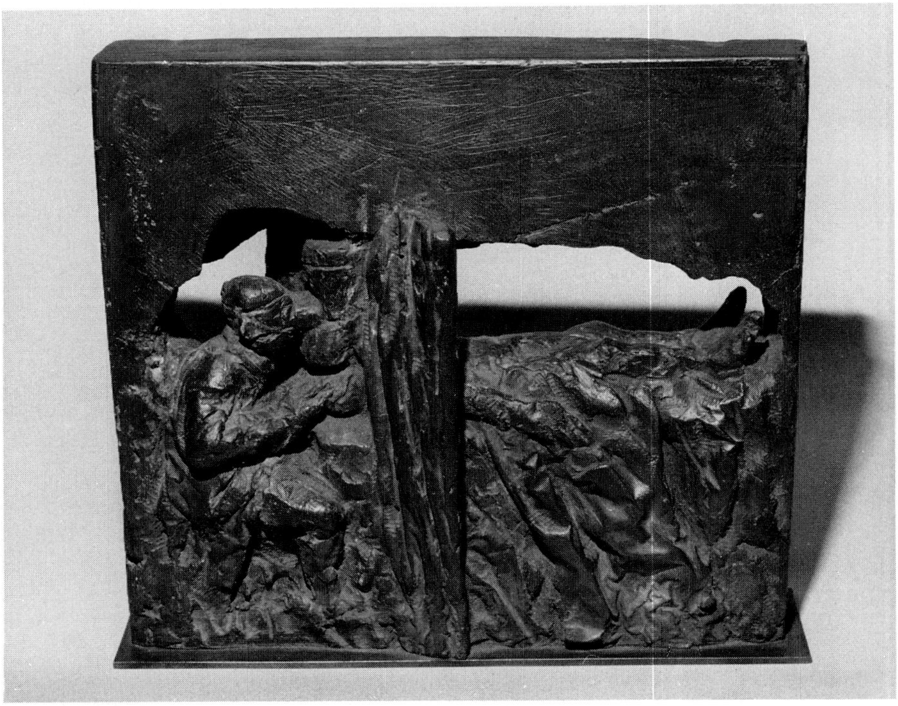

First Sculpture of a Neurosurgeon working with Microscope, created by the famous sculptor Prof. Bernd Altenstein, Academy of Arts Bremen, on the occasion of the 42nd Annual meeting of the German Society for Neurosurgery, Bremen: 5–8 May 1991. Bronze; 34.0 × 30.5 × 8.5 cm. Edition: 1–8 with number and signature (Information: Congress President)

President's Opening Remarks

K. Piscol[1]

Politics and Professional Competence

We recall how the United States of America struggled in its infancy with the selection of a suitable constitution. A major issue in this struggle was the choice between a democracy and a republic. Which model should be followed: that of old Athens, or the fresh ideas of the French Revolution? A key point of discussion was the franchise, for it related to people's right to have a voice. Can and will an itinerant worker make an electoral decision, especially one affecting regional issues, with the same interest and the same sense of responsibility as the informed resident who has a stake in establishing a well-functioning, stable community in the long term? While this question has been answered politically, it remains open philosophically. In any case, even then there was discussion at the national political level about the importance of competence.

I do not wish to be misunderstood. I see no alternative to open democracy and believe that it is the best available option, the best option for the *governing of a state!*

Mankind has undergone an arduous evolution from homo sapiens to homo ludens, having gradually freed itself from the exigencies of a mere creaturely existence. But this progress has imposed a new obligation: as a "zoon politikon," a political animal, man is obliged to develop appropriate rules for societal living, culminating in the modern ideal of universal emancipation. This development has become so generalized and prominent in present-day social awareness that we may lose sight of the fact that homo sapiens must also be homo faber, the skillful man, if humanity is to assert itself.

Can we take a proven, contemporary political principle and apply it to the professional realm? Politics deals with the satisfaction of general needs, while profession is concerned with meeting specific needs. Politics is intended to solve social problems, while professional activity is geared toward individual problems. The modern politician can and must be concerned with equality, the technical expert with specialty. I admit that these distinctions have their limits and that they overlap to a degree. Also, they should not lead to the grotesque characterization that the modern scientist knows more and more about less and less, until he knows everything about nothing, while the modern politician knows less and less about more and more, until finally he knows nothing about everything!

[1] Neurochirurgische Klinik, Zentralkrankenhaus, St.-Jürgen-Str., W–2800 Bremen 1, FRG.

Advances in Neurosurgery, Vol. 20
K. Piscol, M. Klinger, M. Brock (Eds.)

No one has denounced the results of professional overspecialization more vehemently than the extraparliamentary opposition of the 1960s, with their references to "expert idiots." But with due respect for their provocative and stimulating activities, they did our society a disservice. The term, originally applied as a critique for political asceticism, has unfortunately acquired its own dynamic which, at least in the Federal Republic of Germany, has done considerable harm. Subsequent generations developed with a paucity of scientific experts while cultivating a surfeit of "political idiots."

I address these questions not out of deep concern that this trend might permanently damage our society. I believe that the self-healing forces that are unleashed by practical reason and individual needs will ultimately prevail over the current notion that a smattering of knowledge bestows the right to exercise a general voice. My concern, rather, is that the incompetence of nonexperts will infuse needless difficulties and faulty decisions into the professional realm that will have to be accepted or compensated by the experts, with a danger of irreparable harm.

This problem is particularly impressive within the medical profession: When disease strikes, even the "zoon politikon" will call for the medical art and will seek the most competent authority who has mastered all facets of the specialty. Political issues are not a concern.

But the same "zoon politikon," while attending, say, a hospital board meeting, might very well denounce the medical authority as an "expert idiot" and dismiss him with the aid of an incompetent majority vote, all in the name of emancipation.

Democracy misplaced! This is the phenomenon that must be called into question, not only because it is misplaced in the professional realm, but also because it erodes respect for the reasonable underlying idea. I believe that politicians are ill advised when they seek forcibly to apply a national political principle to areas that must function by different principles in order to be effective. In particular, partisan political maneuvering must not become a driving force in these areas simply because resentful currents call for a dismantling of privileges born of professional competence. A society cannot tolerate such tendencies for long if it is to remain competitive. We have long witnessed the spectacle of political omnipresence in the USSR and the so-called people's democracies. The ruin of eastern state socialism was caused – at least in part – by this phenomenon.

Professional excellence should not merely be tolerated but, in a healthy society, should be encouraged as a goal worth striving for! Professional competence must be accorded its due, and it must be the decisive factor in discussions and decisions relating to the particular field.

Given present-day social conditions, this goal can be achieved only through common efforts. In specialist groups whose numbers are limited, such as the Deutsche Gesellschaft für Neurochirurgie (German Society for Neurosurgery) only a focusing of common interests can make our voice heard. This is the challenge that is placed before both our scientific society and our professional association. The articulation of legitimate demands should be permitted not just in panels and committees but also in forums of public interest, including our annual meetings.

Fedor Krause Memorial Lecture

The Influence of Researchers in the German Speaking World on the Development of Neurosurgery

Held at the presentation of the Fedor Krause Medal to Prof. Dr. Karl-August Bushe, Würzburg

Let me express my sincere appreciation for this honor, whose significance is apparent to me and which moves me deeply. Let me also include in this honor those who have gone with me a part of the way in the realization of our goals as neurosurgeons in Göttingen and in Würzburg. Two of them, Hans-Jochim Weber and Horst Wenker, team members in the initial phase, are no longer among us.

At this point my thoughts go especially to my academic teacher, Prof. Dr. Gerhard Okonek, a man of untiring strength with a sensitive nature, an excellent surgeon. Okonek was the oldest student of Wilhelm Tönnis in Würzburg and from 1937 the director and academic chief of neurosurgery in Göttingen. He died at the age of 54 years of a disease whose conquest had been his life's goal.

Die Wissenschaft ist ewig in ihrem Quell,
unermeßlich in ihrem Umfang,
endlos in ihrer Aufgabe,
unerreichbar in ihrem Ziel.

The source of science is eternal,
its extent is immeasurable,
its task unending,
its goal unattainable.

The significance of these words, uttered by the important nineteenth century natural scientist and anthropologist Karl-Ernst von Baer of Königsberg (1792–1876), became increasingly clear to me during the preparation of this lecture. The volume of material available was so enormous that I was forced to take a certain amount of liberty in my choice of contents. This choice was also influenced by the subjective evaluations of the respective scientists, as well as by sympathies for this or that researcher, aspects of local patriotism also playing a certain role.

The first scientific session of this neurosurgical meeting dealt with a difficult topic – the problem of neurosurgical standards. Neurosurgical standards represent the state of the art of our field at as high a level as possible. The present level of our field is not the result of present activities alone, but rather the result of achievements starting with the beginning of skull surgery and continuing up to the present modern state of brain research.

Who were the anatomists, surgeons, neurologists, psychiatrists, and physiologists whose innovative ideas and actions represent the bricks and stones in our present

Advances in Neurosurgery, Vol. 20
K. Piscol, M. Klinger, M. Brock (Eds.)

large building of neurosurgery? Their achievements have frequently been forgotten, or the originality of their discoveries has been attributed to others or been adopted by others, as I will show.

Wer nicht von dreitausend Jahren
sich weiß Rechenschaft zu geben
bleibt im Dunkeln unerfahren
mag von Tag zu Tage leben (Johann-Wolfgang von Goethe)

(Whoever fails to learn a lesson
from three thousand years
remains in darkness
doomed to live from day to day.)

The primitive methods of trepanation which were used 3000 years ago are very interesting, but will not be considered here because the first written descriptions in our standard surgical textbooks do not appear until towards the end of the Middle Ages in the German-speaking world.

Such important men as Hans von Gersdorf, Wilhelm Fabry von Hilden, Johannes Schulthes and Gottfried Purmann were not yet neurosurgeons in the present sense, but did develop the basis upon which modern techniques and scientifically oriented brain surgery could be founded. The demands of the victims of the battlefields on their skills made them into skilful surgeons, developers of innovative operative methods and inventive producers of instruments for skull operations.

Hans von Gersdorf, called Schylhans, from the Alsatian village of Görsdorf, a surgeon in Strasbourg and well-known through his book *Feldbuch der Wundartzney* (1530) (Fig. 1) developed a series of original instruments, particularly two lifting machines with a two-legged and a three-legged apparatus used for impressed fractures. They were intended to avoid further depressing the impressed bone fragment into the skull. He warned against injury to the dura because of the danger of infection.

Fabricius Hildanus (1560–1634) of Hilden near Düsseldorf, city physician in Bern and known beyond the borders of Switzerland in France, England, Denmark and Hungary, improved and modified instruments to raise impressed fractures. These instruments were later imitated by Benjamin Bell in England and Jean Louis Petit in France. Fabry developed a method with which the raised fragment was fixed to the bone with a special apparatus. Furthermore, he thought of new concepts on the cause of wound infections, which in his opinion were maintained by foreign bodies, parasites and traumatized tissue. In his works, consisting of several volumes with more than 400 separate illustrations, he reports on the treatment of skull fractures and even dared to remove traumatized brain tissue. With his book *Von der Fürtrefflichkeit und Nutz der Anatomy*, he prepared the way for the introduction of anatomy instruction, since, as he reported, "the clinical course of a number of cases was fatal only because the treating surgeon had no anatomical knowledge."

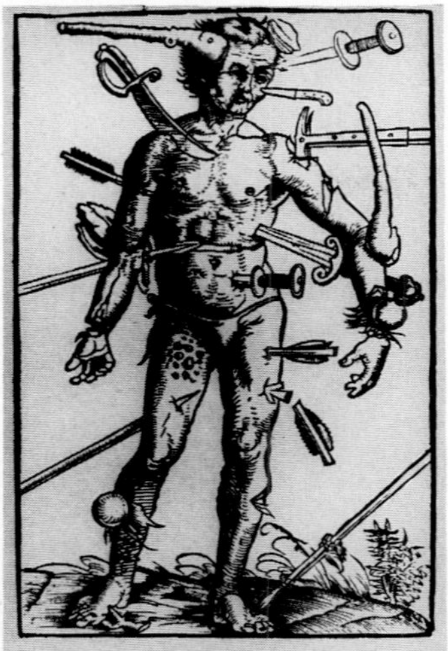

Fig. 1. "Der Wundenmann" from Gersdorf's *Feldbuch der Wundartzney* (1517)

Johann Schulthes (1595–1645), called Scultetus, city physician in Ulm and a skilled surgeon, famous in his time because of his apparatus for the correction of spinal fractures and deformities, created a number of new skull trepans and described the area of application of each instrument, as well as the indications and the techniques of each operation His work, *Armamentarium chirurgicum* or *Wundarzneiy'sches Zeughaus* (1655), was the most important surgical book in his time. It was written in Latin and intended for the academically educated physician. It found wide distribution throughout Holland, France, England and Italy through 15 editions in various languages.

Matthäus Gottfried Purmann (1649–1711), city physician of Breslau and the chief military surgeon of Frederick William, the Great Elector of Brandenburg from 1640 to 1688, published his great surgical work *Wund Artzney*, the first truly *scientific* surgical book, in 1705, 55 years after the death of Schulthes. He achieved unusual skill in skull trepanations, he performed tracheotomies, operated on carotid artery tumours with ligatures, and was the first to perform blood transfusions from sheep to man in Germany. A young man, Mr. Weißlein from Frankfurt on the Main, is said to have survived this.

In contrast to his predecessors, who used ointments, pastes and pus provocation for the healing of wounds, he recommended cleansing, bandaging and fixation of the wound in preparation for pus-free, dry wound treatment.

He directed an assistant to blow away the bony fragments during the trepanation with a small tube constructed by him as these block the view and can thus lead to

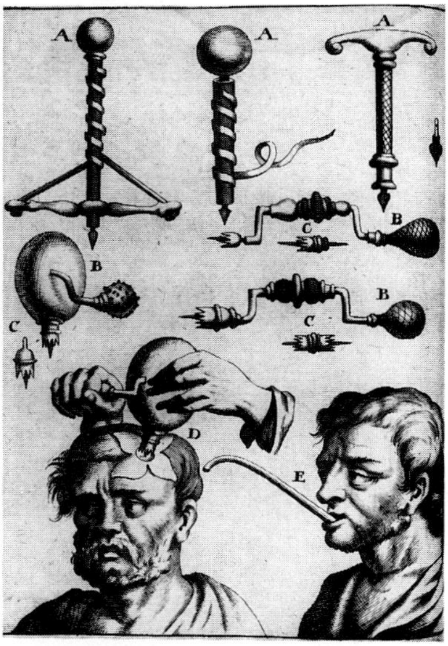

Fig. 2. Group of trepanation instruments from Purmann's *Wundartzney* (1705)

injury of the dura. He invented a mechanical trepanation device enclosed in a case and functioning with a transmission shaft (Fig. 2).

Lorenz Heister (1683–1758), professor at the University of Altdorf-Nuremberg and later in Helmstedt (Fig. 3), differs from the previously named surgeons because of his scientific education, which he received in Gießen, Amsterdam and Leiden, later in France and England, and which enabled him to represent a clinical field in our present-day sense. The instruments he developed were technically superior, particularly his trepanation instrument and those instruments for lifting skull fractures, which found wide distribution.

In 1718 he published his famous textbook *Institutiones chirurgicae*, which was translated into many languages and was valid up to the nineteenth century, setting the standard for surgery in all of Europe.

He gave the tracheotomy its name, as it had been called bronchotomy up to his time. He was offered many chairs at various universities: Tsar Peter offered him a salary of 3000 roubles; he refused the chair of the University of Göttingen; and the Prince Bishop of Würzburg offered him a 1000 thaler salary, a large supply of wine and fruit, as well as freedom of religion. He remained faithful to Helmstedt.

Continuing the efforts of Heister, August Gottlied Richter (1742–1812) made a great contribution to uniting the field of surgery with the scientific parts of medicine. In 1766, at the age of 24, he became professor at the Georg-August University of Göttingen, the famous "Leine Athens" of George II, King of England and Elector of Hanover; he taught there until 1803.

Richter simplified surgical apparatus and disposed of the superfluous instruments of the past. Using the example of travelling oculists, hernia and stone cutters, he

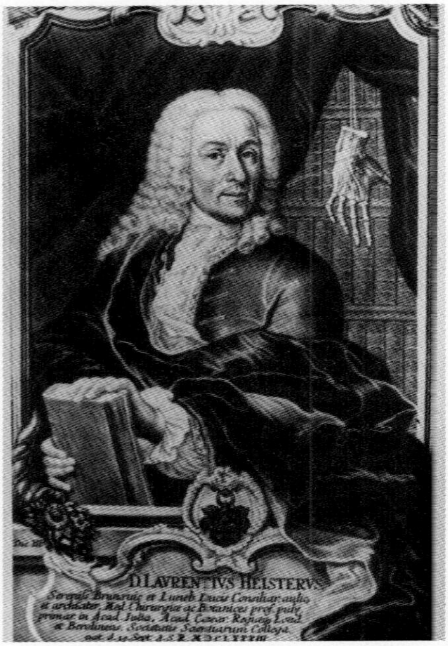

Fig. 3. Lorenz Heister (1683–1758)

showed how little genuine scientific knowledge some operations required. Every idiot could do a trepenation, he felt, but the *evaluation* of head injuries, the detection of the causes of malignant tumours and their removal, these things could only be done by a genuine physician. In his famous book *Chirurgische Bibliothek* and his work *Anfangsgründe der Wundarzneikunde* (1802) which consists of several volumes, he discussed the pathophysiological problems of the brain and classified head injuries into three degrees of severity, just as we do today. His chief merit for the field of neurosurgery was that he described clear indications for trepanation and took a stand against the prophylactic trepanation supported by Percival Pott (1714–1788), thereby limiting the excesses of the practice of trepanation. He had been informed that Prince Philip of Orange had undergone trepanation 17 times and that de la Touche had performed this operation 52 times in one patient within 2 months.

Increased intracranial pressure was the absolute indication for trepanation according to Richter. All other head injuries were to be operated on only if the quality of the pulse, the reaction of the pupils and the general state of the patient indicated a worsening of the brain symptoms. This almost corresponds to modern concepts.

He invented a trepanation instrument in which the pyramid did not have to be removed in the course of the trepanation, but could be moved, and thus improved the rigid system of the tripod for raising impressed fractures. Richter defined the symptoms of cortical epilepsy in the present-day manner. Jackson did not describe these symptoms until decades later, but they carry *his* name.

A similar lack of credit was given to the Swiss anatomist Johannes Jakob Wepfer (1620–1695), who described the circulus arteriosus in 1658; this structure, however, received the name of Thomas Willis (1621–1675) in 1664.

Albrecht von Haller (1708–1777) of Bern, who taught in Göttingen before Richter, activated progress of our field less in the way of operative innovation but rather in that he exerted an influence through his experimental physiological investigations. He is the originator of modern physiology whose results are written up in many works.

Haller based his classical teaching of excitability and sensitivity as the basic qualities of nerves and muscles on hundreds of animal experiments. He described excitability as the ability to react to stimuli and movements – a specific characteristic of muscle fibres. This finding was basic progress over the stand of Francis Glisson, who considered excitability to be a general characteristic of tissues and not dependent on the nervous system. Haller's revolutionary discoveries continue to exert their influence into our day, although most of us do not realize it.

Haller also refuted Thomas Willis' (1621–1675) theories that the cerebellum is the superior organ for heart activity and breathing. In experiments, Haller demonstrated that these functions are localized in the medulla oblongata, although he opposed the localization of brain functions because of inadequate experimental conditions. In his experiments he applied a stimulus with acid swabs and these led to seizures and unconsciousness.

Haller founded a collection of anatomical specimens, many of which he prepared himself, and in 1747 he was the first to detect and describe the lateral exit of the fourth ventricle, although the name for this structure is linked to a later investigator, Herbert von Luschka (1820–1875), who described these foramina in 1855.

Haller's influence on the further development of medicine can only be compared to the great discoveries of William Harvey (1578–1657) and Adreas Vesal (1514–1564). Haller's influence on the anatomists of the founding period in Göttingen continued up to the present as many of these people made decisive discoveries: Johann-Friedrich Meckel the Elder, Alexander Monro (1697–1767), August Wriesberg, and his student Samuel Thomas Sömmering.

Johann-Friedrich Meckel the Elder (1724–1774) was professor of anatomy in Berlin from 1751. His dissertation of 1757 in Göttingen seems up-to-date even now and describes in exact detail the trigeminal nerve, including its end branches (Fig. 4). Meckel showed that the ganglion is surrounded by the dura and is used to press a cavity, the terminal cavity, which has since then been described as Meckel's cave. He was also the first to point to the sphenopalatinous ganglion.

During the same period, anatomists in Vienna were working on the anatomy of the central part of the trigeminal nerve. In 1765, Anton Hirsch called the ganglion there the Ganglion Gasseri, after his teacher Lorenz Gasser, professor of anatomy 1757–1765, although it had been described previously by others such as Santorini (1681–1737).

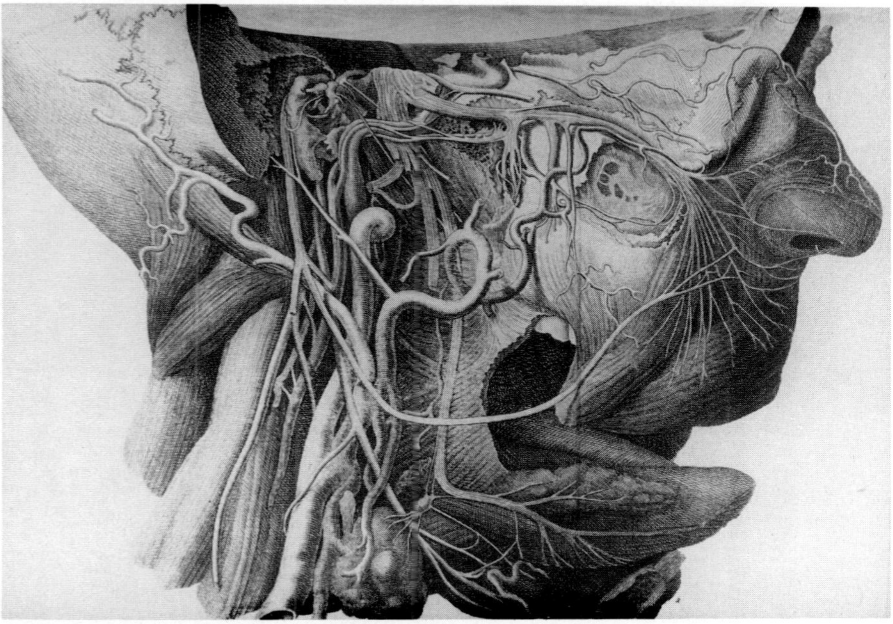

Fig. 4. Anatomical drawing showing the trigeminal nerve from J.F. Meckel's *Dissertatio inauguralis medica anatomica physiological de quinto pare nervorum cerebri* (Göttingen 1748)

August Wriesberg (1739–1808), anatomist in Göttingen, discovered and described the motor branch of the trigeminal nerve, the so-called minor portion, in 1767, 16 years after Meckel. In the same publication he also mentions the intermediate nerve of the seventh cranial nerve for the first time (Fig. 5).

His student Thomas Samuel von Sömmering (1755–1830) was the discoverer of the substantia nigra and the electrical telegraph. In his dissertation at the University of Göttingen, he demonstrated that the facial nerve and the statoacoustic nerve are separate nerves, in contrast to the opinion of Charles Bell (1774–1842). His work has since then been recognized as the first clear classification of the 12 cranial nerves. Willis (1621–1675) had described nine nerve pairs and in Galen's time (129–199 A.D.) there were only seven (Fig. 6).

Sömmering's exact descriptions and drawings on the sensory organs have gained world-wide recognition and have not lost their significance. His book *Das Organ der Seele* (1796) was a great sensation at the time, but was later generally rejected and regarded as a step in the wrong direction for an important scientist. Today, however, it is quite modern because of its explanations about the morphology of the central nervous system, because of the demonstrations about Gestalt recognition, and because of its effort to correlate knowledge about brain research with the areas of psychology and philosophy. Half a century was to pass before the more exact

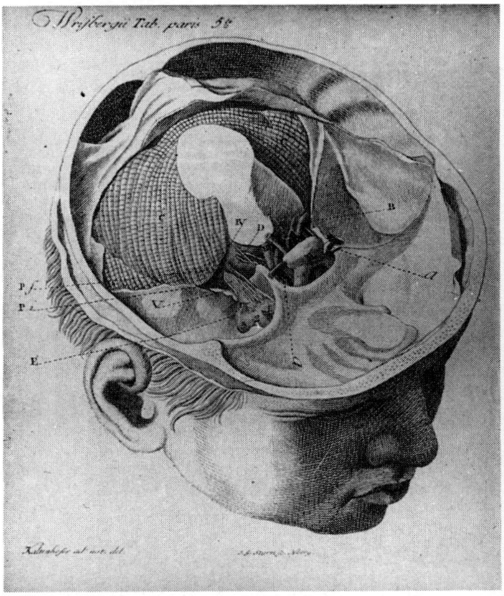

5

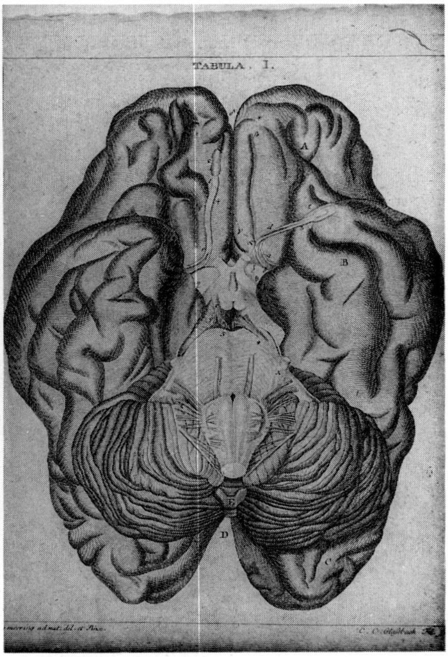

6

Fig. 5. Anatomical drawing showing the portio major and minor from H.-A. Wirsberg's *Obervationes anatomicae de quinto pare nervorum encephali* (Göttingen 1777)

Fig. 6. Anatomical drawing showing the seventh and eighth nerves from Sömmering's *De basi encephali* (Göttingen 1778)

anatomic knowledge of this era were incorporated into the operative treatment of diseases of the nervous system.

The surgeon and anatomist Konrad Johann Martin Langenbeck (1776–1851) developed surgical measures for the treatment of facial pain, according to Fothergill, so-called quinti neuralgia, which were based on the results of Meckel. In his paper "Taractus Anatomico Chirurgicus de Nervis Cerebri in Dolore Faciei Consideratus" (Göttingen, 1803) he reported that the aetiology of this clinical entity was difficult to determine. In particular, it was not an inflammatoray pain since there was a complete lack of a pathological substrate and chiefly the second and third branches of the nerve are affected. Since conservative measures with mercury, belladona and even arsenic did not lead to success, he thought of influencing the pain by surgical procedures on the peripheral branches of the trigeminal nerve. In this way he achieved prolonged freedom of pain in several cases, but he also reports on recurrences. However, Langenbeck also evolved operative techniques in autopsy cases to influence the "tic convulsiv" of the facial nerve by resecting it at the stylomastoid foramen. Technically this was not difficult for him, for he was regarded as a quick and brilliant surgeon. This is confirmed by a surgeon who came from America to see him operate but could not do without a snuff of tobacco during the preparation for the extraarticulation of the shoulder: When he looked up, Langenbeck had already completed the procedure. Despite his hard work and great ability, he was unusually narrow minded and had a very high opinion of himself. It is said that he divided people into two categories, those who could operate and those who were operated on. Even at that time there was opposition from the younger generation in Göttingen, as his students, who knew him to be an early riser, countered with the words "One cannot conquer the world by rising earlier than other people."

It remains to his credit that he gave the initial impulse for the surgical treatment of facial neuralgia. Later this was improved and modified by Dieffenbach and Fedor Krause, as well as by Spiller and Frazier.

The development away from pure skull surgery to brain surgery occurred between the middle of the nineteenth and the beginning of the twentieth century and was made possible through improved knowledge about localization within the brain and the functions of this central organ.

The beginning of this period is marked by Johann Christian Reil (1759–1819), professor in Halle and later in Berlin, the founder of the first scientific journal of this type, the *Archiv für Physiologie*. He made a decisive contribution to our neuroanatomical knowledge. He discovered the individuality of the area of sensation, the cerebellar nucleus, as well as the lenticular nucleus and the boundaries of the sylvian fissure. Using special methods of fixation, he was the first to isolate nerve fibre bundles in order to demonstrate their connections from the midbrain to the spinal cord. On the basis of these studies Bernard Aloys von Gudden (1824–1886), who later drowned in Lake Starnberg together with the mentally ill King Ludwig II of Bavaria, was able to follow the fibrous paths in the chiasm in cases of degenerative disease. He showed that *one* optic nerve has *direct* fibres to the optic tract on the same side, as well as *crossing* fibres passing through the chiasm to the tract on the other side.

Gudden also carried out important studies on the development of the growing skull. His philosophy was "first anatomy, then physiology. If, however, physiology is first, then never without anatomy."

At the same time Franz Josef Gall (1758–1828) and Johann Kaspar von Spurzheim (1776–1832), who worked together in Vienna for 13 years, published their studies on the anatomy and physiology of the brain. They came to the conclusion that the white matter of the brain consists only of nerve fibres, while the gray cortex is the organ of brain activity. On the basis of his anatomic studies, Gall was also able to show that the root of the trigeminal nerve does not originate in the pons alone, but also contains fibres from the medulla oblongata. Gall and Spurheim attempted to localize areas of body representation on the surface of the brain. In this way they paved the way for localization and functional studies of the brain which are indispensible for surgical procedures on the brain. Their studies finally led to phrenology, which was badly misused in later times. Because of this, the early important research of Gall has been forgotten.

In this area the Berlin physiologist Hermann Munk (1839–1912) was the first to report that the recognition of touch was located in the rolandic cortex and that cortical blindness is caused by the destruction of the occipital pole. His concept of "sensory cortical fields" was accepted later in 1870 by Fritsch (1838–1927) and Hitzig (1838–1907), who in turn were able to show that stimulation of the motor centres in the region of the central gyrus led to movements in certain muscle groups.

By performing experiments on dogs in Hitzig's apartment in Berlin – in the bedroom it is said – using an electrode with weak current placed on the anterior surface of the gyrus, they succeeded in eliciting motor reactions on the opposite side. They were successful in determining motor centres for the neck, the front paws, the rear legs and the facial musculature. The resection of these centres led to a contralateral paralysis. Therefore, they called this region the "motor centre". These studies were a vital contribution to the localization of the brain. A few years later their studies were confirmed by the excellent neurophysiologist at King's College London, Sir David Ferrier (1843–1928), who made further developments. At about the same time, the sensational studies of the psychiatrist Karl Wenicke from Halle (1848–1905) were published. In 1874, he discovered the cause for sensory aphasia and was convinced that there are sharply delineated centres for elementary psychic functions on the surface of the brain.

The neurologist Korbinian Brodmann (1868–1918), who was greatly supported by Oskar Vogt (1870–1959), described the cellular structure – the cytoarchitecture – of the brain in 1908 and contributed to the study of brain localization. His fundamental book *Vergleichende Lokalisationslehre der Großhirnrinde* has remained a standard work even up to the present.

The list of such excellent scientists and researchers in the German-speaking world who contributed to the contours of our field of neurosurgery is almost endless and includes such names as Nissl, Alzheimer, Cécile and Oskar Vogt, Edinger, Bielschowsky, Obersteiner, Nonne, Erb, Burdach, Flechsig, Virchow, von Recklinghausen and Queckenstedt.

The progress of neurosurgical research has been influenced by four men in particular: Hermann Ludwig Ferdinand von Helmholtz, Heinrich Irenaeus Quincke, Wilhelm Conrad Röntgen and Hans Berger.

Helmholtz (1821–1894), physician and physiologist in Berlin, was born in Potsdam. As a student he was able to show that every nerve fibre originated in a ganglion cell. For this he has been called the discoverer of the neuron. Later, he measured the depolarization rate of the nerve, which his teacher, the physiologist Johannes Müller, believed to be immeasurably great. Helmholtz found the velocity of nerve conduction to be 27 m/s for the gastrocnemius muscle, the motor nerve of the frog. "That is three times as fast as the flow of the Orinoco river," exclaimed Alexander von Humboldt at the time.

This was followed by his most famous achievement, the invention of the ophthalmoscope in 1850, an instrument which made the first endoscopic examination of a living organ possible. In this way it became possible for the first time to objectively evaluate any increase in intracranial pressure by observing the optic nerve. All his publications, including those in the area of acoustics, were written in precise detail and were easily understandable. Helmholtz himself said, "Many parts of my papers were rewritten four to six times, the layout rearranged repeatedly until I was satisfied. But such careful work is of great advantage for the author. It forces him to check every sentence and conclusion."

As a teacher he was occasionally less inspiring, especially if the material did not fascinate him, and he spoke in a halting manner. This was entirely different in the case of Heinrich Quincke (1842–1922) of Kiel, who held his audience spell-bound with his fascinating topics and his serious way of presentation which, according to Max Nonne, served only the subject he was presenting. His modest report on the lumbar puncture which he presented over 100 years ago as professor of internal medicine in Wiesbaden was one of the greatest discoveries in medicine. Quincke inaugurated the lumbar puncture, acting on a therapeutic consideration. According to Victor von Bruns 1854 in Tübingen, he performed a puncture of the ventricle in two children with hydrocephalus. Quincke himself said, "The performance of a puncture on the normal brain, i.e. without dilatation of the ventricles, is not without danger. For this reason I tapped the subarachnoid space at the level of lumbar vertebrae between the third and fourth vertebrae by inserting the needle and removing the dropwise flow of CSF up to 1 ccm of fluid." This procedure, which every doctor must learn today, was a brave manoeuvre at that time. The many possibilities which this diagnostic procedure offers were already pointed out by Quincke himself and included the recording of CSF pressure as well as chemical and microscopic changes in the CSF.

His fertile imagination meant that his suggestions for the treatment of his patients were often more than his assistants could handle. But he also had his weaknesses. Born in Berlin, he did not succeed in understanding the Holstein Low German dialect in all his years in Kiel, so he had to have the help of assistants and students during his lectures.

Hans Berger (1873–1941), born in Coburg and the grandchild of the famous poet Friedrich Rückert (1788–1866), was an assistant of Otto-Ludwig Binswanger (1852–1929) in Jena together with Brodmann and Oskar Vogt, and he succeeded Binswanger in office. He regarded the chief task of neurology to be the discovery of the physiological background of mental activity. After 20 years of research, he succeeded in recording the first human EEG through a trepanation defect in 1929. Five years later he was able to perform the same study through the intact skull, showing alpha and beta waves (Fig. 7). His method resulted in a complete revision of the classification of epilepsy. On the basis of Berger's discovery, Walter Grey succeeded in localizing brain tumours through the intact skull by way of abnormally slow waves in 1936.

Hans Berger was a strict head of department and chief. All patients admitted the previous day had to be completely examined by the time of the early morning conference, and a written history which he checked had to have been completed. There were *no* scientific discussions. The place for this was Saturday afternoon, from 5 to 7 p.m., the so-called *Klughusten* ("clever coughing"). On Sunday morn-

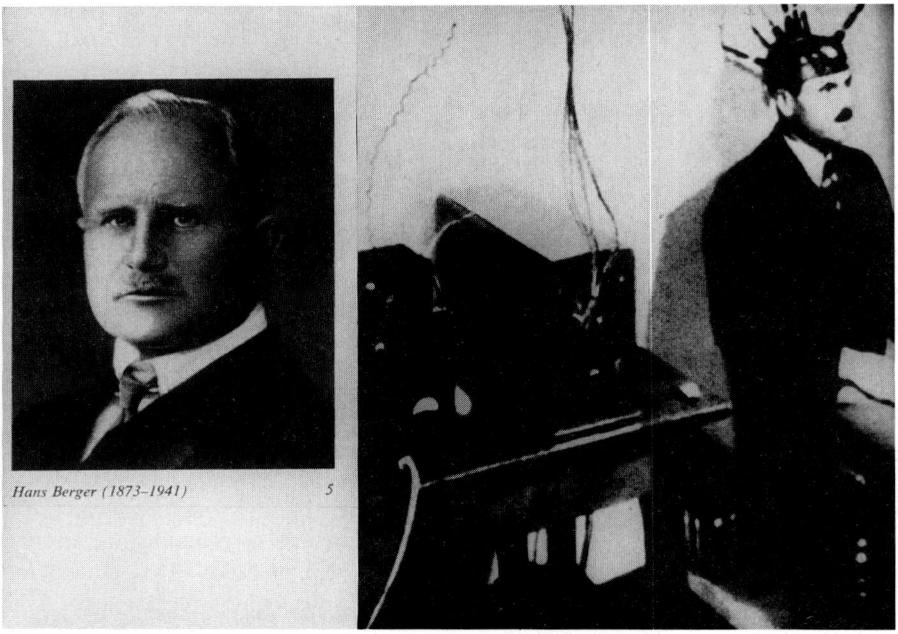

Fig. 7. Hans Berger (1873–1941) (*left*) and one of the first devices for recording the human EEG (*right*)

ings, the doctor on duty had to meet him at the door at the hospital to report to him, so that only Sunday afternoons were genuine free time.

The discovery of X-rays by Wilhelm Conrad Röntgen (1845–1923) almost 100 years ago in 1896 in Würzburg led to a revolution in the diagnostic possibilities in all fields of medicine. This is not the place for a complete assessment of this method of diagnosis, but it was Fedor Krause who first profited from it as a neurosurgeon when he removed a 7 mm revolver bullet demonstrated in the X-ray in the frontobasal region of a young man who had shot himself out of love. For this procedure he used the subfrontal approach to the chiasm, which he had developed. The first X-rays Conrad Röntgen made were of the hand of the leading biologist of this time, Albert von Kölliker (1817–1905), anatomist in Würzburg and originator of cell physiology. The Kölliker collaterals are well-known to neurosurgeons, who still perform open chordotomies. It was Kölliker who created the term "X-rays" for the world (Fig. 8).

After the introduction of anaesthesia by the American Crawford Long (1815–1878) in 1850, the principle of antisepsis by the Englishman Joseph Lister (1827–1912), and the use of aseptic wound treatment by Ernst von Bergmann (1836–1907), the age of *modern surgery* began (Fig. 9). This had a particularly great effect on progress in brain surgery. By the First World War, the "surgery of removal" had almost been perfected. In later times, new techniques were added through antibiotics and chemotherapy, as well as anaesthesia and shock treatment. The daredevil era

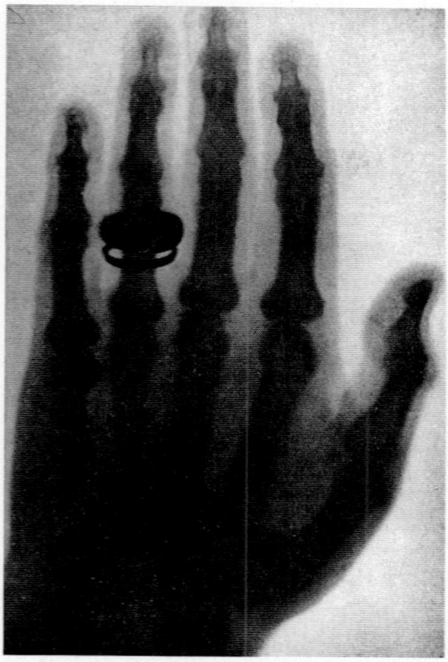

Fig. 8. One of the first Roentgen ray photographs showing the hand of the famous Würzburg anatomist Albert von Kölliker (1817–1905)

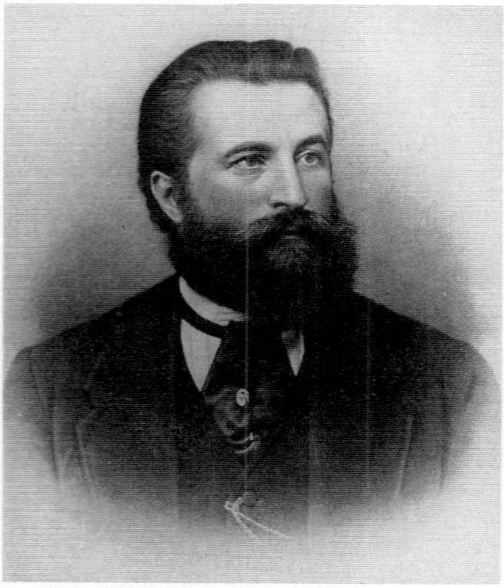

Fig. 9. Ernst von Bergmann (1836–1907)

was thus dominated by the thoughts of physiologists, which is why this is called physiological surgery.

The surgical texts of this new era pointed out that a rise in systolic and pulse pressure as well as bradycardia are dreaded signs of increased intracranial pressure which can lead to decerebration. Bergmann was also the first to realize a fact that was unknown until then, namely that the pressure and flow in intracranial veins is of great importance, and he performed experiments on the dependence of venous pressure on the increase of arterial pressure. Together with his assistant Cramer, he also observed the veins directly through a glass window which was built into the skull, registering the effect of physiological saline injected into the carotid artery on veins.

In John Fulton's well-known biography on Cushing, we read, "Because of the ingenious method of building a small window into the skull of the animal, Cushing was able to see the effect of intracranial pressure directly." This led to the impression that Cushing was the first to use this method, but even before Bergmann, the Italian physiologist Ravina had observed the pulsation of the brain using the same method.

In order to study the problems of pressure which Fulton mentioned, Harvey Cushing performed experiments on the increase of intracranial pressure with Theodor Kocher (1841–1917) in Bern in 1909, because the latter worked intensively with these problems. Although they were more elegant than those performed 30 years before by Bergmann, they were in principle identical with them. Cushing's work was published in the *Mitteilungen aus den Grenzgebieten der Medizin und Chirurgie.* The publisher, an important physician for internal medicine and a researcher on metabolism, Bernard Naunyn of Strasbourg, remarked that, "There is no progress over our work." However, the continuous surveillance of blood pressure and pulse in clinical practice for the follow-up of patients with intracranial lesions – this must be accredited to Cushing.

Taking a stand on such questions of priority as described here, the American neurosurgeon Eben Alexander Jr said at the opening lecture of the 1981 Combined Meeting of the American Academy and our German society in New York, "If you think you have a new idea or *original* idea, it's probably because you can't read German."

Returning to Bergmann, it should be mentioned that he was responsible for the survival of patients after intracranial procedures by inaugurating the concept of asepsis. He did without carbol spray, introduced stream sterilization, and emphasized careful disinfection of the hands. When asked by visiting surgeons who came to watch him, "What's new in surgery?" he would answer, "Today we wash our hands *before* the operation."

A remarkable number of excellent surgeons came from his school, including such personalities as Nicolai Gulecke (1878–1958), who worked closely with Ernst Berger in Jena and published an excellent textbook on neurosurgical operations, Fritz Gustav von Bramann (1854–1913), the inaugurator of the corpus callosum puncture to relieve intracranial pressure, and Fritz König (1860–1952), who paved the way for the independence of neurosurgery.

It was a very productive period for neurosurgery as a whole. Ulrich Rudolf Kroenlein (1881–1910) from Potsdam and a student of Langenbecks, professor in Zürich, became well-known because of his innovative work on meningeal bleeding. Similar to Kocher, he invented a craniometer which is named after him. He found new ways for resecting the trigeminal nerve and developed the approach to the retrobulbar space which we still use today, the so-called Kroenlein operation.

Much of the preparation for the shunt operation in infantile hydrocephalus which was inaugurated by Spitz, Nulsen and Pudenz in the 1950s was done by Erwin Payr (1871–1946), professor of surgery in Leipzig. Following the suggestion of Gustav Gärtner from Vienna in a paper delivered at a medical meeting in Lübeck, he was the first to drain CSF into a blood vessel in 1908. He connected one lateral ventricle to the sagittal sinus by way of a calf artery or a section of the saphenous vein. Later, he drained the lateral ventricle into the jugular vein or the facial vein.

The Renaissance of the transnasal approach to the pituitary gland in the 1960s by the introduction of an operation microscope is a reminder that Hermann Schloffer (1868–1937) had, in Vienna, already carried out a successful transnasal operation of a pituitary tumor in 1908 after Fritz König (1866–1952) had worked out the approach via the sphenoid sinus on an autopsy case in 1898. Harvey Cushing used this approach in 1914, but later discarded it again because operative treatment using the intracranial approach was more effective at that time.

It was a tremendous technical step forward when the surgeon Wilhelm Wagner (1848–1900), who worked in Könighütte in Silesia, developed the "temporary resection of the skull" in 1889 after extensive previous studies on autopsy specimens. This procedure supplanted trepanation and represented the birth of the classical osteoplastic craniotomy which we still use today.

While Johann Friedrich Dieffenbach (1792–1847), who was known as the "brave surgeon," reported discouraging results following the trepanation of head injuries because of infection, Richard von Volkmann (1830–1889), the famous surgeon from Halle and one of the most successful introducers of antisepsis and asepsis in Germany, reported on 36 trepanations for head injuries with excellent results.

When Fedor Krause (1857–1937) (Fig. 10) born in Friedland, Silesia, entered the surgical department in Halle, which was directed by Richard von Volkmann, his future professional life was at a decisive point. Krause, who was a gifted pianist and had received prizes in his youth, was undecided as to whether he should return to music at the beginning of his time in Halle. The impression which Volkmann's personality made on him led him to favour the field of surgery.

Throughout his professional life from Halle, where he obtained his "Habilitation" and became professor through his work on the field of malignant neurinomas, to Altona, where he was chief of surgery until 1900, up to his time as chief of surgery in the Berlin Augusta Hospital, he made extremely important contributions to brain surgery, although his training was general surgery – as documented by the Krause flap.

Impressed by his work and ideas on the trigeminal nerve, the Berlin neurologist Hermann Oppenheim (1858–1919) indicated to Krause the approach to the ganglion gasseri which is used till today: along the base of the skull remaining outside the dura, lifting the closed dura, coagulating the middle meningeal artery, visualizing the third and second branch, and then exposing the ganglion. Initially he was content with the exposure of the second and third branches, but since there were not enough successful improvements with this method alone, he performed the first resection of

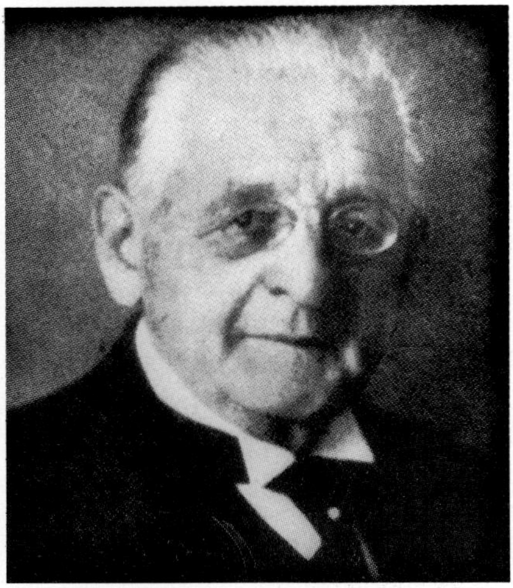

Fig. 10. Fedor Krause (1857–1937)

the ganglion in 1913. His book *Die Chirurgie des Gehirns und Rückenmarks*, which was published in 1911, described over 70 cases of ganglion removal. In this unique book, he described all the approaches to the various areas of the brain which he had developed and which are still used throughout the world today. As previously mentioned, these include the transfrontal approach to the chiasm. In 1913 he and Hermann Oppenheim presented the first case of a successfully removed tumour of the colliculi, which they removed approaching from the posterior fossa with the patient in a sitting position.

The otologist Güttich wrote in his obituary, "Krause was the first person who looked into the fourth ventricle of a living human being." In addition, he laid the ground for the approach to the cerebellopontine angle and to the visualization of the eighth nerve. He was the first to operate on patients with angiomas of the brain successfully, and the first to remove a medial lumbar disc. Together with Oppenheim he published a paper on the "compression or strangulation of the cauda equina" in 1909. A patient with paraplegia of acute onset regained his ability to walk following the removal of a bean-sized "tumour" which Krause removed after a laminectomy on 23 December 1918. It was a medial lumbar disc, which was called an enchondroma in the terminology of that time. In the literature Mixter and Barr are thought to have been the first to perform the operation on a lumbar disc, according to their publication in 1933.

Hermann Oppenheim took part in many important procedures and decisions on indications and planning of the operative approach. He is one of the initiators of modern German neurosurgery, which Krause realized in an entirely unique manner. The continuing developments in the specialty came very close to the present state of the art. The excellent work of the main representatives of this period,

Otfrid Foerster (1873–1941) and Wilhelm Tönnis (1898–1978) are honoured by the memorial lectures of the Deutsche Gesellschaft für Neurochirurgie.

"Fern sind wir davon, uns in unseren Leistungen überheben zu wollen" (It is not our intention to praise ourselves because of our achievements) – this remark comes from Ernst von Bergmann, who was very much against nationalistic overtones in medicine. It is my intention, however, merely to point out that a large number of small building stones in the form of discoveries by excellent researchers in the German-speaking area played their parts in forming the international mosaic of neurosurgery as we know it today.

It remains my wish that those who come after us may solve the unsolved scientific and clinical problems, in the sense of Karl Ernst von Baer, "Die Wissenschaft ist endlos in ihrer Aufgabe, unerreichbar in ihrem Ziel."

When Fedor Krause, 80 years old, learned about the independence of neurosurgery in his domicile in Rome shortly before his death 22 September 1937, he wrote to Wilhelm Tönnis "Nur vorwärts auf dem eingeschlagenen Wege. Er führt zum Ziel" (Forward on the chosen path. It will lead to the goal).

K.-A. Bushe (em.)[1]

[1] Neurochirurgische Universitätsklinik und Poliklinik im Kopfklinikum, Josef-Schneider-Str. 11, W–8700 Würzburg 16, FRG.

Neurosurgical Standards

Neurosurgical Standards and Quality Assurance

W. J. Bock[1]

In a survey of physicians and medically versed lawyers on the definition of medical standards, the response was almost always the same: "The treatment of a disorder in accordance with the current norm." The medical expert appearing in court is asked by the judge or defense attorney, "Did this treatment conform to medical standards?"

In the United States, for example, it was "standard" practice until 1985 to perform an extracranial-intracranial bypass procedure for transient ischemic attacks (TIAs). When the results of a double-blind study on the operative and nonoperative management of TIAs were presented at the Eighth International Congress of Neurological Surgery in Toronto, overnight it became "standard" to withhold this operation, since the study showed no significant difference between the treatment methods. These few examples show how difficult it is to standardize measures and thus invest them with a certain general validity.

In the first part of this report I shall discuss standards and quality assurance in general, and in the second part I shall illustrate how these principles apply to an area of neurosurgical practice.

Defined in mathematical or statistical terms, a standard represents the arithmetic mean of a statistical series. We all know the standard deviation as the mean square deviation characterizing the distribution of values in a statistical series about its arithmetic mean. The standard deviation tells us whether a calculated mean value is typical of the series as a whole. When we speak of error theory and the gaussian distribution curve, the standard deviation is taken to represent the deviation from the normal curve. If I now attempt to apply these mathematical and statistical concepts to clinical treatment, the difference from the usual concept of a standard as a consistent quality becomes clear.

Why is it necessary to grapple with these concepts? Since the early 1970s, there has been broad international interest in the concept of quality assurance in medical treatment. At the 91st Congress of German Physicians in Frankfurt in 1988, the concept of quality assurance was incorporated into the model professional code for practitioners. Section 7a stated that every physician should participate in the quality measure of the Medical Council. On December 20, 1988, lawmakers passed Social Legal Code V (SBG V), whose provisions for quality assurance in medicine were initially given too little notice by the medical community. In Section 2, dealing with services, it states: "The quality and effectiveness of services shall conform

[1] Neurochirurgische Universitätsklinik, Moorenstr. 5, W-4000 Düsseldorf, FRG.

Advances in Neurosurgery, Vol. 20
K. Piscol, M. Klinger, M. Brock (Eds.)

to the generally accepted state of the medical art and shall take due account of medical progress." Again, there is reference to a general standard without defining exactly what it is. Section 12, dealing with economic feasibility, states that medical services which are unnecessary or uneconomical cannot be demanded. Section 66 regulates the support of insured parties in the event of faulty treatment, while Section 70 states that health insurance funds and care providers, i.e., physicians and hospitals, shall guarantee consistent, need-oriented care that conforms to the general state of the medical art. Even more significant is Section 112, which includes bilateral agreements and framing recommendations on hospital treatments. Item 3 in that section prescribes "procedural and testing principles" for testing quality and economy. Sections 135 and 137 regulate the quality assurance of ambulatory and inpatient care. According to these sections, hospitals are to participate in the measures of quality assurance: "The measures shall be extended to the quality of treatment, care structuring, and treatment outcomes. The measures shall be structured in such a way that comparative testing is possible." It is further stated that "The agreements shall specify the cases in which second opinions should be sought prior to major surgical interventions." It is noteworthy that the medical service of the health funds is charged with testing the essential prerequisites, and that the actual attending physicians are nonexistent as far as lawmakers are concerned. This has the effect of excluding competent physician consultation, at least for the neurosurgical specialty, since competent specialists generally are not represented in the medical services of the health funds.

Lawmakers and the professional code force us, then, to deal with the concepts of "standard" and "quality assurance." We must ask what is meant by the quality of medical services. What are its prerequisites, and of what does it consist?

Donabedian recognizes three types of quality: structural quality, process quality, and outcome quality. Structural quality includes the quality of physician training, the setup of practices, the condition of hospitals, technical facilities, and the accessibility of physicians to patients and nursing staff. It is obvious that a high technical standard is not synonymous with sound medical care. Similarly, good structural quality in the hospital or office setting does not automatically result in healthier patients. Thus, a high technical standard is not the same as a high standard of treatment.

Physicians' services are much more a matter or process quality, with "process" referring to all diagnostic and therapeutic measures. Today, many factors play a role, including not just objective diagnostic findings but also subjective data. Some determinants of process quality are the patient-doctor relationship, waiting times, physician responsiveness to patients' questions, and the availability of the same physician on different visits, which is not always possible at many hospitals. The same applies to nursing and technical personnel.

Outcome quality, or the quality of the result of a medical action, is no less difficult to assess. As a rule of thumb, we might say that a satisfied patient indicates a good-quality result, but this represents a subjective impression rather than a statistically founded standard value.

Selbmann states that quality assurance consists of five steps, starting with the recognition of problem areas and the setting of priorities. From this comes the identification of the goals of quality assurance and the definition of quality in the selected problem area. This second definition phase is followed by a detailed observation phase with documentation and data collection. Next come analysis and proposals for alternative solutions. The final step is implementation of the proposals followed by an assessment of the efficacy of the measures. Selbmann states: "Only a closed-loop system of this kind, repeatedly processing the same problem or changing problems, can rightly be termed quality assurance."

There is a pressing need, then, to deal more intensively with the concept of *standards* as the basis for quality assurance. Schäfer considered the difference between the concepts of "norm" and "standard." Industrial norms, for example, deal with the standardization of products of their manufacture in order to achieve the compatibility of products, permit their general use, and obtain products of consistent quality. A norm, then, refers to things, while a standard refers to people. There is no clear definition of the term "standard" in the sense of an industrial norm but rather, as noted earlier, in a statistical sense. Schäfer stipulates that goal setting is a necessary prelude to effectively achieving an intended goal. This goal setting corresponds to the established standard. However, this standard must also be measured in terms of feasibility; it must be determined whether the requirement is justified in that particular form. Additionally, a standard must meet the criterion of acceptability to the physicians who apply it, and it must be possible to revise an established standard when needed. This ensures that the standard does not embody outdated knowledge. Another requirement is comparability. Schäfer states: "The goal of standardization is to establish consistency of professional training at a uniformly high level."

Überla, identifying conformance to a standard as one dimension of quality, stresses the need to formulate standards for the individual structural processes involved in outcomes so that deviations can be recognized. This would ensure reproducibility of the process in question. He also calls for ways to define the temporal structure of processes, placing special emphasis on the availability of the physician to the patient.

More difficult is his call for a physician-specific quality dimension. How can one measure knowledge and experience, observational skills, and intuitive thinking? How can one judge critical detachment with respect to one's own performance or evaluate the multiplicity of a physician's skills?

Überla believes that quality improvement, and thus the raising of a standard, is tied to improvements in medical education and training at all levels. The availability of equipment and pharmaceutical agents is cited as a resource example. Critical, though, is the degree of help that the patient experiences from the measures and the patient's personal satisfaction with his or her therapy.

Überla cites various options for enhancing the quality of medical services. One is the formulation of standards for common disease situations. Because most standards in medicine are unarticulated, improperly defined, or misunderstood, they are contradictory and open to attack. It is advisable, therefore, to have representative specialists define the standards for specific diagnostic and therapeutic steps in a given field, instead of having persons outside the field formulate ostensible "standards," as is commonly done today.

Überla states that quality can be positively influenced by improving the time structure of physician-specific quality and improving available resources. As part of this, he calls for greater involvement of the consumer (i.e., the patient) in the quality assurance process. He also recognizes the need for collegial support by other members of the specialty.

To evaluate a quality assurance measure, I can follow the practice of van Eimeren and assign an effect to a particular measure, or I can perform a cost-benefit analysis with regard to health, as is the practice of the health insurance funds. But the latter approach does *not* take into account the acting parties, i.e., the physicians – the same exclusion that is made in the Social Legal Code.

So far we have neither a definition of quality nor of suitable standards in medicine. Implicit in this is a recognition that there are limits to what we can do to influence quality, due in part to education-related issues. Although a change of licensing requirements is currently under discussion in various circles, including the curtailing of formal education and the omission of large areas of factual knowledge, I believe this is a negative example that would result in a quality decline. Lack of funding, lack of empirical data, and the expanding presence of legal issues and bureaucracy in medicine are factors that oppose a positive influence, combined with a justified fear among physicians of even more administration.

The programs previously instituted in neurosurgery can be measured by the quality assurance activities of Seelos or the phased approach proposed by Selbmann, who recognizes three phases: phase I, consisting of scientific study with method development; phase II, a study phase with broad effect; and phase III, routine implementation. The last phase includes the regulation of finances and the testing of long-term effectiveness in routine use.

In 1978 the German Society for Neurosurgery founded a Quality Assurance Committee at their annual meeting in Munich. The concept was presented at various meetings. Herniated lumbar disc, cerebral convexity meningioma, and anterior communicating branch aneurysm were selected as tracer diagnoses because a certain standardization of procedures was ensured for these disorders.

Despite the length of time that has passed, "herniated lumbar disc" is the only diagnosis for which an adequate number of patients have been recruited. When the results were presented, one interesting conclusion was that the average hospital stay in these cases was much too long.

Although many felt that their own patients were discharged more quickly, the critics were unable to support their contention with statistical data. We neurosurgeons still have a long way to go to reach phase III, or the routine program phase.

There are few data for which we can compare actual and desired values. The same applies to the definition of standards and the selection of quality criteria. Thus, we cannot yet develop the strategies that will ultimately lead to quality improvement. Even in the phased approach of Selbmann, the tracer method should continue to be used in the future for the development of neurosurgical standards.

I would like to illustrate this development using lumbar root compression as an example.

The study should include individual data relevant to quality, such as (1) patient data in encoded form, (2) diagnostic measures, (3) therapeutic procedures, (4) complications, and (5) findings at discharge. It would also be desirable to have a long-term result in the form of a 6-month follow-up examination. It is important to issue both the collective statistics from which the individual standards are derived as well as the statistics for the individual hospital so that each participating hospital can evaluate its position relative to the mean value for all participating centers. When a deviation from the standard value is noted, appropriate corrections can be made.

Looking at the individual steps listed above, the general patient data should include standard encoded data along with pertinent data on the patient's history. The most difficult and time-consuming phase is the formulation of diagnostic standards. This includes a standardized technical examination in addition to accurate neurological findings. This poses the question, which of the methods is standard and which is also standardized? Individual procedures have *not* been evaluated using this approach. It is likely, for example, that myelography, already showing a downtrend in favor of the lower-risk modalities of computer tomography (CT) and magnetic resonance (MR) imaging, will soon no longer represent the diagnostic standard.

I see even greater difficulties in developing standards with regard to therapeutic procedures. Treatment options range from conservative measures to open surgery. But the value of a different procedure has not yet been assessed. Presumably it will be possible, with suitable evaluation of diagnostic standards that have yet to be devised, to establish tendencies in the recommendation of therapeutic procedures. If we pick out a single treatment modality such as open surgery, we need to differentiate it further according to whether exposure is gained by a laminectomy, hemilaminectomy, or fenestration, whether a complete evacuation of the intervertebral space was performed, and whether it was necessary to open or extend the root canal.

The *findings at discharge* are always a critical concern in quality assurance measures. These findings are stated in comparison with the findings on admission. They should be reported in an honest, objective fashion, and they should include recommendations for further treatment. Upon discharge, an *immediate* report should be forwarded to the next attending physician. Consideration should be given to neurosurgical aftercare and provision made for feedback at 6 months regarding the quality of the outcome.

Plausibility is essential in the reporting of discharge data if the quality of results is to be improved. A previous pilot study showed that some centers never reported complications, and that paralysis cases invariably improved. This type of conduct is a serious obstacle to the formulation of standards. Also, apparently not all patients were included in the study. A multicenter study can only be as good as the candor of the participating centers in filling out the data sheets.

What is the place of quality assurance in neurosurgery compared with other specialties and other nations? The most advanced study is that of the German Society for Surgery, which is also based on the principle of tracer diagnoses. This study is so respected by the public health industry that its broad implementation is planned. Oldest and best known is the perinatal study, which was conducted throughout the Federal Republic of Germany and has led to a significant reduction in perinatal mortality. I shall limit international comparisons to Holland and the United States. The Union of Dutch Specialists is the official advisory body in terms of quality assurance measures and the establishment of medical standards and criteria. In 1989 more than 90% of all patients were covered in 75% of all hospitals. The various models in the United States are not directly applicable to the Federal Republic of Germany, although the second opinion has since become a legal option in Germany as well. However, individual hospitals in the United States must fulfill certain quality assurance measures as a condition for receiving financial assistance.

I believe that, in the future, methods of quality assurance should be institutionalized within the framework of the specialty area. It would be advantageous to have both internal and external processing in an on-line type of system.

I cannot close without offering a critical evaluation of legally prescribed quality assurance measures. Because all techniques and procedures in medicine are problem oriented, those working on the problems must be involved. Only competent specialists have the expertise needed for the definition of individual standards. Quality assurance is tied to persons rather than organizations, so it cannot be defined and carried out by administrative organs. Current legal regulations specified in Social Legal Code V do not ensure cooperative collaboration because they exclude competent specialists. Yet professional societies are called upon to develop respective standards. I consider this to be self-contradictory. One can only hope that lawmakers will make the necessary and appropriate corrections, for otherwise the introduction of "quality assurance" will tend to result more in therapeutic restriction. We are all called to raise the standard of every neurosurgical measure, especially in conditions that could be treated by other physician groups.

The Concept of Neurosurgical Standards from the Clinician's Perspective

R. Wüllenweber [1]

When we first delved into the problems of neurosurgical standards in Würzburg 2 years ago, legal experts and neurosurgeons agreed that reducing a standard to the "lowest common denominator" in a defensive therapy, influenced by legal liabilities, cannot be the optimum solution because it discourages innovation [12].

At that time Mr. Schreiber made it clear that risk assessment in neurosurgical diagnosis and treatment is of critical importance, but that there may be situations in which there is no valid standard that would prohibit taking a risk. As evidence that standards are still a matter of pressing concern, I again quote Mr. Schreiber: "A 'standard' does not prescribe a particular method once and for all; rather, it is adaptable, leaving room for the testing of other methods whose prospect for success is in reasonable proportion to the associated risks. The danger of standardization lies in the regressive prescription of outdated methods" [7].

It is important, then, to further develop the concept of a standard for a given clinical situation by testing a given, valid standard in a current clinical situation against the latest scientific developments and clinical experience, including risks.

Mr. Schreiber paraphrased the American literature by noting that: "Standard implies reference to a normal behavior that is practiced and accepted in real life." But when we equate "standard" with "normal behavior," we are merely simplifying our task by replacing a somewhat imprecise term with one that is even less precise. If we wish to define standards in a meaningful way, we must go into details, and in this sense I would extend the title of my report by adding the subtitle: "With special reference to the treatment of cerebral gliomas."

Getting back to *risk assessment*, I wish to cite two examples that illustrate the *risks of diagnosis*. First there is the question of whether angiography is still appropriate for the differential diagnosis and localization of brain tumors and the evaluation of their blood supply. Despite the risks of iodinated contrast media, we cannot categorically answer "no," because computer tomography (CT) and magnetic resonance (MR) imaging may leave specific questions unanswered. Another example is stereotaxis biopsy for the tissue diagnosis of mass lesions of the cerebrum.

Therapeutic risks include direct operative risks, which in turn relate to tumor location and blood supply, as well as general surgical risk factors such as age, general health, and coexisting disorders. Risks also include side effects such as those associated with adjuvant chemotherapy or radiotherapy.

[1] Haager Weg 69, W–5300 Bonn 1, FRG

Advances in Neurosurgery, Vol. 20
K. Piscol, M. Klinger, M. Brock (Eds.)

Typical complications, like those discussed by Mr. Franzki in his talk in Würzburg on preoperative consultation [4], cannot be disregarded if we, as practicing physicians, do not wish to expose patients to an exorbitant risk. And we cannot ignore the question of securing informed consent from a patient with altered mentation, which occurs with many cerebral tumors.

I see additional risks in the *interpretation of therapeutic results*, especially in retrospective studies. The danger of standards prescribing outmoded methods, as noted by Mr. Schreiber, is certainly present in "retrospective studies." In a study on the treatment of astrocytomas and glioblastomas, initiated by Mr. Kuhlendahl nearly 20 years ago [6], we attempted to offset this danger by having all the histologic findings reviewed and confirmed by a panel of competent neuropathologists. With regard to prospective randomized studies, it is important to evaluate the selection process, the criteria for inclusion and exclusion, which might be called the "stumbling blocks of statistics."

Cohadon began his paper "Indications for Surgery in the Management of Gliomas" [3] by quoting a remark by Percival Bailey: "About the group of gliomas it is difficult to say anything intelligent concerning them." To learn whether this attitude has changed during the past decade, we must look to the results of large studies published in recent years.

First I shall look at a controversial issue raised by Cairncross and Laperriere in an article titled "Low-Grade Glioma, to Treat or Not to Treat?" [1], a title that is rather provocative for neurosurgeons. The authors ("neuro-oncologists" and "radio-oncologists") point out that neurosurgery indeed plays a significant role in the treatment of certain types of low-grade glioma, such as cystic astrocytoma of the cerebellum in children, and of extensive hemispheric tumors or cysts in which surgery can prevent a life-threatening intracranial herniation. Neurosurgical procedures can cure medically untreatable epileptic seizures caused by a low-grade glioma. The authors further emphasize that neurosurgical treatment is *not curative* for most patients with diffusely infiltrating hemispheric tumors, but that it offers the advantage of establishing a diagnosis in equivocal cases, even though it is not considered justified in all cases to incur the risk of a surgical procedure just to render a diagnosis.

It should be noted that some difficulties undoubtedly stem from the WHO grading system, which classifies pilocytic astrocytoma as a grade I astrocytoma. These tumors grow so slowly that their "natural course" (spontaneous course not subject to therapeutic influence) can be traced over many years, indicating that these are "semibenign" lesions that, when well demarcated, are amenable to cure by total extirpation. The same applies to subependymomas, many of which are noted incidentally on CT scans without producing clinical symptoms.

The use of radiotherapy is a major controversy with these tumors. The side effects of radiotherapy at high doses, especially with whole-skull irradiation, require that the potential benefit to the patient be weighed against the toxic effects.

Chemotherapy of low-grade gliomas is strictly contraindicated due to the acute toxic effects and possible long-term complications. The authors conclude that the optimum treatment of low-grade gliomas remains doubtful, that retrospective studies on radiotherapy should be viewed as suggestive rather than conclusive, and that all therapeutic effects with regard to tumor growth, malignant transformation, and impairment of cognitive functions must be compared with the "natural course" of the disease.

Following this publication, the editor, Mr. Hachinski, apparently had difficulty attracting an opposing viewpoint, which finally was presented 1 year later (1990) by Shaw [9]. A radiologist, Shaw stresses the value of radiotherapy and notes that a 10-year survival rate of 40% can be achieved. He states that complications of radiotherapy can be largely prevented by a proper irradiation technique. There are reports of good results in a prospective randomized study at the Mayo Clinic, but so far the numbers are too small to permit a definitive evaluation.

The controversies are finally apostrophized as a "controversial consensus." Hachinski points out that a "consensus can remain a consensus only until it is called into question." Not surprisingly, all authors have reached the conclusion that large, prospective, controlled studies are needed to advance our knowledge in this area.

The study of the Brain Tumor Cooperative Group (Shapiro et al.), published in the *Journal of Neurosurgery* in 1989 [8], focuses on three chemotherapeutic regimens and two radiotherapeutic regimens in the *postoperative* treatment of malignant gliomas. The authors of this study conclude that the standard treatment of malignant gliomas should consist of a maximal tumor resection followed by combined radiation therapy and chemotherapy with BCNU. I find it significant that this study applies psychometric tests (Karnofsky index) in an attempt to evaluate the quality of survival. In the majority of patients who survived longer than 1 year, there was a higher numerical incidence of anaplastic astrocytomas than glioblastomas – a fact previously documented in Kuhlendahl's 1973 study of astrocytomas and glioblastomas, in which anaplastic astrocytomas, designated as grade III or IV astrocytoma by the old grading system, were found to be associated with better survival than histologically confirmed glioblastoma multiforme.

Mr. Ostertag and Mr. Bock will report at this conference on the glioma studies of the neuro-oncologic study group of the German Cancer Society. The results of the EORTC study (European Organization for Research and Treatment of Cancer) were published by Hildebrandt and Thomas in a recent issue of the *Journal of Neurology, Neurosurgery and Psychiatry* [5]. This study was the subject of an editorial published by Whittle and Gregor in the same journal [11]. Taking issue with the widely accepted multimodal therapy of medulloblastoma and primary cerebral lymphoma, the authors of the editorial claim that there is still much diversity of opinion regarding the diagnosis and treatment of low-grade and high-grade gliomas. Although the mortality associated with computer-controlled stereotaxic biopsy is less than 1% according to this study, the risks of this examination should not be disregarded, and the procedure should be done only if it will have specific therapeutic implications, i.e., deep-seated tumors that cannot be accurately diagnosed by CT or MRI, and cases where interstitial brachytherapy is the only reasonable treatment option. The resection of low-grade, well-demarcated tumors is confined to lesions located in "silent brain regions" where extirpative surgery will not result in speech disturbances or motor deficits. Successful radiotherapy can be provided only if side effects such as necrosis and leukoencephalopathy are controlled through reduction or focusing of the dose. There is still controversy with regard to the chemotherapy of low-grade astrocytomas. The cytotoxic effects are so significant, however, that this therapy cannot be recommended as a standard for low-grade gliomas. The authors of the editorial close by emphasizing that all therapeutic options for malignant gliomas are palliative, and that the most important criterion for treatment must be the prolongation of life of acceptable quality.

The large study of Cohadon [3] is based on comprehensive clinical experience. This author extensively reviewed the literature of recent years, critically evaluated it, and compared it with his own neurosurgical experience. He concludes that the neurosurgical treatment of gliomas is at best incomplete due to the location of the tumor and its infiltrative behavior. He attributes this to the hidden actively neoplastic cells that are detected histologically within a radius of 2 cm outside the limits of a "total resection." Given this biological fact, Cohadon believes that some so-called major advances in neurosurgery are naive, even if they are "technically impressive."

Despite its palliative nature, surgical treatment is indicated in many cases; but in all cases, cautious patient selection is needed to ensure that surgery and adjuvant therapy do not merely prolong life by a few weeks while failing to enhance its quality. Cohadon places hope in advances in molecular biology that will permit the development of substances that can seek out and destroy neoplastic cells.

Is Bailey's statement still true today? When we compare the results of current studies with those of 20 years ago, it is clear that there are no grounds for optimism in the neurosurgical treatment of gliomas.

It was my intention to demonstrate that standards in the treatment of cerebral gliomas are still very difficult to define, and that the primary issue relates to the assessment of risks, i.e., a meticulous patient selection process for every diagnostic and therapeutic measure. Technical competence is as important a basis for decision making in patient selection as free individual responsibility.

References

1. Cairncross JG, Lapperriere NJ (1989) Low-grade glioma, to treat or not to treat? Arch Neurol 46:1238–1239
2. Cairncross JG, Lapperriere NJ (1990) A reply. Arch Neurol 47:1139–1140
3. Cohadon F (1990) Indications for surgery in the management of gliomas. Advanc Tech Stand Neurosurg 17:189–234
4. Franzki HH (1990) Neuere Entwicklung in der Rechtsprechung zur Aufklärung. In Bushe KA, Brock M, Klinger M (eds) Advances in neurosurgery, vol 18. Springer, Berlin Heidelberg New York Tokyo, pp 299–305
5. Hildebrand J, Thomas DGT (1991) Report of a workshop sponsored by the European Organisation for Research and Treatment of Cancer (EORTC) on the treatment of primary malignant brain tumours. J Neurol Neurosurg Psychiatry 54:182–183
6. Kuhlendahl H, Miltz H, Wüllenweber R (1973) Die Astrozytome des Großhirns. Acta Neurochir 29:151–162

7. Schreiber H-L (1990) Risiko und erforderlicher Standard in der Neurochirurgie – Überholtes, Notwendiges, Unerprobtes – (Juristisches Referat). In: Bushe KA, Brock M, Klinger M (eds) Advances in neurosurgery, vol 18. Springer, Berlin Heidelberg New York Tokyo, pp 294–298
8. Shapiro WR et al. (1989) Randomized trial of three chemotherapy regimens and two radiotherapy regimens in postoperative treatment of malignant glioma – Brain Tumor Cooperative Group Trial 8001. J Neurosurg 71:1–9
9. Shaw EG (1990) Low-grade gliomas: to treat or not to treat? Arch Neurol 47:1138–1139
10. Shaw EG, Daumas-Duport C, Scheithauer BW et al. (1989) Radiation therapy in the management of low-grade supratentorial astrocytomas. J Neurosurg 70:171–176
11. Whittle IR, Gregor A (1991) Editorial. The treatment of primary malignant brain tumours. J Neurol Neurosurg Psychiatry 54:101–108
12. Wüllenweber R (1990) Risiko und erforderlicher Standard in der Neurochirurgie – Überholtes, Notwendiges, Unerprobtes – (Neurochirurgisches Referat). In: Bushe KA, Brock M, Klinger M (eds) Advances in neurosurgery, vol 18. Springer, Berlin Heidelberg New York Tokyo, pp 288–293

Medical Treatment Standards from a Legal Perspective

H.-L. Schreiber [1]

I. From a medical perspective, a "standard" is of interest to the neurosurgeon chiefly as a guide: What treatment is medically indicated for a given patient when one considers the prospects for recovery, advantages, risks, and hazards? What does the current state of medical science and practical experience tell us when we take into account current technical capabilities in diagnosis and treatment? Looking beyond the individual case, what can be said with regard to the same or similar cases of disease?

A standard is also an instrument for evaluating the potential accountability or liability of a physician. One danger of this interpretation is that a "standard" might become the "lowest common denominator of a defensive medicine," as Wüllenweber so aptly put it. This would be wrong for medicine and would undermine the principle of physician accountability, the purpose of which is to protect the patient by holding the physician liable for improper conduct. It would debase the purpose of this principle – and I grant that this may be a side effect of the expansion of liability – if, as a defense against potential liability, we were to "standardize" medicine by keeping to traditional methods instead of choosing innovative procedures that, especially in neurosurgery, might entail a greater risk.

Thus, a medical treatment standard serves both as a guide to orient the physician and as a means of evaluating the physician's conduct from the standpoint of accountability. Standards of care give substance to the general, fundamental rule of accountability for negligence. The law contains no more concrete provisions than the rule concerning the "necessary diligence" that must be exercised if one is to avoid liability. It is defined as that which the physician can and must do in a specific situation. The threshold of liability is negligence on this point, not failure: one is made liable by deviating from the standards of medical science and practice. These standards are formed in general terms by the scientific and practical state-of-the-art that is available to the physician at the time of treatment. Obviously, this is a medical interpretation and not a legal one. "Standard" implies reference to a normal mode of conduct that is followed and accepted in real-life situations. It does not prescribe adherence to traditional medical practices. A standard carries a general connotation, but generalization does not always work in medicine. There are broad areas of medicine in which minimum treatment standards can be defined, but there

[1] Juristisches Seminar der Universität, Platz der Göttinger Sieben 6, W–3400 Göttingen, FRG.

Advances in Neurosurgery, Vol. 20
K. Piscol, M. Klinger, M. Brock (Eds.)

are many areas in which they cannot. Medical procedures cannot be stipulated by a committee of the the DIN (German Institute for Standardization): there are still areas of controversy, and much remains undefined.

I will not, like Wüllenweber, speak of the standard that is valid for a specific, individual clinical situation. But this is largely a matter of semantics: The current level of research and clinical experience will basically dictate the therapeutic approach in any given case. Science seeks to limit generalizations while deriving principles that can be profitably applied to other, similar cases. A standard can become dangerous if it develops into an instrument for maintaining adherence to previous methods. But that is not its function: No one is obliged to maintain traditional practices if there is another approach that promises greater rewards with fewer risks.

II. Since the conference in Würzburg, "standards" has reemerged as a topic of discussion not because of these general questions but because of the difficult problems that arise in specific questions dealing with the proper treatment of diseases – the question of defining standards for specific disease groups.

Wüllenweber has spoken of the frequent "imponderability" of assessing treatment prospects. Today let us try to address the question of a standard by way of examples, as it relates to particular therapeutic approaches for specific diseases, and let us consider examples that can help us determine what constitutes a standard.

III. Wüllenweber first spoke about cerebral gliomas and their management, dealing initially with the question of standards in diagnosis. What does it include, and what are the reasonable limits of diagnostic inquiry? A legal distinction has been drawn between diagnosis and mere curiosity. It has been stated that a diagnostic investigation should include all possibilities, even if they are remote, but that it should not cover possibilities that are *very* remote. Obviously this is not a useful, manageable differentiation. Who would argue that a diagnostic procedure should depend upon whether a given possibility is remote or *very* remote? The limits of a diagnostic workup are drawn by the potential value of the workup in supplying new information. Invasive diagnostic procedures should be avoided if, to all intents and purposes, they can have no therapeutic implications in terms of deciding whether to operate or initiate chemotherapy, or in determining whether a biopsy is indicated. It has been debated whether CT and MRI have eliminated the need for angiography in the localization and further evaluation of brain tumors. What constitutes the standard here? I cannot answer this question from a legal perspective, and there is probably still no consensus about what is required. This is a case where a standard is lacking and still needs to be developed. The question of whether traditional diagnostic modalities should continue to be used again illustrates the danger that standards may bind us to conventional practices.

With regard to the neurosurgical treatment of gliomas, little can be said from a legal perspective.

1. Chemotherapy for low-grade astrocytomas continues to be controversial due to the toxic side effects. If one treatment modality is not unequivocally preferable to another, both modalities are acceptable from a legal standpoint. The degree of risk and possible advantages should be considered in each individual case.
2. Regarding the controversy over radiotherapy for low-grade gliomas, we can add these comments to those of Wüllenweber: If prospective, controlled studies are needed to clarify questions that are still controversial, a standard cannot be said to exist, for such studies presuppose a comparable uncertainty over the preferability of one treatment over another. As long as this uncertainty persists, we are not bound by a "standard procedure."
3. If a cerebral glioma is amenable only to palliative surgery because of its location and infiltrative spread, the standard would require consideration of the therapeutic value for the individual patient. This is the decisive criterion. Another factor is the patient's quality of life in cases where life can be prolonged for only a short period (say, a few weeks). Thus, treatment planning in these cases is highly individualized and cannot follow a fixed, standardized scheme.

Even the most persuasive conference lecture cannot establish a standard. Generally, a standard does not develop all at once but evolves gradually through a process of trials and discussions.

Occasionally, legal decisions that are made today in liability judgments involving cases treated in prior years must be based upon a different, earlier standard. This has occurred, for example, in decisions involving the use of thromboprophylaxis in cases dating from the early 1980s. Here the courts have refused to designate the prophylactic use of heparin as a standard treatment, despite the fact that this prophylaxis has become standard during the past few years. Thus, when legal decisions are made involving cases from prior years, there is a danger that the judgment may imply that it is not standard practice to institute medical thromboprophylaxis. This is another situation where a standard can abet the stagnation of medical progress. Present-day treatments must be based on the standard of today, not those of yesterday, if we are to continue to define liability in terms of deviation from a standard. It must always be remembered that standardization in medicine is an open-ended process. It is easy to speak of standards with respect to, say, the setup of hygienic and organizational facilities. When it comes to therapeutic standards, it must be considered that there can be no unconditional adherence to current, conventional procedures. This would cripple medical progress. The standard can be useful for orientation in fields of activity where uncontested or widely accepted procedures have been introduced. In this sense it designates a particular level that should be maintained under all circumstances. But the standard is not unconditionally binding; it must not impede the advance of medicine or the introduction of new surgical procedures if they offer better prospects for success.

References

Deutsch E (1991) Arzt- und Arzneimittelrecht. 2nd edn. Springer, Berlin Heidelberg New York Tokyo

Laufs A (1988) Arztrecht, 4th edn. NJW Schriftenreihe H. 29. Beck, München

Schreiber H-L (1984) Rechtliche Maßstäbe des medizinischen Standards. Langenbecks Arch Chir 364:295ff

Schreiber H-L (1986) Arzthaftung. Perspektiven der Rechtswissenschaft. Beitr Gerichtl Med XLIII:2ff

Cerebral Aneurysms

Endovascular Treatment of Berry Aneurysms by Endosaccular Occlusion

J. Moret, A. Boulin, and L. Castaings[1]

Although the surgical experience in treatment of aneurysms in tremendously large versus the endovascular one, it becomes possible to have a good idea of what the future will be as far as we have a better approach to the endovascular treatment possibilities and results. To avoid comparing "apples and potatoes," this study will take into account only what is commonly called berry aneurysms, i.e., typical surgical aneurysms whose sizes are equal or inferior to 1.5 cm and which extend intracranially and in almost all cases totally in the subarachnoid space (Table 1).

The specificity of our study is double: First, it is indeed strictly comparable to the neurosurgical series regarding the material as it has been described above. Second, all the aneurysms have been treated by the same team, using the same endovascular technique, and the same rules of follow-up (first control angiogram 4–6 months after the endosaccular occlusion, second control angiogram 1 year after the first one). All the aneurysms underwent an endosaccular occlusion using a latex balloon filled

Table 1. Anatomical localizations

Intracavernous (partialla)	7
Carotido-ophthalmic	33
Post. communicating artery	11
Carotid bifurcation	12
Basilar artery (tip or trunk)	31
Middle cerebral artery	10
Ant. communicating or cer. art.	13
Post. cerebral art.	3
PICA	5
Subarach. vert. art.	3
	128

PICA, proximal internal carotid artery

[1] Department of Interventional Neuroradiology, Fondation A. de Rothschild Hospital, 25–29 Rue Manin, F-75940 Paris, France.

Advances in Neurosurgery, Vol. 20
K. Piscol, M. Klinger, M. Brock (Eds.)

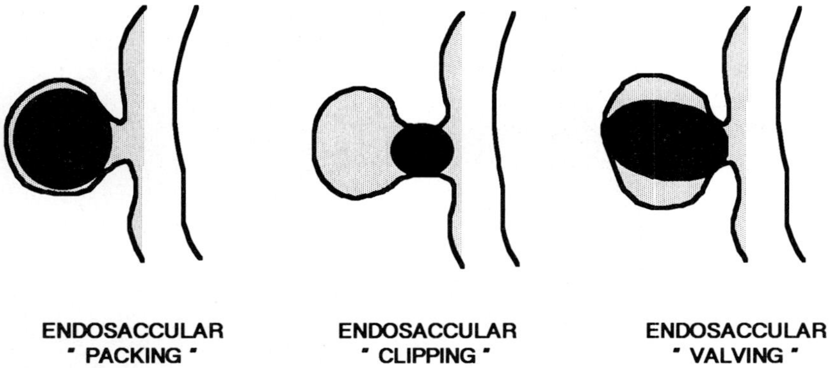

Fig. 1. Schematic drawings of endosaccular techniques for aneurysm occlusion

with 100% polymerizing substance (Polymeran from Balt Company). Navigation, positioning, and detachment of the balloon were performed using a catheter especially designed for that use (Magic BD 2L from Balt Company). Endosaccular occlusion is achieved according to three different methods: endosaccular clipping, endosaccular packing, and endosaccular valving (Fig. 1).

Treatment was attempted for 128 aneurysms in 124 patients: 22 cases were acute patients who bled within 48 h before treatment; 45 cases were nonacute patients (bleeding 10 days to some weeks before treatment); 61 patients had never hemorrhaged.

Because of arteriosclerosis, impossibility of occluding the aneurysmal sac, or impossibility of entering the aneurysmal neck, the endosaccular treatment failed in 36 cases (10 of those failures have been treated by parent vessel occlusion). In one case although the balloon was perfectly occluding the aneurysm, we decided to quit because the anchorage of the balloon was suspected to be borderline and we did not want to take any risk in an asymptomatic patient, especially because it was an easy localization for neurosurgical treatment. Finally, 101 of the 128 cases (79%) were successfully treated. Of these 101 treated cases, 91 underwent a selective occlusion of the aneurysmal sac and 10 an occlusion of the aneurysm and the parent vessel. Four patients had two aneurysms treated by endosaccular occlusion.

The long-term follow-up shows 18 recurrences among the 91 aneurysms treated by selective occlusion of the sac (20%). Each time the parent vessel occlusion was associated with the aneurysm occlusion (ten cases), we never observed any recurrence. A retrospective analysis of those recurrences demonstrates in almost all of them a small remaining neck appearing as a small crescent or triangle of contrast medium at the base of the aneurysm on the immediate control angiogram. Of the 18 recurrences 9 underwent a second endovascular treatment (6 of the 9 retreated cases were successfully occluded, 1 patient died from secondary clotting complications after retreatment). Of the 18 recurrences 2 underwent surgical treatment. Three recurrences are scheduled for a second endovascular treatment. Four patients bled and died some days or some weeks after the endosaccular treatment and were obviously recurrences. Four patients are just being kept under angiographic controls because the remnant is small and stable according to time. These "time-stable aneurysmal remnants" set a new concept regarding the understanding of the postendovascular treatment evolution. When a remnant ist stable after several control angiograms, we consider it a posttreatment deformation and no longer a recurrence.

We observed 19 complications among the 128 cases (15%), which in fact represent 137 different attempts at treatment because of the 9 retreated cases after recurrence. Analysis of those complications reveals 9 deaths and 10 neurological deficits: 8 of the 9 deaths involved posterior fossa localizations, 3 brainstem ischemia, and 5 aneurysm rupture (1 rupture occurred during treatment, the 4 other ruptures occurred some days or weeks after treatment because of early recurrence). One death was related to a middle cerebral artery embolus which occurred 4 weeks after the endosaccular occlusion. Because no other etiology was demonstrated, we have decided to impute that death to the endovascular treatment. Seven of the ten neurological deficits were related to clotting phenomena despite the fact that all the treatments were performed under full heparinization. Because of these problems of clotting, we have decided since July 1990 to perform the endovascular treatment under full heparinization associated with an aspirin therapy (500 mg i.v. immediately before the procedure) even when the patient is treated in the acute phase of the bleeding. Since this association between aspirin and heparin has been used, we have not observed any other complication related to clotting phenomena. Two of the ten neurological deficits were related to a secondary migration of the balloon (in one case we did not reposition the balloon, in the other one we failed to reposition it). One of the ten neurological deficits occurred after migration of the polymerizing substance because of rupture of the balloon before total solidification of that substance (this was related to the use of a wrong HEMA which had degraded the latex balloon at the beginning of our experience).

Analysis of complications we have avoided is also very important as it shows that although we are working remote from the aneurysm itself, we have the possibility of escaping from dangerous situations. Repositioning of the balloon after detachment is one of the major technical tricks that makes the technique safer. In 11 cases a secondary migration of the balloon occurred (it was always some minutes to 1 h after detachment), leading to the occlusion of the parent vessel. In one case (the first one in our experience) we did not reposition the balloon and we encountered an ischemic complication. In all of the ten other cases we repositioned the balloon using a second nondetachable balloon catheter. In nine of those ten cases, repositioning was successful without complication. In the only case where repositioning failed, the patient experienced an ischemic complication.

Looking at the complications on the basis of their percentage of occurrence, one must take into account all the attempts of treatment, i.e., 137 procedures (128 cases + 9 retreatments). The risk of complications is therefore 14%, including 6.5% mortality and 7% morbidity, whatever the localization of the aneurysms is. If we want to compare our results with the neurosurgical ones, the anatomical localization is very important insofar as it is the only strictly identical parameter between both techniques of treatment. Carotido-ophthalmic and basilar aneurysms are known to be either difficult or dangerous or both regarding the neurosurgical approach. We must consider that those two latter localizations represent 26% and 30%, respectively, of the aneurysms we have treated, which means that neurosurgical treatment for the same population of patients might have been tricky and/or dangerous in 56% of our cases. Looking at our statistics in more detail, one can notice that 39 cases of vertebrobasilar aneurysms (31% of the total number of our aneurysms) were responsible for 58% of the total number of complications, while 89 cases of aneurysms in other localizations were responsible for 42% of the total number of complications. If we are now able to avoid complications related to clotting phenomena during the treatment (and it seems that this is possible since we associate heparin plus aspirin), it means that we can expect a reduction of almost 40% (7 of 19 complications) of the overall rate of complications, which represents a great improvement.

At that stage of our experience the timing of treatment regarding the onset of the hemorrhage versus the clinical results cannot be reliably taken into account because 22 cases treated by endosaccular occlusion in an emergency is too small a series. However, six of the nine deaths we have to deplore occurred during emergency treatment, but five of them were related to clotting complications which have no special relationships with emergency conditions. Nevertheless, the therapeutic traumatism of the endovascular treatment is without doubt much less important than the neurosurgical one. As a rough conclusion, we can say that according to our experience 71% of intracranial berry aneurysms can be treated by endosaccular occlusion, while 79% can be treated by an endovascular approach if we add to the endosaccularly treated cases those cases where parent vessel occlusion can be performed.

Finally, behind the statistical numbers which are absolutely necessary to evaluate the performance of a given technique, it is the philosophy of treatment of berry aneurysms which has changed. Endosaccular occlusion is definitely an alternative treatment whose indications must be discussed with priority for carotido-ophthalmic and basilar aneurysms whatever the circumstances of discovery are. In asymptomatic aneurysms a careful attempt at endovascular treatment carries few risks and seems to be also the first choice of treatment, especially because its failure can be immediately followed by a surgical procedure. In emergency cases, except for the carotido-ophthalmic and basilar localizations, our experience with endosaccular treatment needs to be larger for a more appropriate analysis.

Strategies of Endovascular Treatment of Large and Giant Intracranial Aneurysms

H. C. Nahser and D. Kühne[1]

Introduction

The purpose of this brief communication is to outline possibilities and frontiers of the endovascular treatment of large and giant aneurysms of the carotid and cerebral arteries.

Balloon occlusion was introduced by Serbinenko [2] and was further developed by the French Neuroradiological School. Later advances were suggested by Higashida [1]. Up to now we have treated 55 large or giant cavernous and parasellar aneurysms, 12 large or giant aneurysms of the vertebrobasilar system, and 10 giant aneurysms of other intracranial sites. Recently, we changed our approach from selective occlusion of aneurysms to embolization with coils.

Treatment with Microballoons

Cavernosal Carotid Artery Aneurysms

The majority of our 55 cavernosal and parasellar large and giant carotid aneurysms presented with ocular nerve lesions and visual disturbances due to compression of the oculomotor and optic nerves. If the aneurysm enlarged into the subarachnoid space, even in the cases of large and giant aneurysms, bleeding was recorded. Rarely, transient ischemic events have been recorded due to thromboemboli from aneurysms. Only symptomatic aneurysms were treated by us. In this report, traumatic and spontaneously dissecting aneurysms are not considered.

The possibility of selective balloon occlusion in these locations depends on the form, size, and location of the aneurysm neck. Initial diagnostic angiography is complemented by cross-compression studies to outline anterior and posterior collateralization and followed, if collateralization is present, by a 20-min test balloon occlusion of the affected carotid artery. If the occlusion is not tolerated and occlusion of the carotid artery is mandatory for therapy, EC-IC bypass (superficial temporal to middle cerebral artery) precedes the interventional procedure. Pre-embolization MRI investigation is essential to demonstrate the amount of preformed thrombus in the aneurysm. Selective occlusion of large and giant carotid aneurysms is not

[1] Abteilung Neuroradiologie, Alfried-Krupp-Krankenhaus, Alfried-Krupp-Str. 21, W-4300 Essen 1, FRG.

Advances in Neurosurgery, Vol. 20
K. Piscol, M. Klinger, M. Brock (Eds.)

always possible, depending on the form and size of the neck of the aneurysm. Even if there is good collateralization, a selective occlusion may not always be the goal because expansion of remnants of the neck or emboli out of such expansions have been recognized. In all these cases a definitive result was achieved by occlusion of the carotid artery in combination with the aneurysm neck. Endovascular trapping was needed when there was residual influx into the aneurysm via the ophthalmic artery. Especially in the case of ophthalmic artery aneurysms, endovascular trapping was performed by occlusion with two balloons, one just proximal and the other distal to the aneurysm. When, after a thorough analysis, selective occlusion of the aneurysms is possible, the detachable balloon system is introduced under local anesthesia, sedation, and systemic heparinization. The balloon is navigated into the aneurysms under road mapping fluoroscopy. There, it can be inflated to the required size. During detachment, stabilization of the size of the balloon can be provided by a second nondetachable balloon system.

Out of 55 cases, selective permanent occlusion was achieved in 18. In 37 cases permanent selective occlusion was not possible, in three of these cases a previously performed selective occlusion resulting in balloon migration into thrombosed parts of the aneurysms. Residual filling of parts of the aneurysm made carotid balloon occlusion necessary. An occlusion was performed primarily in 34 carotid arteries, eight with trapping and seven after EC-IC bypass. According to our observations, it was unnecessary for carotid occlusion to follow immediately after the bypass operation.

Regarding complications in these procedures, we recorded reversible ischemia in three cases. In one particular case it originated from an embolus to the middle cerebral artery which was treated with local urokinase before the aneurysm was occluded. In all cases except one, in which severe optic nerve dysfunction turned into complete amaurosis of the afflicted eye, local symptoms resolved completely within 6–12 months after treatment due to shrinkage of the thrombosed aneurysm. This correlates with the findings of MRI follow-up. MRI follow-ups were performed in 27 patients over a period of up to 4 years. There was a 50% reduction of the mass effect in the first 6 months after treatment, and of 75% after the first year. In those patients (treated either selectively or nonselectively) who were studied after 2 years ($n = 17$), remnants of the aneurysms were not visible. In the cases with carotid occlusion, no late ischemic events were recorded in the observation period of up to 8 years, and there were no MRI T2 changes resulting from ischemia in the affected hemisphere.

Fig. 1a, b. Large aneurysm of the origin of the basilar artery with acute growth of the thrombosed part, leading to acute brain stem insufficiency. **a** Anteroposterior, **b** lateral view. The aneurysm has a large thrombosed part and only a small nonthrombosed part

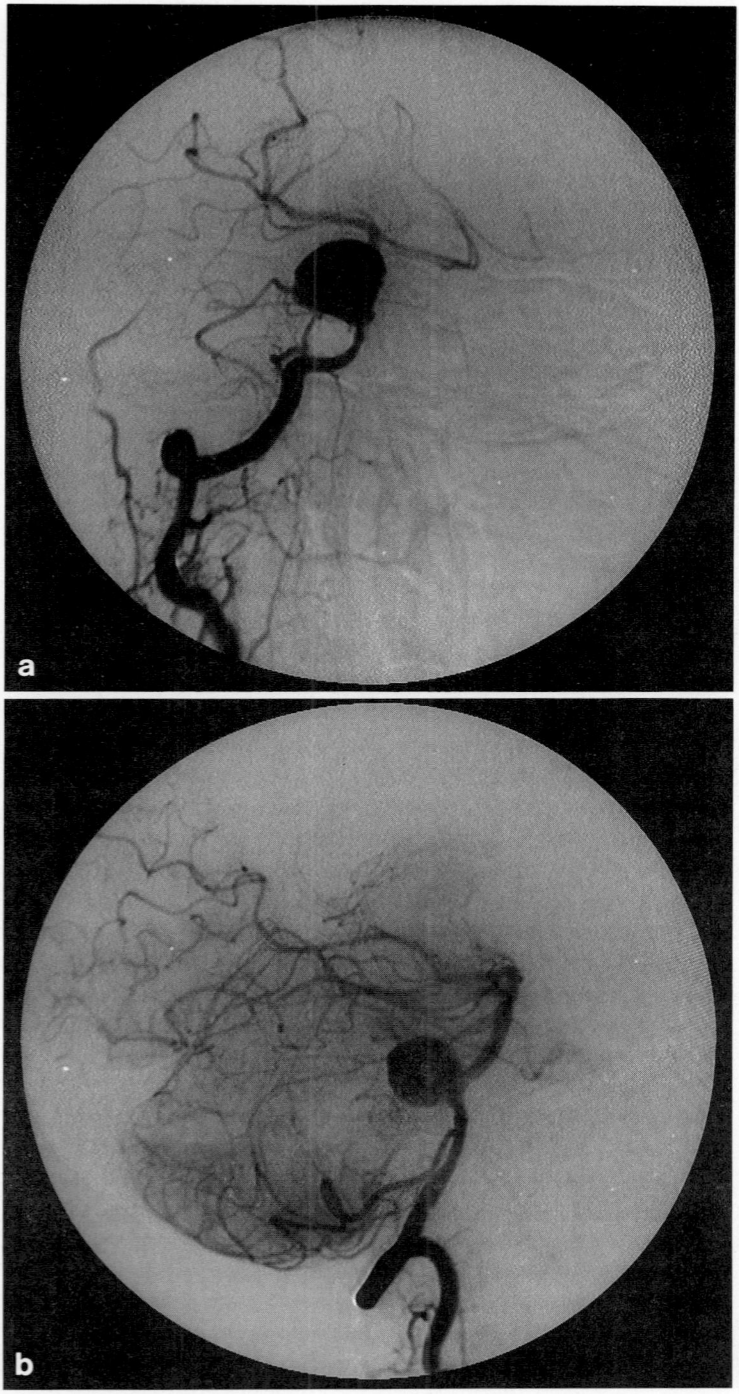

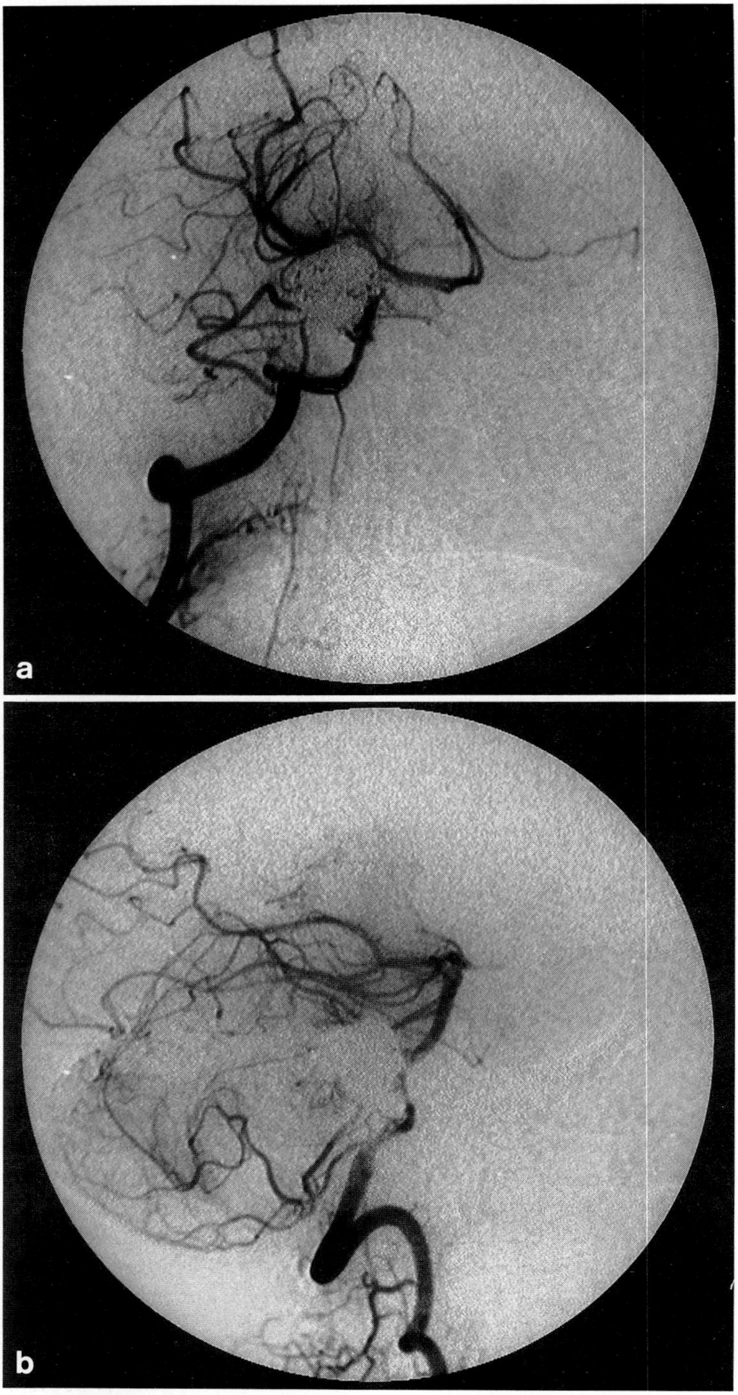

Aneurysms of the Basilar Tip and Other Locations

Compared to the results with the cavernosal carotid aneurysms, the results with the large basilar aneurysms were poor. Eleven aneurysms at the basilar tip and one at the middle basilar artery were treated. Seven of these can be classified as large and five as giant. Six patients presented with subarachnoid hemorrhages and five with neurological disturbances due to the mass effect of the aneurysm. In all cases, despite one balloon, selective occlusion with preservation of the perforating arteries of the basilar tip was achieved.

In two patients, 6–12 h after successful balloon implantation a basilar thrombosis occurred, leading to progressive brain stem dysfunction. Local fibrinolysis with urokinase was successful only in one of these cases. Two patients developed clinical signs of an expanding mass at the basilar tip after complete obliteration of the aneurysms. Angiography in neither case showed any filling of the aneurysm. Further growing of the thrombosed aneurysm was disclosed by MRI. Both patients died from rebleeding. A valve mechanism produced by the balloon must be considered as the cause in these cases, allowing influx of blood into the aneurysm in systole. In two other cases early balloon deflation led to refilling of the aneurysm: one of these was later successfully treated with microcoils.

The following aneurysms at other intracranial sites were also treated with balloons: five at the anterior communicating artery, two at the carotid bifurcation, and three at the posterior communicating artery. In all cases, primary selective balloon occlusion could be achieved. On follow-up we observed a shrinking of the anterior communicating artery aneurysms in three cases. In one case recurrent subarachnoid hemorrhage occurred after early balloon deflation, and surgical clipping of the aneurysm was performed. There was reopening of one of the PCA aneurysms, too, after balloon deflation: this partient was later treated with coil embolization (see below). All other patients have had an uneventful course up to now and no further hemorrhages.

Treatment with Microcoils

Coil implantation was performed as an alternative to balloon embolization in eight patients. In these cases, although surgery was performed in three cases, selective clipping was considered to be too risky. In two cases attempted balloon embolization failed. The lesions treated were two aneurysms at the basilar tip, one aneurysm of the middle basilar artery, one posterior communicating artery aneurysm, one aneurysm of the cranial carotid bifurcation, two giant cavernosal carotid aneurysms,

Fig. 2a, b. Due to the acute course of the disease, a one-stage coil embolization had to be performed. **a** Anteroposterior and **b** and lateral views show complete closure of the nonthrombosed part of the dome and the neck with preservation of the parent and neighboring arteries and one anterior communicating artery aneurysm. Three of these were classified as large (< 2.5 cm) and five as giant (> 2.5 cm). In each case, embolization was performed in stages due to the grade of secondary thrombosis. In the first stage a basket was built in the giant aneurysms by using larger Cook Hilal Coils in which Dacron-coated Target Coils were packed. Near the neck, simple coils without Dacron fiber (Target) were used, to prevent secondary occlusion of the parent artery. Up to four sessions were needed. In two patients a transitory ischemic episode occurred during or shortly after the intervention. In all cases the aneurysms could be obliterated, in some cases leaving a small remnant at the neck. Neurological deficits caused by the mass effect of the aneurysms resolved. A simultaneous decrease of edema was demonstrated in low-field MRI (0.3 T) in a follow-up period of up to 1 year. No new or further hemorrhage occurred. All these patients remain in follow-up, utilizing neurological investigation, MRI, and, if indicated, angiography.

In a further case an emergency coil embolization was performed. Progressive acute brain stem dysfunction occurred in a patient with an aneurysm at the origin of the basilar artery. The aneurysm had bled 2 years before and there was a slow growth of the aneurysm, documented by MRI. The aneurysm could be completely obliterated, with preservation of the parent artery. The patient's symptoms slowly decreased in a short follow-up period.

Discussion

Successful obliteration of large and giant skull base and intracranial aneurysms with balloons depends upon the site of the aneurysm. In our series, aneurysms of the cavernous parts of the carotid artery could be managed with minimal risk and no permanent deficits using detachable balloons. An improvement in the symptoms of paracavernous space-occupying aneurysms was achieved in all but one case. The patency of the carotid artery was preserved in one-third of cases. The pathophysiological background of this is that in this anatomical situation the jet effect into the aneurysms is sufficiently altered. This is, in our experience, not always possible in other intracranial sites and may lead to dangerous situations. For instance, a valve mechanism can develop at the neck of the aneurysm and lead to expansion of the aneurysm and final bleeding.

Detachable microcoils promise a safer way to obliterate the aneurysms at these locations. In an early series of nine patients with follow-ups of up to 1 year, there was regression of the mass effect by organization of the thrombosed parts of the aneurysms. Further advances in this technique can be expected with the introduction by electrically detachable coils.

References

1. Higashida RT, Halbach VV, Barnwell SL. Treatment of intracranial aneurysms with preservation of the parent vessel: results of percutaneous balloon embolization in 84 patients.
2. Serbinenko FA (1974) Balloon catherization and occlusion of major cerebral vessels. J Neurosurg 41:125–142

Endovascular Treatment of Basilar Bifurcation Aneurysms

M. Schumacher and W. Radü[1]

Introduction

Treatment of cerebral aneurysms, in particular giant aneurysms of the vertebrobasilar system, has been changed since Serbinenko [6] and 1 year later Debrun [1] introduced detachable balloons for aneurysm occlusion. The endovascular approach has been advanced additionally by the development of a thermoplastic microcatheter with double lumen and progressive suppleness [3]. In giant aneurysms, balloon occlusion has been combined with occlusive coils, allowing the number of balloons for packing the lumen to be reduced [2, 4, 7].

Both techniques have been used for endovascular obliteration in our patients with tip of the basilar artery aneurysms.

Materials and Methods

Within the last 2.5 years eight patients with aneurysms of the basilar bifurcation were admitted to our hospital (Table 1). The patients ranged in age from 18 to 69 years, three males and five females. The maximum diameter of the aneurysm sac varied from 8 to 50 mm. Only one was situated medially, all the others were placed eccentrically in reference to the top of the basilar artery.

In all patients the risk of surgical treatment was estimated to be excessively high due to the site and/or size of the aneurysm. In one 69-year-old patient with a giant aneurysm there was additionally an inability to tolerate general anesthesia.

The interventional procedures were performed with standard equipment (high-resolution DSA, road-mapping technique, measuring of activated clotting time, systemic anticoagulation).

For balloon occlusion, a distal 1.8-F microcatheter (Balt Magic BD 2L) and latex Balt balloons number 1–3 were used. Detachable balloons were filled with Polymeran, an acrylic mixture solidifying within 20–30 min. Placement of platinum flower coils of different sizes (Target Therapeutics, ranging 2–6 cm in length in introducer and an unrestrained outside diameter of 2–4 mm) was carried out with a Target microcatheter.

[1] Abteilung Neuroradiologie, Universität Freiburg, Hauptstr. 5, W–7800 Freiburg, FRG.

Advances in Neurosurgery, Vol. 20
K. Piscol, M. Klinger, M. Brock (Eds.)

Table 1. Aneurysms of the basilar bifurcation, size and clinical state before and immediately after treatment

Patient	Size	Signs and symptoms before treatment	Signs and symptoms after treatment
B.M.	Giant	Internal ophthalmoplegia, mental deterioration	Mental deterioration
S.H.	8 mm	Normal	Hemiparesis, hemianopsia
R.G.	10 mm	Normal	Normal
R.J.	Giant	III, walking disab.	Walking disab.
P.E.	13 mm	Dysarthria	Dysarthria, diplopia
S.J.	18 mm	Normal	Tetraparesis, PC infarction
L.M.	10 mm	VI	Normal
H.A.	Giant	Walking diasab. dizziness	Coma

Table 2. Therapy and clinical outcome of aneurysms of the basilar bifurcation

Patient	Treatment	Outcome
B.M.	Occlusion l. vertebral a.	Mental deterioration
S.H.	No balloon surgery	Perman. deficit
R.G.	Balloon	
R.J.	Balloon	Normal
P.E.	Balloon	Normal
S.J.	Coils	Perman. deficit
L.M.	Balloon, coils	Normal
H.A.	SAH prior to b. occl.	Exitus

Results

As listed in Table 2, three patients could be treated by balloon exclusively, two of them in the acute phase, one patient in the late subacute period (Figs. 1 and 2). Though the final clinical outcome in these patients was good, in one patient (R.G.) hemiplegia occurred 8 h after endovascular occlusion of the aneurysm. Angiography immediately employed after clinical deterioration revealed a dislocation of the balloon blocking the basilar bifurcation. With a second nondetachable balloon, the dislocated balloon could again be pushed into the aneurysm sac. Within 1 h the neurological deficit disappeared completely, leaving the patient in an excellent condition up to now (1 year after treatment).

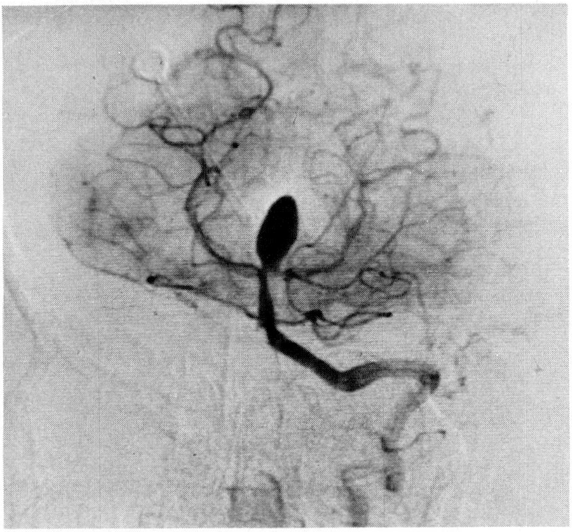

Fig. 1. Frontal view of left vertebral angiogram shows 5- to 12-mm aneurysm midsagittal positioned at the top of the basilar artery; neck is clearly visible

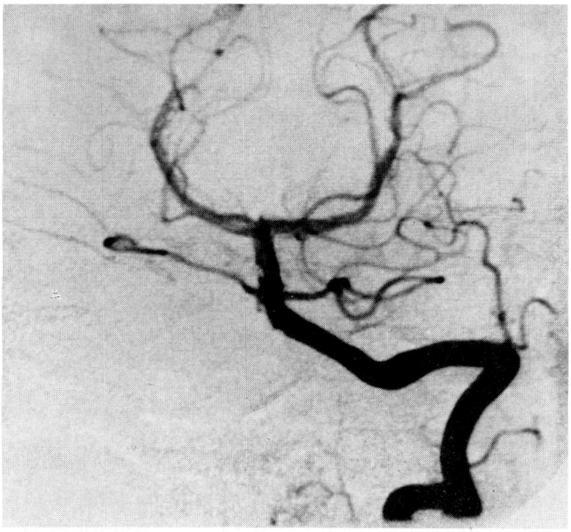

Fig. 2. Same patient as in Fig. 1 after placement of a single detachable latex balloon demonstrating complete obliteration of aneurysm with preservation of the basilar and both posterior cerebral arteries

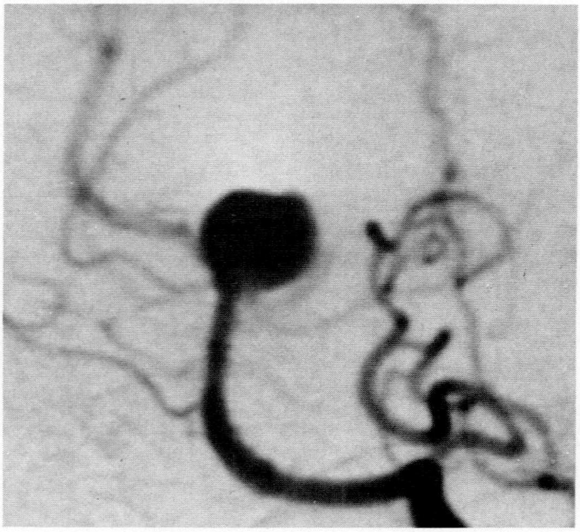

Fig. 3. Left vertebral angiogramm (frontal view) shows 12- to 14-mm aneurysm at basilar bifurcation slightly eccentrically positioned. The left posterior cerebral artery (PCA) originates directly from the ICA (not shown)

By occlusion of the vertebral artery in one 69-year-old patient (B.M.), an incomplete thrombosis of a giant aneurysm could be achieved. Because of severe arteriosclerotic stenotic process including the distal portion of the basilar artery in front of the aneurysmal neck, no attempt was made to pass a balloon into the aneurysm.

A complication directly associated with the placement of coils in an 18-mm aneurysm (S.J.) occurred when the end of the last coil dislodged into the top of the basilar artery, followed by thrombosis.

In one case regrowth of an incompletely occluded aneurysm took place, requiring a second procedure. Since the first balloon prevented insertion of further balloons, it was necessary to pack the residual lumen with coils passing the first balloon (Figs. 3 and 4).

Subarachnoidal rebleeding occurred in one patient during the balloon advance via the vertebral artery into the proximal internal carotid artery (PICA), immediately followed by coma and several days later by death. It is still an open question whether blocking of the PICA contributed to the recurrence of the hemorrhage.

In one patient (S.H.), we decided not to detach the balloon, though from the angiographic point of view the aneurysm could be completely excluded from the circulation, and patency of the entire vertebrobasilar system could be confirmed. Testing different positions and filling volumes, several neurological deficits occurred such as deterioration of consciousness, hemiparesis, deviation of the eyes, and disorientation which normalized after the deflated balloon had been removed.

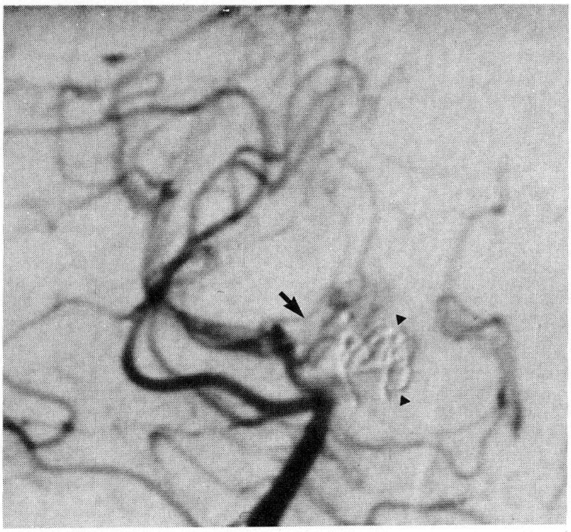

Fig. 4. Same patient as in Fig. 3 after final treatment. The aneurysm initially had been subtotally occluded by a latex balloon, leaving behind a small crevice between the balloon and aneurysm neck. A follow-up angiogram showed a regrowth of the neck remnant (not demonstrated). The recurrent aneurysm portion then was occluded by intrasaccular placement of five flower coils (*arrowheads*), preserving the basilar artery, perforating arteries, and PCA. The previous, detached balloon is still in place (*arrow*)

After clipping of the aneurysm, the patient developed a severe hemiparesis, hemineglect, and hemianopia.

Discussion

Endovascular balloon occlusion of aneurysms of the posterior circulation is an alternative method in cases in which surgery seems to be risky. Generally this is true in giant aneurysms, in which direct surgical approach is still difficult or impossible. Balloon embolization also is accepted as a primary treatment particularly in aneurysms of the basilar bifurcation since the majority of poor surgical results occurred in this localization [5].

Technical problems still exist in the usage of balloons as well as coils, e.g., incomplete obliteration of the aneurysm, premature loss of balloon, and thromboembolic complications. However, the main advantage of this method is that it is performed on conscious patients and that aneurysms can be reached without much effort also in difficult surgical locations such as vertebrobasilar and carotido-ophthalmic.

References

1. Debrun G, Lacour P, Caron JP, Hurth M, Comoy J, Keravel Y (1975) Inflatable and released balloon technique experimentation in dogs: application in man. Neuroradiology 9:267–271
2. Hilal S (1988) Synthetic fiber coated platinum coils successfully used for the endovascular treatment of arteriovenous malformations, aneurysms, and direct arterio-venous fistulae of the central nervous system. 26th Annual Meeting of the American Society of Neuroradiology. Chicago, Ill., May
3. Moret J, Picard L, Lepoire J, Castaings L, Boulin A (1988) Endovascular treatment via the endovascular approach of the so-called surgical subarachnoid aneurysms: a new technique. In: Nadjmi M (ed) Imaging of brain metabolism. Spine and cord. Interventional neuroradiology free communications. Springer, Berlin Heidelberg New York Tokyo, pp 267–276
4. Nakahara J, Taki W, Nishi S, Shibata O, Kikuchi H (1990) Treatment of giant anterior communicating artery aneurysm via an endovascular approach using detachable balloons and occlusive coils. AJNR 11:1195–1197
5. Perless SJ, Drake CG (1985) Posterior circulation aneurysms. In: Wilkins RH, Rengachary SS (eds) Neurosurgery. McGraw-Hill, New York, pp 1422–1437
6. Serbinenko FA (1974) Balloon catherization and occlusion of major cerebral vessels. J Neurosurg 41:125–145
7. Yang PJ, Halbach VV, Higashida RT, Hieshima GB (1988) Platinum wire: a new transvascular embolic agent. AJNR 9:547–550

Embolization of Large Aneurysms with Detachable Balloons

F. Brassel[1], L. Solymosi[2], E. Lins[1], J. Wappenschmidt[1] and W. Becker[1]

Introduction

The evolution of intravascular embolization techniques during the last 20 years has offered a new approach in the therapy of large intracranial aneurysms [1–8]. Improvements in microcatheter and microballoon technology, steerable micro-guidewires, and high-resolution digital subtraction angiography with road-mapping capability allow access to nearly all cerebrovascular territories.

Patients and Methods

Since 1979, interventional procedures were performed in 22 patients having large intracranial aneurysms which were not easily accessible neurosurgically. Balloon embolization was carried out in 20 of these cases. The aneurysms were located in the intracavernous portion of the internal carotid artery in 8, at the level of the origin of the ophthalmic artery from the internal carotid artery in 9, at the internal carotid artery bifurcation in 1, at the distal end of the basilar artery in 4, and in the trifurcation of the middle cerebral artery in 1. One patient showed a large intracavernous aneurysm bilaterally. The maximum outer diameter of the aneurysms ranged from 10 mm to 80 mm. Nineteen patients showed symptoms due to mass effects. Five cases presented with a subarachnoid hemorrhage, one with an intracerebral hemorrhage, two with oral bleeding from traumatic pseudoaneurysms of the intracavernous internal carotid arteries, and one with a ruptured intracavernous aneurysm resulting in a carotid cavernous sinus fistula. Interventional therapy was performed because of surgically inaccessible anatomical location, broad-based or fusiform aneurysms without a well-defined surgical neck, and failed neurosurgical clipping of the aneurysm.

Iso-osmotic, contrast-filled detachable latex or silicone balloons which underwent progressive shrinkage were used, except in one case which was embolized with a nondeflating silicone polymer-filled latex balloon. Prior to embolization all patients underwent a four-vessel cerebral angiography with appropriate views of

[1] Abteilung für Neuroradiologie, Medizinische Hochschule Hannover, Konstanty-Gutschow-Str. 8, W–3000 Hannover 61, FRG.
[2] Neurochirurgische Universitätsklinik, Sigmund-Freud-Str. 25, W–5300 Bonn, FRG.

Advances in Neurosurgery, Vol. 20
K. Piscol, M. Klinger, M. Brock (Eds.)

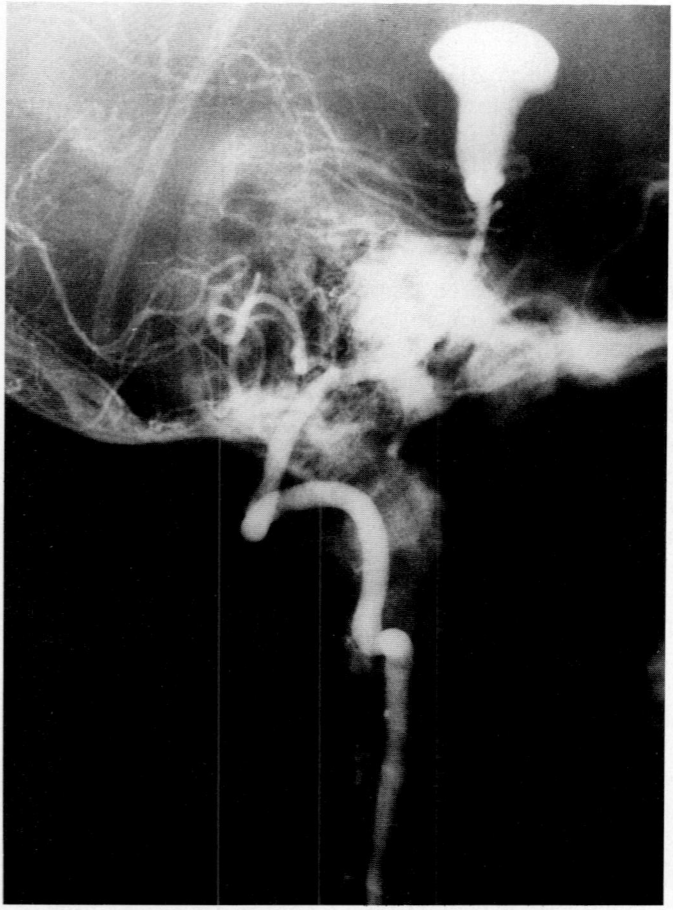

Fig. 1. Left vertebral artery angiogram with large basilar artery bifurcation aneurysm in a 48-year-old female before treatment

the aneurysm and a functional angiographic investigation of the cerebral circulation to evaluate the adequacy of the circulation in the circle of Willis. At a second sitting, transfemoral embolization was performed under continuous neurological monitoring, using standby anesthesia, neuroleptic analgesia, or sedation and in three patients, under general anesthesia.

Results

Embolization could be carried out in 20 of 22 aneurysms. In 10 cases, the parent vessel was occluded along with the aneurysm; in 7 patients, primary occlusion of the aneurysm was achieved with preservation of the patency of the parent artery; in 3 cases, the balloon failed to occlude the aneurysm. The size of the 20 embolized aneurysms remained unchanged in 4, decreased in 13, and showed total shrinkage simultaneously with deflation of the contrast-filled balloons (Figs. 1 and 2) in 3 cases. In the follow-up from 2 months to 12 years, neurological symptoms have improved in 9 patients to date, improved transiently in 3, remained unchanged in 4, and deteriorated in 4. The 3 patients who showed temporary improvement died because of rebleeding. One of the cases died 3.5 weeks after a successful embolization of a basilar tip aneurysm, despite no change in size and location of the contrast-filled latex balloon. The possible site of the bleeding was the neck of the aneurysm. Another primarily successfully embolized basilar tip aneurysm showed premature deflation of the latex balloon with reopening of the aneurysm. Subtotal embolization in another institution resulted in a lethal rerupturing of this aneurysm 3 months after the second treatment. The third case, a middle cerebral artery aneurysm, rebled fatally 3 months after a successful packing of the aneurysm with a silicone balloon. The aneurysm had reopened despite an unchanged size of the contrast-filled balloon.

Discussion and Conclusion

From our experience, embolization with detachable, iso-osmotic contrast-filled balloons proved valuable in the treatment of neurosurgically inaccessible, large intracranial aneurysms. All but one patient had been treated with detachable latex and silicone balloons, filled with iso-osmotic contrast material. All contrast-filled latex balloons showed progressive deflation over a period of 3 weeks to 4 months after the embolization. In four patients, this phenomenon led to reperfusion of the aneurysm, necessitating a second embolization. Therefore, balloon size and location must be carefully monitored during the first 6 months after embolization with the help of either plain radiographs or CT. If the balloon exhibits a change in its location or axis, suggesting a migration away from the neck of the aneurysm, an immediate reangiography should be performed to exclude reperfusion of the aneurysmal cavity. If the aneurysm is reperfused, a reembolization of the aneurysmal lumen should be carried out. Alternatively, when the patient's intracerebral circulation is satisfactory, occlusion of the parent vessel at the level of the neck of the aneurysm (balloon trapping) offers a second therapeutic option. Embolization of large aneurysms with iso-osmotic contrast-filled latex balloons which show progressive shrinkage in the course of time allows, in certain cases, not only the occlusion of the aneurysm, but also its simultaneous shrinking, thus avoiding the tumorous effect of the "plegic aneurysms" (Figs. 1 and 2).

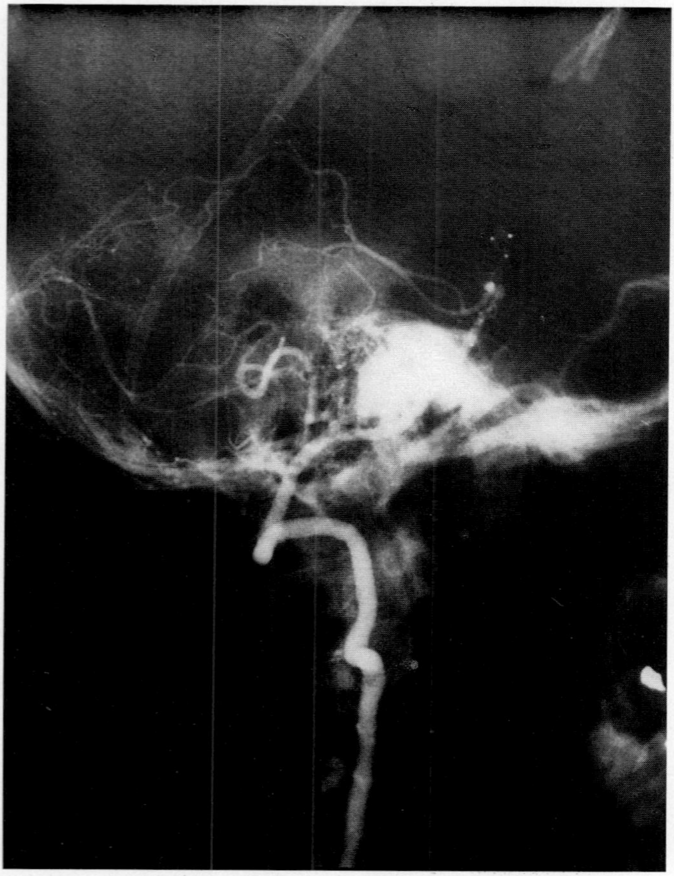

Fig. 2. Left vertebral artery angiogram 5 months after embolization with three iso-osmotic contrast-filled latex balloons. Note the three deflated balloons with radiopaque gold markers in the neck of the totally shunken aneurysm (confirmed by CT)

References

1. Berenstein A, Ransohoff J, Kupersmith M, Flamm E, Graeb D (1984) Transvascular treatment of giant aneurysms of the cavernous carotid and vertebral arteries. Surg Neurol 21:3–12
2. Debrun G, Fox A, Drake C, Peerless S, Girvin J, Ferguson G (1981) Giant unclippable aneurysms: treatment with detachable balloons. AJNR 2:167–173
3. Higashida RT, Halbach VV, Dowd CF, Barnwell SL, Hieshima GB (1991) Intracranial aneurysms: interventional neurovascular treatment with detachable balloons – results in 215 cases. Radiology 178:663–670
4. Negoro M, Kageyama N, Ishiguchi T (1983) Cerebrovascular occlusion by catheterization and embolization: clinical experience. AJNR 4:362–365

5. Romodanov AP, Shcheglov VI (1983) Intravascular occlusion of saccular aneurysms of the cerebral arteries by means of a detachable balloon catheter. In: Krayenbühl H (eds) Advances and technical standards in neurosurgery, vol 9. Springer, Berlin Heidelberg New York Tokyo, pp 25–49
6. Scialfa G, Vaghi A, Vasecchi F, Benardi L, Tonon C (1982) Neuroradiological treatment of carotid and vertebral fistulas and intracavernous aneurysms. Neuroradiology 24:13–25
7. Serbinenko FA (1974) Balloon catheterization and occlusion of major cerebral vessels. J Neurosurg 41:125–145
8. Triebelk H-J, Grzyska U, Frehrking M, Zeumer H (1989) Klinische und MRT-Verlaufskontrollen von Karotisaneurysmen nach Ballonembolisation. Radiologe 29: 427–431

Endovascular Treatment of Internal Carotid Artery Aneurysms

V. Olteanu-Nerbe[1], G. Dürr[2], A. Piepgras[1], P. Schmiedek[1], F. Marguth[1], and H.-J. Reulen[1]

Introduction

Until 1988, difficult aneurysms of the proximal internal carotid artery (ICA), particularly those located within the cavernous sinus (CS), were treated in our department by combined occlusion of the internal carotid artery and extra-intracranial bypass surgery. However, due to further improvements of interventional neuroradiological techniques, the management of patients with these lesions has since been changed.

In this study, we present our preliminary experience in patients with carotid artery aneurysms who where treated with detachable balloon embolization.

Clinical Material and Methods

Over a 2-year period between 1988 and 1990, a total of four patients were treated. Clinically, one patient was admitted following a subarachnoid hemorrhage, two presented with a cavernous sinus syndrome, and one patient had a history of recurrent transient ischemic attacks. Angiography disclosed an intracavernous aneurysm in two patients, a large ophthalmic aneurysm in one, and a proximal internal carotid artery aneurysm located at the extracranial-petrosal segment, close to the skull base in another patient. Since all aneurysms were thought to be unsuitable for a direct surgical clipping procedure, it was decided to perform endovascular treatment.

Embolization Procedure

All procedures were performed under local anesthesia. For prevention of thrombus formation systemic anticoagulation was used. The embolization procedure was done using an ITC (Interventional Therapeutic Corporation, San Francisco, USA) detachable balloon microcatheter system. Secondary balloon deflation after aneurysm occlusion was prevented by using HEMA, a hydrophilic liquid polymer. To make sure that during the embolization procedure a possible occlusion of the internal carotid artery would not result in ischemic deficits, an initial 60-min test occlusion

[1] Neurochirurgische Universitätsklinik, Klinikum Großhadern, Marchioninistr. 15, W–8000 München 70, FRG.
[2] Radiologische Universitätsklinik, Klinikum Großhadern, Marchioninistr. 15, W–8000 München 70, FRG.

Advances in Neurosurgery, Vol. 20
K. Piscol, M. Klinger, M. Brock (Eds.)

was done. Continuous neurological evaluation as well as measurements of carotid back pressure [8, 9] and transcranial Doppler studies [10], including the Diamox test, were done before and after occlusion to assess the sufficiency of the cerebral collateral circulation.

Representative Case Reports

Case 2

This 27-year-old male presented with orbital pain and intermittent diplopia. Cerebral angiography demonstrated a giant left-sided intracavernous aneurysm (Fig. 1). Although selective aneurysm embolization could have been tried, a carotid balloon occlusion was done because of additional large ectasia of the adjacent carotid artery, which was felt to possibly present a permanent source for thromboembolic events. The clinical follow-up over a 26-month period was uneventful.

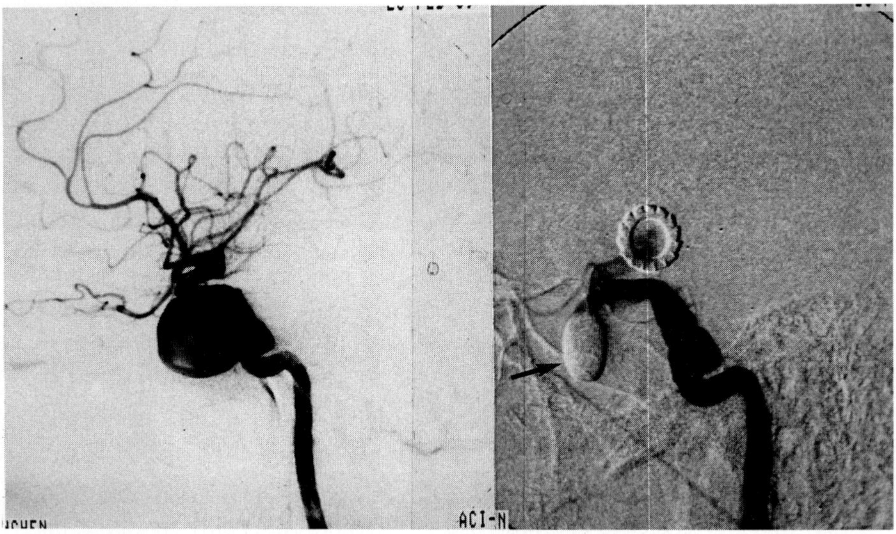

Fig. 1. Case 2. *Left,* internal carotid angiogram, lateral view, demonstrating a large intracavernous aneurysm of the internal carotid artery. *Right,* follow-up angiogram after placement of a single detachable balloon (*arrow*) demonstrating obliteration of the aneurysm as well as additional large ectasia of the internal carotid artery

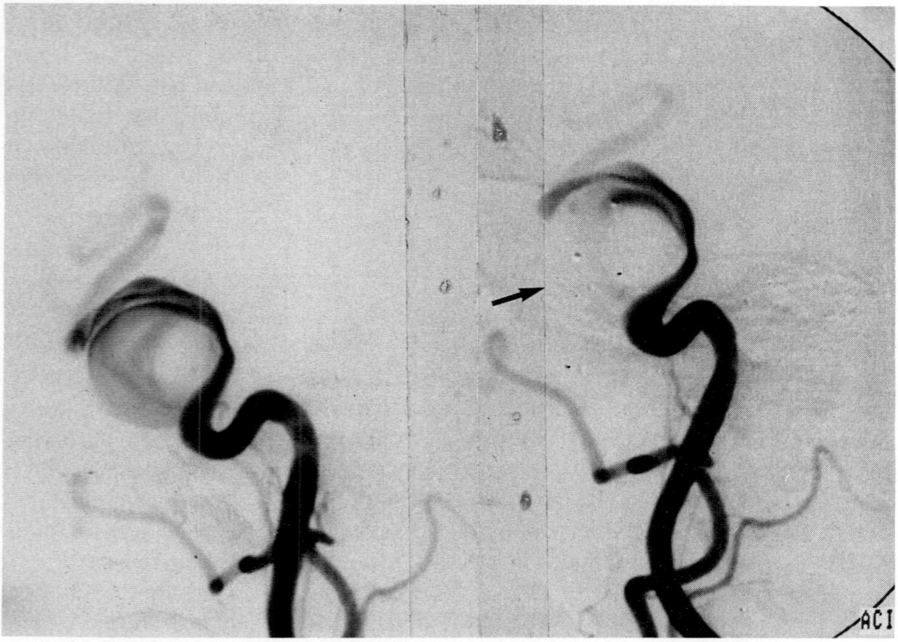

Fig. 2. Case 3. *Left*, internal carotid artery angiogram, lateral view, showing a giant aneurysm of the cavernous internal carotid artery and additional narrowing of the parent vessel. *Right*, follow-up angiogram after placement of two detachable balloons, which are subtracted out (*arrow*), demonstrating obliteration of the aneurysm as well as a preservation of the internal carotid artery

Case 3

This 62-year-old woman presented with headache, diplopia, and trigeminal pain. Cerebral angiography revealed a giant left-sided intracavernous aneurysm and an additional narrowing of the carotid close to the aneurysm possibly due to compression by the aneurysm sac (Fig. 2). Due to the size of the lesion, two detachable balloons were used for selective occlusion. On the 2nd postembolization day, transient deterioration and mild aphasia occurred. A follow-up angiogram revealed an occlusion of the internal carotid artery. At 21 months after treatment the patient remains asymptomatic.

Case 4

This 32-year-old man presented with a history of transient cerebrovascular ischemia including aphasia and right-sided sensomotoric deficits. Cerebral panangiography revealed as a thromboembolic source a left-sided internal carotid artery aneurysm which was located at the extracranial-petrosal junction area (Fig. 3). Since direct surgical repair of the lesion was not possible, selective balloon embolization was done. Two months later, severe cerebral ischemia with aphasia and hemiparesis occurred. Cerebral angiography revealed an occlusion of the internal carotid artery. Subsequently, the patient's condition improved, and he is now able to live an independent life.

Results

Table 1 summarizes results in this series of four patients. Selective occlusion of the aneurysm with preservation of the carotid artery patency was achieved in three cases. In one case, due to an additional ectatic carotid artery, primary occlusion of the vessel was done. Only one patient (case 2) in whom indirect aneurysm obliteration after occlusion of the internal carotid artery was done had an excellent and uneventful follow-up. In the remaining three patients various complications occurred during the follow-up period. In one patient (case 1) severe subarachnoid hemorrhage occurred 3 months after selective occlusion of an ophthalmic aneurysm because of migration of the balloon through the aneurysm wall with refilling of the aneurysm. This patient was treated surgically thereafter with occlusion of the aneurysm and removal of the balloon from the contralateral carotid cistern. In both remaining patients in whom also selective aneurysm embolization was performed, 2 days (case 3) and 2 months (case 4) after the procedure, signs of cerebral vascular insufficiency occurred as a result of secondary occlusion of the internal carotid artery.

Discussion

The optimal treatment of patients with aneurysms within or close to the skull base remains a matter of controversy [3]. Whereas overall encouraging results were obtained in several small series using occlusion of the internal carotid artery with simultaneous institution of an additional extra-intracranial arterial collateral [2, 11, 13, 14], evolving interventional procedures hold promise for the successful treatment of these patients as well [1, 4–6, 12]. One result of this admittedly small series is the finding that using microcatheter balloon techniques the aneurysm can be selectively occluded with preservation of the patency of the internal carotid artery in the majority of cases. However, less favorable was the observation that patients who initially seemed to have an excellent result are obviously prone to develop secondary thromboembolic complications resulting in brain ischemia as seen in two of our patients. Although it is difficult to speculate on the exact mechanism of this secondary deterioration following balloon embolization, one reason could be that in the cases with a fairly wide aneurysm neck the contact surface of the arterial blood and the balloon may promote the formation of emboli.

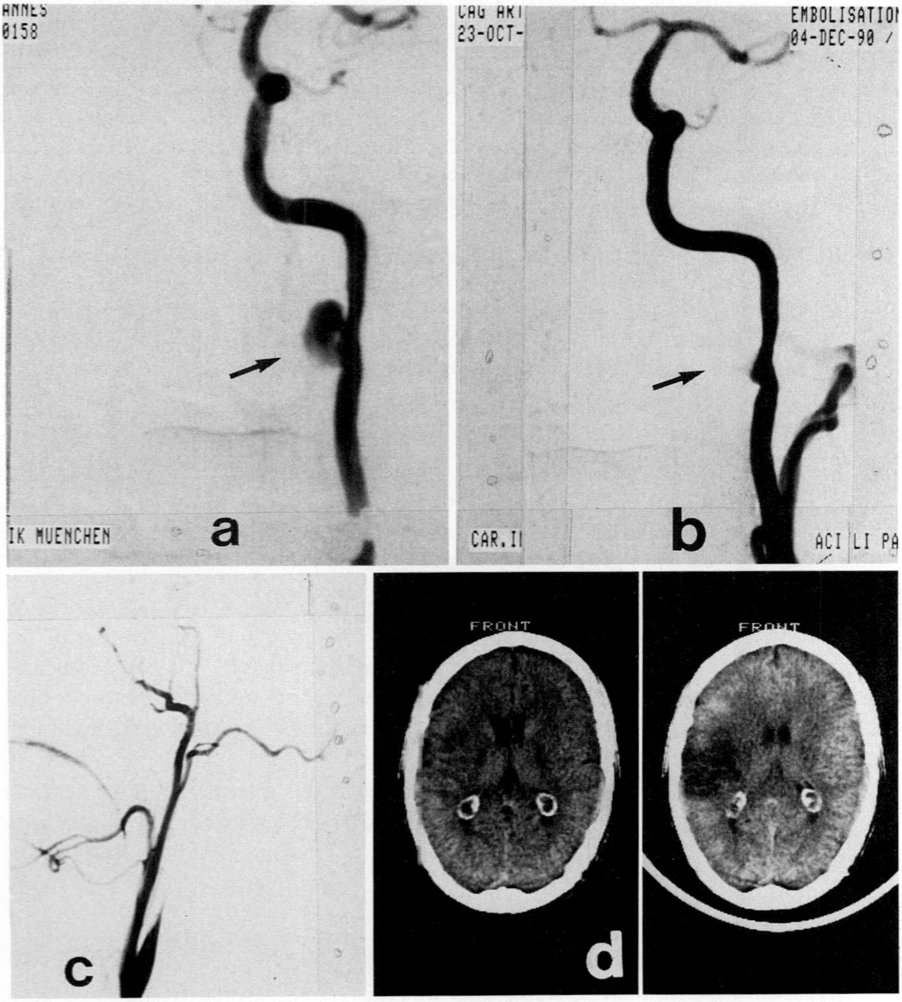

Fig. 3a–d. Case 4. **a** Carotid angiogram, frontal view, showing an aneurysm (*arrow*) of the internal carotid artery at the extracranial-petrosal junction area. **b** Follow-up angiogram after placement of a detachable balloon, which is subtracted out (*arrow*), demonstrating obliteration of the aneurysm and preservation of the parent vessel. **c** Follow-up angiogram 2 months after endovascular procedure, demonstrating occlusion of the internal carotid artery. **d** Cranial computer tomography 6 months (*left*) and 1 week (*right*) after internal carotid artery occlusion, demonstrating brain infarction of different degrees in the left middle cerebral artery territory

Table 1. Presentation of four patients with aneurysms of the ICA treated with balloon embolization

Case	Age, sex	Presentation	Aneurysm location/size[a]	Treatment	Complications (interval)	Follow-up and results
1	57, F	SAH	rt, ophthalmic/ large	Selective occlusion	SAH (3 months)	28 months, good after surgery
2	27, M	Mass effect	lt, cavernous/ giant	Occlusion of ICA	None	26 months, excellent
3	62, F	Mass effect	lt, cavernous/ giant	Selective occlusion	TIA (2 days)	21 months, excellent
4	32, M	TIA	lt, EPJA/large	Selective occlusion	PRIND (2 days) ICA occlusion	4 months, good recovery of CVI

ICA, internal carotid artery; EPJA, extracranial-petrosal junction area; SAH, subarachnoid hemorrhage; TIA, transient ischemic attack; PRIND, prolonged reversible ischemic neurological deficit; CVI, cerebrovascular insufficiency.
[a] Size = large (12–25 mm), giant (> 25 mm).

In addition, the unusual complication seen in one case with a migration of the balloon and refilling of the aneurysm and another hemorrhage [7] clearly indicates that long-term follow-up observations in these patients are necessary before a final statement can be made concerning the effectiveness of this rather new treatment modality.

Although balloon embolization represents an attractive alternative to the surgical treatment in patients with difficult aneurysms, it should be applied only in carefully selected patients.

References

1. Berenstein A, Ransohoff J, Kupersmith M (1984) Transvascular treatment of giant aneurysms of the cavernous carotid and vertebral arteries. Functional investigation and embolization. Surg Neurol 21:3–12
2. Diaz FG, Auseman JI, Pearce J (1982) Ischemic complications following internal carotid occlusions combined with intracranial-extracranial anastomosis. Neurosurg 10:563–570
3. Diaz FG, Ohaegbulam S, Dujovny M, Ausman JI (1988) Surgical management of aneurysms in the cavernous sinus. Acta Neurochir (Wien) 91:25–28
4. Debrun G, Fox A, Drake C (1981) Giant unclippable aneurysms: treatment with detachable balloons. AJMR 2:167–173
5. Higashida RT, Hieshima GB, Halbach VV (1986) Intravascular detachable balloon embolization of intracranial aneurysms: indications and techniques. Acta Radiol 369:594–596
6. Higashida RT, Halbach VV, Cahan LD; Hieshima GB, Honishi YK (1989) Detachable balloon embolization therapy of posterior circulation intracranial aneurysms. J Neurosurg 71:512–519

7. Hodes JE, Fox AJ, Pelz DM, Pearless SJ (1990) Rupture of aneurysms following balloon embolization. J Neurosurg 72:567–571
8. McKay RD, Sundt TM, Michenfelder JD, Gronert SA, Messin JM, Sharbrough FW, Piepgrass DG (1976) Internal carotid artery stump pressure and cerebral flow during carotid endarterectomy: modification by halothane, enflurane and innovar. Anesthesiol 45:390–398
9. Moore WS, Hall AD (1969) Carotid artery back pressure. A test of cerebral tolerance to temporary carotid occlusion. Arch Surg 99:702–710
10. Piepgras A, Schmiedek P, Leinsinger G, Haberl RL, Kirsch CM, Einhäupl KM (1990) A simple test to assess cerebrovascular reserve capacity using transcranial Doppler sonography and acetazolamide. Stroke 21:1306–1311
11. Roski RA, Spetzler RF, Nulsen FE (1981) Late complications of carotid ligation in the treatment of intracranial aneurysms. J Neurosurg 54:583–587
12. Serbinenko FA (1974) Balloon catheterization and occlusion of major cerebral vessels. J Neurosurg 41:125–145
13. Serbinenko FA, Filatov JM, Spallone A, Thurilov MV, Lazarev VA (1990) Management of giant intracranial ICA aneurysms with combined extracranial-intracranial anastomosis and endovascular occlusion. J Neurosurg 73:57–63
14. Sundt TM, Piegras DG, Marsch WR, Fode NC (1986) Saphenous vein bypass grafts for giant aneurysms and intracranial occlusive disease. J Neurosurg 65:439–450

Possibilities and Limitations of Endovascular Techniques for the Treatment of Craniocerebral Aneurysms

B. Richling and G. Bavinzski[1]

Introduction

In recent years the skepticism of neurosurgeons regarding endovascular techniques for the treatment of craniocerebral aneurysms has given way to vivid interest in this topic. However, among those neurosurgeons who have operated craniocerebral aneurysms regularly there are still some doubts about reports on larger groups of patients with solely endovascularly treated cerebral aneurysms. Most recent reports [4] on outstanding results obtained in the endovascular treatment of small to minute cerebral aneurysms and those on the endovascular treatment of giant extradural and intradural aneurysms with microcoils and balloons raise questions as to the approach indicated for treatment that cannot be solved by the purely surgically trained neurosurgeon alone.

This article intends to show to what extent endovascular techniques may form a part of strategies for the treatment of craniocerebral aneurysms. A concept is presented that provides for endovascular techniques in cases where the surgical approach poses increased risks, while priority is attached to surgical interventions in all those cases where the endovascular approach (still) involves increased risks.

Case Reports

The various types of aneurysms require grossly different approaches, both with regard to endovascular therapy and surgical intervention. Therefore, aneurysms are categorized here into *extradural aneurysms* (mostly in the form of infraclinoidal intracavernous aneurysms of the internal carotid artery), *giant intradural aneurysms* (more often than not with thick and sclerosed walls and partially thrombosed), and *small berry aneurysms.*

Extradural aneurysms of the internal carotid artery often do not have a neck, which determines the therapeutic approach to be chosen. Their symptoms, i.e., the impairment of cranial nerves, develop on account of the pulsatile pressure of the arterial blood flow in the cavernous sinus. Subarachnoidal bleeding is rare and limited to cases in which a relevant part of the aneurysm extends into the cranial cavity.

[1] Neurochirurgische Universitätsklinik Wien, Währinger Gürtel 18–20, A–1090 Wien, Austria.

Advances in Neurosurgery, Vol. 20
K. Piscol, M. Klinger, M. Brock (Eds.)

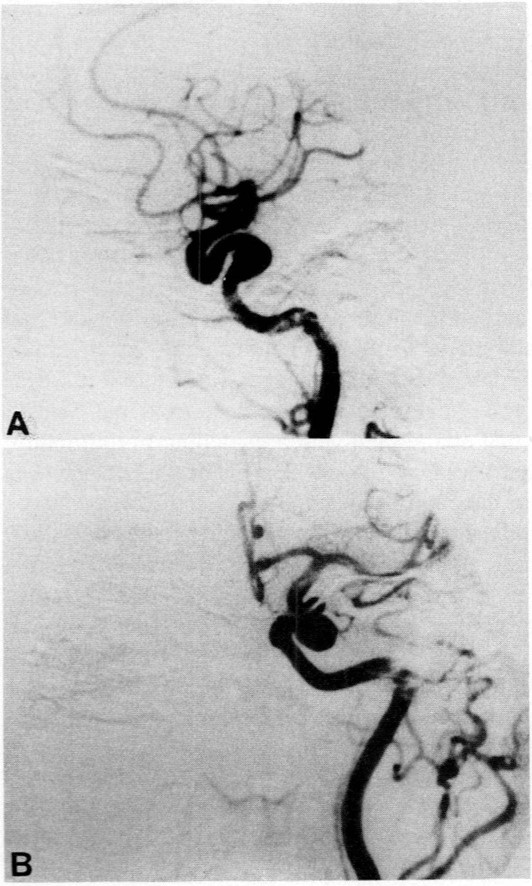

Fig. 1A, B. Infraclinoidal intracavernous aneurysm of the left internal carotid artery

Case Study 1

A 53-year-old patient complained about double vision for the first time some 1.5 years ago. An ophthalmologic examination showed a left abducens paralysis. Examination showed an infraclinoidal intracavernous aneurysm of the left internal carotid artery (Fig. 1). After additional computed tomography (CT) and magnetic resonance imaging (MRI), a balloon-type 8-F catheter was placed into the left internal carotid artery via a transfemoral access under local anesthesia. A guide wire-supported microcatheter (Tracker 18, Target Therapeutics) was advanced into the aneurysm through this catheter. The selective angiogram showed the aneurysm without a neck. This indicated an occlusion with a detachable balloon of the internal carotid artery close to the aneurysm.

The microcatheter was replaced with a detachable microballoon (ITC, DSB 1.8 M) that was advanced along the internal carotid artery close to the aneurysm. The balloon, inflated below the aneurysm, temporarily occluded the internal carotid artery, and the occlusion test period commenced. During this 30-min test period, the blood in the left internal carotid stump was heparinized, and the patient was administered one additional unit of heparin for each milliliter of rinsing liquid in the catheter system. During this test period, the clinical neurological condition of the patient was monitored; somatosensory evoked potentials (SSEP) and the flow in the two middle cerebral arteries were measured with transcranial Doppler (TCD) sonography (Fig. 2). Another 7-F Head-Hunter catheter advanced via a second femoral access demonstrated the angiographic cross-flow from the right internal carotid artery and the right vertebral artery to the left hemisphere (Fig. 3). Since the patient did not show any neurological deficit or changes with regard to SSEP and TCD and in the light of the good angiographic cross-flow from the right to the left, the microballoon was emptied and refilled with a hardening fibrin mixture [1] to its original volume. After hardening of the fibrin mixture the balloon was detached. To secure the occlusion of the carotid, a second balloon of the same type was placed into the proximal internal carotid artery, filled with fibrin, and detached. The session was completed with angiographies from both carotid and vertebral arteries. During the subsequent weeks the cranial nerve symptoms receded, and there were no new neurological defunctionalization symptoms in the sense of ischemic complications.

The surgical treatment of *giant intradural aneurysms* may be problematic: due to partial thrombosis or sclerosis their large sacs are hard to manipulate or to clip. In such cases the aneurysm or the still unobstructed lumen of the aneurysm may be filled by placing one (if required also more) detachable balloon(s). The smaller the neck of the aneurysm, the safer the placing of the balloon within the aneurysm or the detaching of the balloon from the catheter.

Case Study 2

In the course of several months, a 48-year-old patient developed aggravating brainstem symptoms caused by a giant aneurysm of the basilar tip (Fig. 4). Though CT and MRI showed the partial thrombosis of the lumen and calcific deposits in the wall of the aneurysm, it was at first explored surgically and an attempt at surgical treatment was made. During the intervention, however, it became evident that due to the stiffness of the wall of the aneurysm it could not be manipulated in such a way that it was possible to place a clip. Only additional surgical measures involving high risks (hyperthermia, cardiac arrest) could have been resorted to or the basilar artery could have been throttled via a loop. In this situation it was decided to choose an endovascular approach: under local anesthesia a balloon-type 7-F catheter was placed into the left vertebral artery via the femoral artery. A detachable latex balloon (Ingenor, Gold-Valve) was advanced through this catheter and guided into the sac of the aneurysm via the basilar artery. While the inflating of the

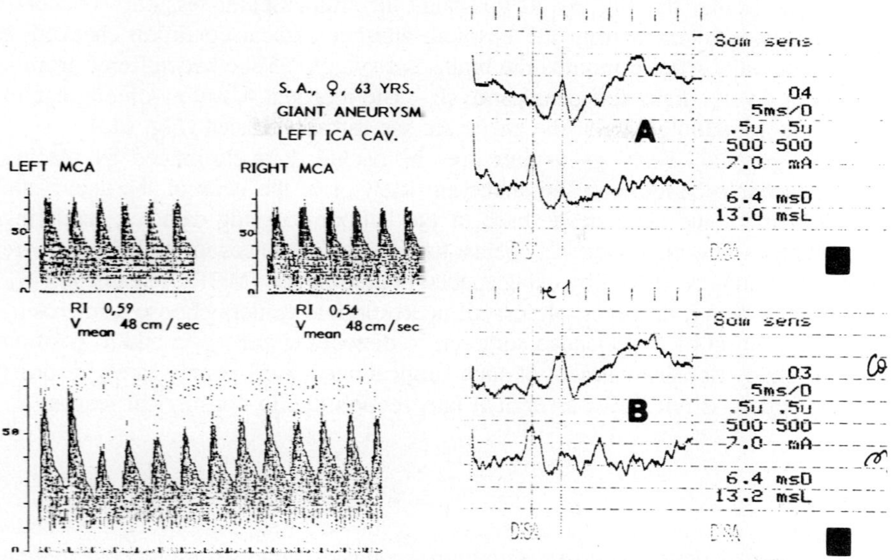

Fig. 2. Transcranial Doppler sonography (*left*) and somatosensory-evoked potentials (*right*) before *A* and during *B* test occlusion of the left internal carotid artery

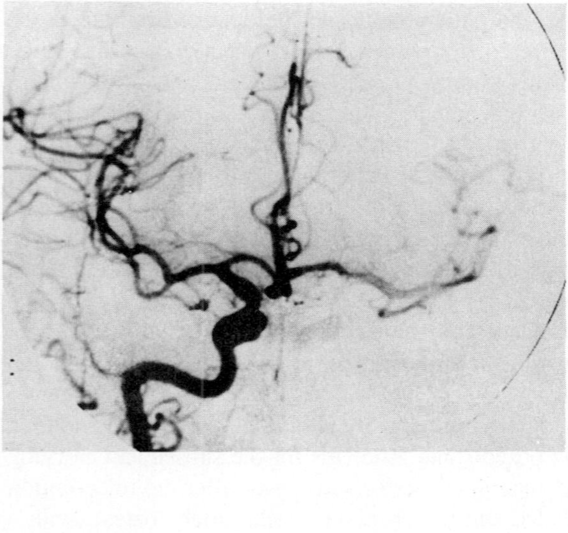

Fig. 3. Cross-flow from the right to the left hemisphere during balloon occlusion of the left internal carotid artery

balloon and the hardening with homologous fibrin did not pose any problems, the typical shape of the balloon led to an only incomplete filling of the lumen of the aneurysm. At the same time, it was impossible to advance a further balloon through the remaining lumen close to the basilar tip on account of its form and the proximity to the basilar tip (Fig. 5). At this point the endovascular session was ended, the patient was released from the hospital, and her clinical condition checked at regular intervals. After 6 months the brainstem symptoms she had suffered from – apart from a very slight abducens paralysis – had receded. A follow-up angiogram showed the remaining part of the aneurysm sac further reduced (Fig. 6).

Small "surgical" *berry aneurysms* may be occluded or eliminated by placing small detachable balloons in the aneurysm itself or in the neck of the aneurysm. The problem of the large dead space of the balloon-carrying catheter, rendering the exchange of contrast medium against hardening substances in the balloon more problematic, may be solved by using special double-lumen (MORET) catheters [4]. For the time being, however, almost all neurosurgical centers choose a microsurgical intervention by experienced surgeons to dissect the aneurysm and to position the clip. Endovascular treatment of such surgical aneurysms is only rarely resorted to if the patient is not fit for a surgical intervention due to nonsurgical reasons.

Case Study 3

A 21-year-old patient was hospitalized on account of acute severe subarachnoidal bleeding of stages III–IV according to Hunt and Hess. The angiogram showed an aneurysm of the proximal basilar artery (Fig. 7). As a secondary finding a marked thrombopenia (40 000) due to hepatopathy was established.

While from a technical point of view, surgical treatment of the aneurysm certainly would have been possible, the patient could not be operated on due to the high-degree thrombopenia he suffered from. An endovascular approach had to be chosen. After administration of a thrombocyte concentrate, increasing the number of thrombocytes to 50 000, an 8-F catheter was placed into the right vertebral artery after puncture of the femoral artery. A detachable balloon (ITC, DSB 1505), in size and shape like the aneurysm, was advanced through the catheter into the right distal vertebral artery. Moving the balloon closer to the aneurysm a spastic stenosis could only be overcome with difficulties (Fig. 8). The balloon was then placed in the sac of the aneurysm, filled at first with contrast medium, and inflated. The angiogram showed that the aneurysm was cut off from the bloodstream while the flow in the basilar artery could be maintained; the balloon was emptied again and filled to the same volume with a hardening fibrin mixture. After hardening of the fibrin mixture, the balloon was detached by dosed and slow microcatheter pulling. Figure 9 shows the angiogram immediately after the session. The patient's continued chronic thrombopenia posed some problems for the subsequent carrying out of angiograms. A follow-up angiogram performed 1 year after the intervention showed the aneurysm still occluded and the proximal basilar artery patent (with a slight constriction of the lumen).

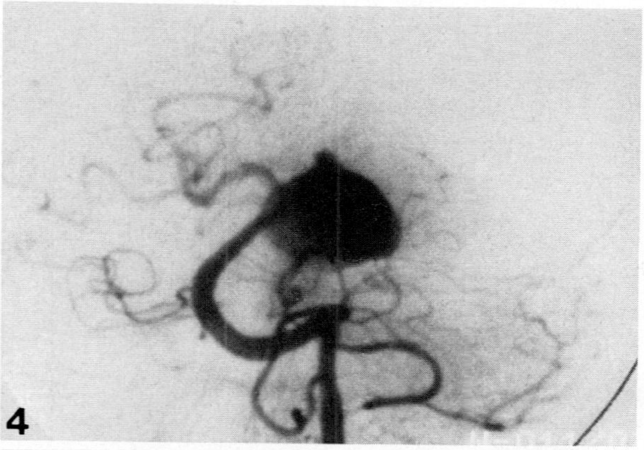

Fig. 4. Giant aneurysm of the basilar tip (case report 2)

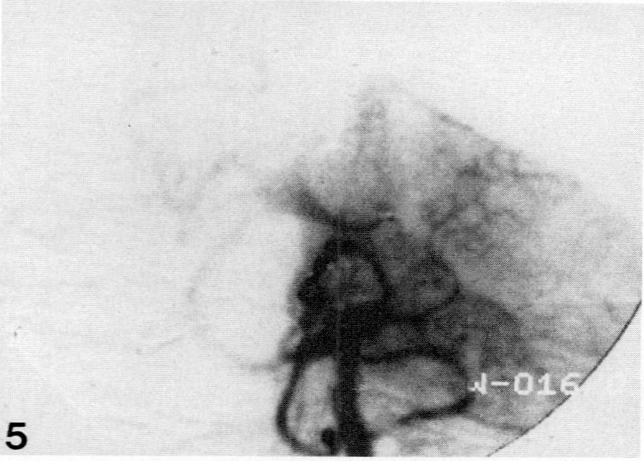

Fig. 5. Detachable balloon inside the aneurysm sac; neck and remaining lumen of the aneurysm patent

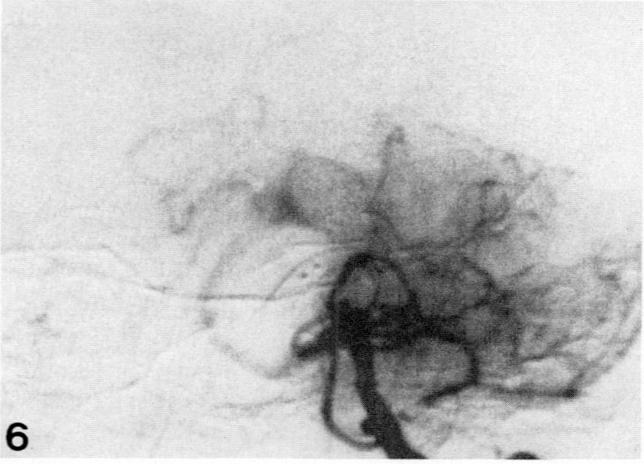

Fig. 6. Follow-up angiogram after 1 year (case report 2). Remaining lumen still patent

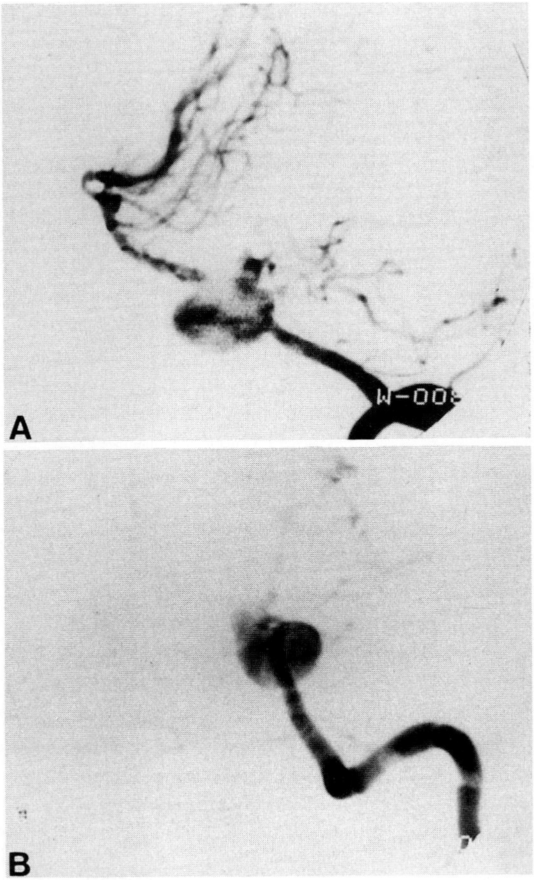

Fig. 7A, B. Aneurysm of the basilar artery (case report 3)

Discussion and Summary

Since the first accounts of detachable balloons guided into cerebral arteries by Serbinenko [7], reports on the selective elimination of cerebral aneurysms with balloons while maintaining the vessels' lumina are increasingly common. The frequency of this therapeutic approach to treating cerebral aneurysms against the number of surgical interventions published was low, while the risk involved in each such intervention and the rate of ensuing complications was high. Comprehensive experience gathered by therapists, improvements in the material of microcatheters and balloons, and the higher quality of digital substraction angiography have generally increased the safety of endovascular interventions. Recently, reports by individual authors have appeared on larger series of successful endovascular treatments of cerebral aneurysms [4].

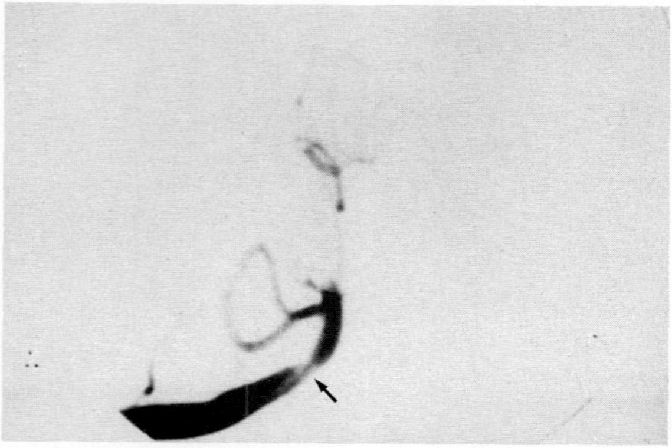

Fig. 8. Detachable balloon (partially inflated) overcoming a stenosis in the right vertebral artery (*arrow*)

The original rejection of endovascular techniques by purely surgically oriented neurosurgeons has given way to a certain degree of interest in this approach. This increased attention, however, is often not reflected in an increased inclusion of endovascular considerations into strategic treatment plans: this is due to the lacking availability of an experienced endovascular team and, above all, to the understandable skepticism of replacing surgical routine work that has been practiced for years by a newly emerging approach. The authors of this report, both long experienced in the microsurgical treatment of cerebral aneurysms and lucky enough to gather experience in endovascular techniques, are faced with the same strategic decision with each individual case. For the time being, however, the high degree of safety for the surgical treatment of the majority of cerebral aneurysms with a diameter of less than 1 cm cannot be expected from endovascular treatment. While this is not so much due to the intervention as such, which (if carried out properly) is completely atraumatic for the patient, the placing of a balloon in the sac of the aneurysm can only be compared with the safety a properly placed clip provides if the further penetration of blood into the fundus of the aneurysm can be absolutely ruled out by proper balloon-placing techniques. Mechanisms such as the enlargement of the aneurysm around the balloon or the movement of the balloon within the aneurysm may lead to a partial refilling of the aneurysm, posing the risk of a late rupture despite balloon occlusion. As emphasized by authors with extensive experience in placing balloons in aneurysms [4], overall importance has to be attached to either totally filling the aneurysm with the balloon or trying to select the proper type of balloon, or even producing balloons to fit the form of the aneurysm established.

The process of thrombosing aneurysms with microcoils involves the problem of the precise placing of the coils within the aneurysm without their protruding into the vessel's lumen and the danger of a thromboembolic scattering during the process of thrombosing. The most recent techniques of electrothrombosis via electrolytically detachable microcoils make it easier to carefully place and rate the scattering of the coils, reducing the danger of thromboembolic scattering due to

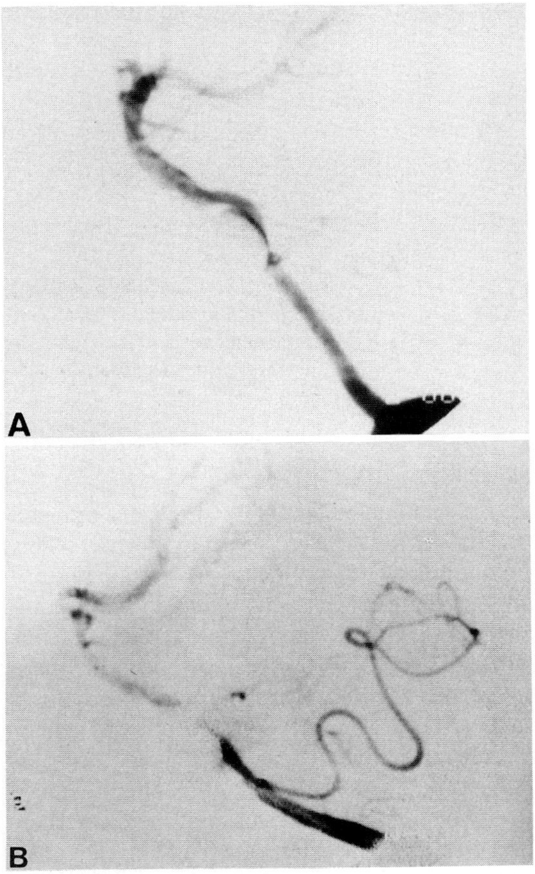

Fig. 9A, B. Follow-up angiogram immediately (**A**) and after 1 year (**B**) after balloon occlusion of the basilar aneurysm

quick electrothrombosis. These techniques [2, 3] are being clinically tested and appear to be very promising.

For the time being, the authors consider the inclusion of endovascular techniques into the treatment strategy of cerebral aneurysms expedient to such an extent that promises to bring the greatest benefit to the patient, weighing all the risks involved. The treatment of *infraclinoidal intracavernous aneurysms* requires major surgical interventions. Surgery of the internal carotid artery in the cavernous sinus and bypassing operations alike require extensive special experience of the operating surgeon and patients who can be put under some strain. With these patients an occlusion with detachable balloons of the internal carotid artery close to the aneurysm after a test period of at least 30 min will be chosen. If the occlusion of the carotid artery is not tolerated, the affected hemisphere may be fed with blood via extra-intracranial bypass operations to finally render the occlusion of the carotid artery possible.

With *intradural aneurysms* preference will be given to endovascular techniques if a surgical intervention poses excessive strain on the patient due to partly thrombosed or sclerosed aneurysm walls. With these *giant intradural aneurysms* in many cases satisfactory results may be obtained by employing endovascular techniques.

Small *berry aneurysms* (diameter less than 1 cm) involve a low morbidity and mortality rate if treated by experienced surgeons. This large group of patients is usually operated on since a properly placed clip provides a higher degree of safety for the patient than he could be offered by the balloon technique (see above). Endovascular treatment will only be performed in isolated cases (case study 2) where increased risk poses problems to a surgical intervention.

References

1. Bavinzski G, Richling B, Saringer W (in press) Experimental comparison between homologous fibrin, Hydroxyaethyl-Metacrylat (HEMA) and contrast dye for permanent solidification of different detachable balloons. Neuroradiology
2. Guglielmi G, Vinuela F, Sepetka I, Macellari V (1991) Electrothrombosis of saccular aneurysms via endovascular approach, Part 1: Electrochemical basis, technique, and experimental results. J Neurosurg 75:1–7
3. Guglielmi G, Vinuela F, Dion J, Duckwiler G (1991) Electrothrombosis of saccular aneurysms via endovascular approach, Part 2: Preliminary clinical experience. J Neurosurg 75:8–14
4. Moret J (in press) Endovascular treatment of berry aneurysms by endosaccular occlusion. Acta Neurochirurgica (Suppl 53)
5. Richling B (1982) Homologous controlled-viscosity fibrin for endovascular embolization. Part I: Experimental development of the medium. Acta Neurochirurgica 62:159–170
6. Richling B (1982) Homologous controlled-viscosity fibrin for endovascular embolization. Part II: Catheterization technique, animal experiments. Acta Neurochirurgica 64:109–124
7. Serbinenko FA (1974) Ballon catheterization and occlusion of major cerebral vessels. J Neurosurg 41:125–145

Technical Possibilities and Aids in Treating Aneurysms in Open Surgery

H. Meyer, G. Bertram, M. Nadji-Ohl, W. Wagner, A. Henssler, F. Schröder, and K. Piscol[1]

Introduction

To be able to make a statement concerning open surgery in the treatment of aneurysms at the Department of Neurosurgery in Bremen, a computer-aided analysis was done on 450 of 511 cases operated on between 1972 and 1990.

These aneurysms had the following localizations: anterior cerebral artery, 41.3%; middle cerebral artery, 26.0%; internal carotid artery 26.0%: posterior circulation, 6.0%.

Of the surgical interventions 87% involved a single aneurysm. In 10% of the cases two or more one-sided aneurysms were surgically treated during the same session. In one case a two-sided aneurysm of the middle cerebral arteries was clipped in one session. In 3% of the cases multiple aneurysms were treated in two sessions. Multiple aneurysms occurred in 11.5% of the patients.

Applied Methods of Operative Treatment

With respect to the operation procedures, the analysis determined that 85% of the aneurysms could be eliminated directly by clipping and 11% by means of trapping. Only 4% had to be treated without the use of clips. Figure 1 shows the percentages of the definitive ways of treatment.

All aneurysms with a relatively narrow neck were occluded with only one clip which was chosen from an assortment of different sizes and shapes according to the individual necessity. Two or more clips were preferred in partially thrombosed, inflexible, or largely domed aneurysms. Combinations of clips were used in aneurysms with a broad neck and critical localizations incorporating arterial bifurcations. In 1.5% of the patients large tangential clips were used in lateral fusiform aneurysms. A combination of clip plus ligature was generally used when the neck of the aneurysm had already been reined and narrowed with the aneurysm thread or when a leakage made a further intervention necessary. Additional wrapping was indicated when ruptures of the neck had extended proximally to the clipping site or when fastening of the clip was desirable. Plain ligature passed around the neck of the aneurysm was used when clipping could lead to damage of adjacent structures. The so-called bipolar shrinking was done to reduce the width of the neck or

[1] Neurochirurgische Klinik, Zentralkrankenhaus St.-Jürgen-Str., W–2800 Bremen 1, FRG.

Advances in Neurosurgery, Vol. 20
K. Piscol, M. Klinger, M. Brock (Eds.)

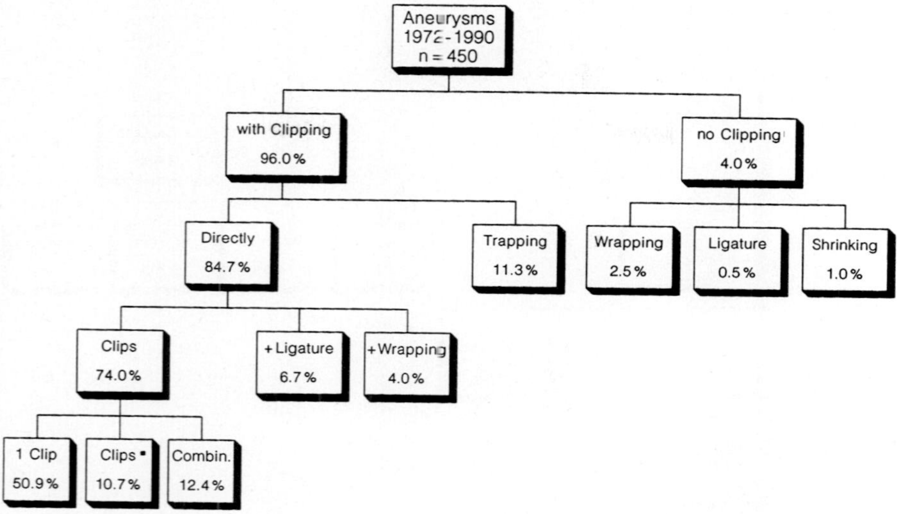

Fig. 1. Techniques for obliteration of aneurysms in 450 cases of open surgery from 1972 to 1990

to remove small and flat aneurysms completely, most often in combination with wrapping.

Trapping was only used in anterior communicating artery aneurysms where no possibility of direct clipping existed. In cases with malformations that were not amenable to clipping or ligation the only possibility was plain wrapping.

Small aneurysms with a maximal diameter of 4 mm, which occurred in 14% of our patients, often were treated with plain or additional shrinking and wrapping, whereas medium- and large-sized aneurysms, which accounted for 71%, were almost exclusively clipped. The remaining 6.4% of giant aneurysms were mainly occluded by clipping. Only when a long passage with bifurcation was involved was wrapping used.

In another study we distinguished two time periods because of different operative considerations: era 1 (1972–1981) was dominated by delayed surgery and era 2 (1982–1990) was dominated by early surgery (see Chap. Pinz et al.). This differentiation will also be used here for our special interest belongs to possible changes in the management of aneurysms between era 1 and era 2 (Figs. 2 and 3). Due to an improvement in direct clipping of the neck, trapping decreased from 19% to 8%, the combined treatment with clip and ligature was reduced from 16% to 2.5%, and the combined procedure of clipping and wrapping fell from 6% to 3.5%. The overall rate of direct aneurysm clipping rose from 74% to about 90%. The treatment without a clip decreased from 6.9% to 2.8%.

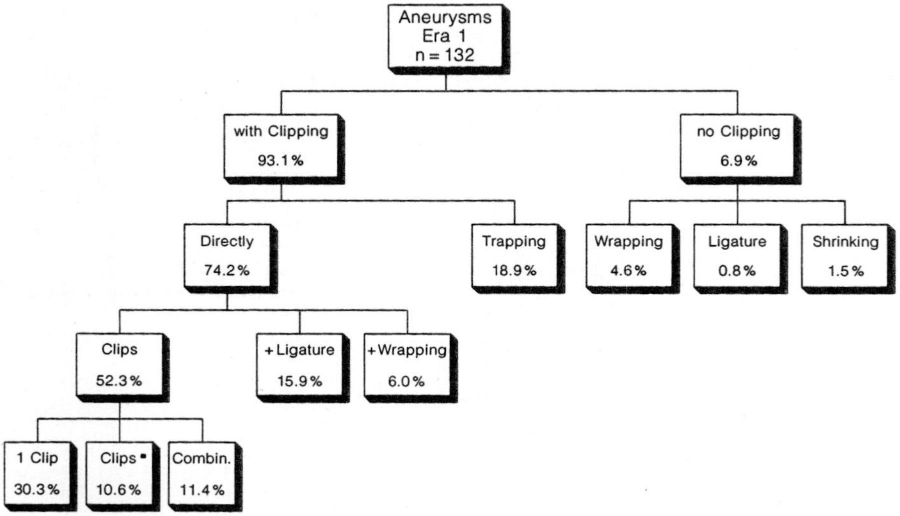

Fig. 2. Techniques for obliteration of aneurysms in 132 cases of open surgery from 1972 to 1981 (era 1)

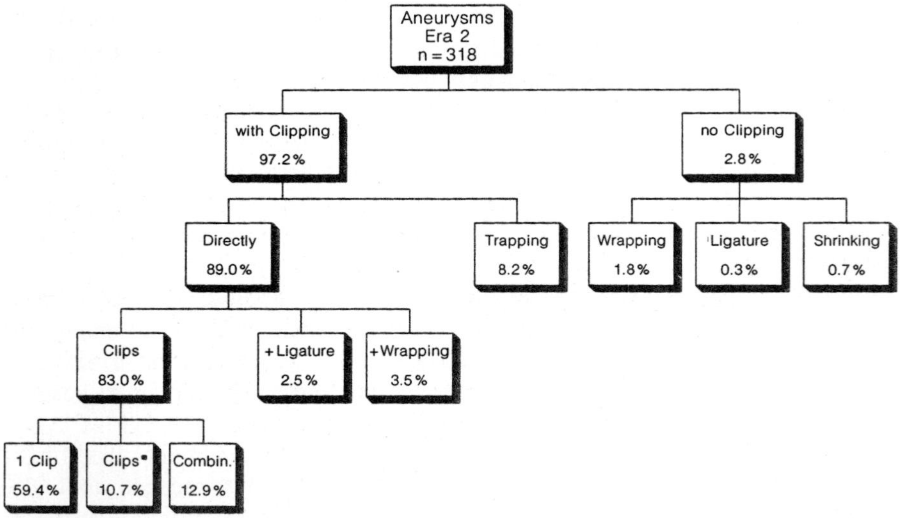

Fig. 3. Techniques for obliteration of aneurysms in 318 cases of open surgery from 1982 to 1990 (era 2)

Additional Methods

Various helpful techniques and measures were used to obtain adequate clip placement, to avoid alterations of adjacent structures, and to prevent complications. For some of them statistically meaningful data were found in our analysis, which shall be noted here.

Auxiliary techniques for the elimination of aneurysms were:

1.	Bipolar shrinking of neck or fundus	8%
2.	Controlled compression and suction	15%
3.	Temporary clipping of the fundus	15%
4.	Temporary clipping of the parent vessel	11%
5.	Use of the armored aneurysm thread	25%

The percentage only reflects the frequency of use, not the real percentage of cases, for the different methods were often used together in the same patient. Bipolar shrinking of the neck was the procedure to be chosen in broad-based aneurysms to ensure better acceptance of the clip or the ligature; shrinking of the whole sac in some small and flat aneurysms led to disappearence of the malformation [1]. Controlled compression and suction and the two types of temporary clipping were necessary if premature rupture occurred in the course of dissection. With regard to the periods compared the event of intraoperative rupture decreased from 19.7% in era 1 to 12.5% in era 2. Our data demonstrate that ruptures which were controlled immediately did not result in a negative outcome.

The *armored aneurysm thread* that was developed in our department [2] is especially effective. In combination with a special holder, the buttoned and flexible metal pin can be used for preparation, subsequently encircling the neck, and finally narrowing and reining it with the thread. At present we are developing a special aneurysm thread with a slit base in which the stretched thread can be retained and finally held through melting (Fig. 4). The advantages are preparation of the neck and obliteration of the aneurysms in one stroke, no projecting parts, and no remaining metal.

So-called *final measures* were employed after clipping to relieve neighboring structures. In nearly 20% of the cases with space-occupying aneurysms, the procedure of choice was to puncture or incise the fundus, evacuation, and subsequent bipolar shrinking. Resection of the fundus or extirpation of the sac was done in thick-walled or thrombosed or giant aneurysms in an additional 18% of the cases. Another form of decompression or liberation was reached by dissection of stronger adhesions or neurolysis; the frequency of this measure was about 15% but again intermingled with the other percentages. In era 2 despite early surgery adhesions were seen in altogether 33% of our cases (compared with 61% in era 1). Intensive lavage of basal cisterns in cases with stronger subarachnoid hemorrhage (SAH) was carried out in nearly 47% of the cases, optionally supported by local application of nimodipine. All these measures should lead either to a reduction of mechanical alterations or to a release of vascular reactions, especially of vasospasm.

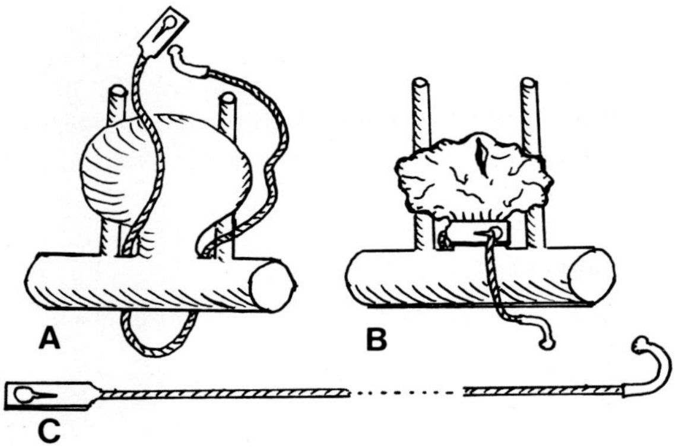

Fig. 4A–C. "Armored aneurysm thread" with slit base (small slit-bearing plastic plate at the end of the thread; C). **A** Manipulation to reinforce the slit base. **B** Reinforced slit base, aneurysm exlcuded and incised

The well-known *adjunctive measures* were:

1.	Simultaneous drainage of ventricles, era 1	13%
	era 2	39%
2.	Extirpation of intracranial hematomas	18%
3.	Extra-intracranial arterial bypass (EIAB)	3%
4.	Flow reduction in feeding vessels or occlusion of feeding vessels	3%

Some highlights of era 2 should be mentioned: two successful sutures of vessels, one intraoperative extra-intracranial anastomosis and, the most spectacular case, an intraoperative embolectomy. In the latter case a clot from debris originating in the saccular aneurysm occluded the main branch of the middle cerebral artery during the clipping (the clip had to be transposed once). After a typical microsurgical embolectomy there was a good flow rate within the vessel.

Conclusion

Open surgery allows a great variety of procedures which can be dealt with individually. Especially the development of numerous aids has helped to increase the percentage of direct aneurysm obliteration to more than 90%, in spite of the great number of early surgeries in the past years.

Open surgery permits a great number of additional relief, auxiliary, and preventive measures that can influence the final outcome to a decisive degree. The comparison of two periods between 1972 and 1990 has shown an impressive development in the tactics and strategies of aneurysm treatment.

There is every reason to expect that further such developments will appear in the future.

References

1. Piscol K (1972) Intracranielle Gefäßnaht-Embolektomie-Versorgung breitnasiger Aneurysmen. Therapiewoche 22:2151
2. Piscol K (1975) Armoured aneurysm thread: A new aid for the surgical treatment of intracranial aneurysms. Advanc Neurosurg 2:411

Surgical Procedure in Multiple Cerebral Aneurysms

W. I. Steudel[1], R. Lorenz[2], D. Rosenthal[2], and A. Ricco[2]

Introduction

There has been a major change in views with regard to surgical treatment of multiple aneurysms in the course of recent decades. As late as 1973, Paterson and Bond asserted that operation on the unruptured aneurysm was not indicated [4]. In 1970, Heiskanen and Marttila suggested that the unruptured aneurysm should be operated on when it can be eliminated via the same approach [2]. Subsequently, it was generally accepted that all unruptured aneurysms accessible to surgery should be operated on, even if a second operation became necessary [1, 3]. At present, this is the view of most authors.

The problem of the surgical procedure in multiple aneurysms continues to be of interest since many questions are still open and subject to controversy: Which aneurysm is ruptured? Which aneurysms are first discovered as a result of the operation? When does the second operation take place? Which aneurysms should be operated on in one session from the same approach? Which aneurysms should be eliminated from two different approach routes? Are there differences between patients with multiple aneurysms and patients with a single aneurysm with regard to the clinical features and the course?

Patients and Methods

From 1980 to 1990, 403 patients with an aneurysm were operated on at the Neurosurgical Department, University of Frankfurt/Main (Table 1). Of these, 42 (10.4%) had multiple aneurysms. These patients comprised 32 women and 10 men (age range 29–72 years, median age 49 years).

Four groups were formed with regard to the surgical procedure: group 1, patients whose aneurysms were operated on in a single session; group 2, patients with two-stage operation; group 3, patients in whom only the ruptured aneurysm was operated on; group 4, patients who were not operated on (Table 2).

A one-stage operation was carried out on aneurysms which could be reached via one approach or which were adjacent: these were mainly middle cerebral and

[1] Neurochirurgische Universitätsklinik, W–6650 Homburg/Saar, FRG.
[2] Neurochirurgische Universitätsklinik, Schleusenweg 2–16,
W–6000 Frankfurt/M. 71, FRG.

Advances in Neurosurgery, Vol. 20
K. Piscol, M. Klinger, M. Brock (Eds.)

Table 1. Frequency of patients with multiple aneurysms

Neurosurgery Division, University of Frankfurt/Main
Of 403 patients operated on since 1980,
42 had multiple aneurysms (10.4%)
2 aneurysms were present in 31 cases
3 aneurysms were present in 9 cases
4 aneurysms were present in 1 case
5 aneurysms were present in 1 case
Neurosurgery Division, University of the Saarland, Homburg [7]
Of 573 patients operated on since 1975,
63 had multiple aneurysms
2 had angiomas in addition (altogether 11% of the total)
2 aneurysms were present in 50 cases
3 aneurysms were present in 9 cases
4 aneurysms were present in 7 cases
2 aneurysms were present in 2 cases

internal carotid artery aneurysms which were combined with middle cerebral artery or with internal carotid artery aneurysms. A two-stage operation was carried out in group 2, in which a middle cerebral artery aneurysm or an internal carotid artery aneurysm was involved six times on the contralateral side. As a rule, these operations were carried out 6 months after the first operation: in two cases after 1 year, in two cases after 1 month, and in one case on the 4th day. In this latter patient, the unruptured aneurysm was dealt with in the acute operation. For this reason, the second operation was carried out immediately. Besides the improvement of the clinical symptoms, the criterion for the time of the second operation was the normalization of the focal changes in the EEG. In the group of the 42 patients with multiple aneurysms, the operation was carried out within the first 3 days in ten cases.

Results

The preoperative state as defined in the classification of Hunt and Hess does not enable a major distinction to be made between patients with single or multiple aneurysms (Table 2). Patients with grades II and III predominate.

The ruptured aneurysm was mainly situated in the region of the middle cerebral artery and the anterior communicating artery. The unruptured aneurysms were mainly located in the region of the middle cerebral artery on the contralateral side and the internal carotid artery (Table 3).

We did not find any difference with regard to the postoperative results as defined by the Glasgow Outcome Scale as compared with the group with a single aneurysm.

Table 2. Preoperative clinical state in multiple aneurysms and the surgical procedure

	Clinical condition according to Hunt and Hess					
	I	II	III	IV	V	n
Mulitple aneurysms						
Group 1 (one-stage operation)	1	8	7	2		18
Group 2 (two-stage operation)	1	7	4			12
Group 3 (operation on the ruptured aneurysm)		2	1	7 (2)		10 (2)
Group 4 (no operation)				1 (1)	1 (1)	2 (2)
Single aneurysms	66	118	98	66	13	361 (27)

( ) died.

Table 3. Location of ruptured and unruptured aneurysm

Multiple aneurysms		Location of the unruptured aneurysm				
Location of the ruptured aneurysms		Middle cerebral artery	Anterior communi-cating artery	Internal carotid artery	Anterior cerebral artery	Basilar artery
Middle cerebral artery	16	10	2	3	4	
Anterior communicating artery	16	2		2		1
Internal carotid artery	4	6	3	9		
Anterior cerebral artery	2	2			1	
Basilar artery	4	3	1	1		
		23	6	15	5	1

The result substantially depends on the prior damage. Two patients in grade IV stage died, and two further patients in the same stage who were not operated on also died (Table 4).

Only the ruptured aneurysms were operated on in ten cases. Two patients died, and seven patients refused the second operation. In one case, the aneurysm was located infraclinoidally and was not operated on.

Table 4. Outcome of patients with multiple and single aneurysms (Glasgow Outcome Scale)

Multiple aneurysms	*n*	Good recovery	Moderate impairment	Marked improvement	Died
Group 1 (single-session operation)	18	18			
Group 2 (two-session operation)	12	12			
Group 3 (operation on the ruptured aneurysm)	10	2	5	1	2
Group 4 (no operation)	2				2
Single aneurysms	361	96	120	39	27

Discussion

Highly divergent clinical frequencies of multiple aneurysms are found in patients reported in the literature. According to a compilation of Fox (1989), the percentages range from 6% to 31.9% [1]. The reference figures of the Frankfurt/Main and Homburg/Saar University Hospitals (Table 1) indicate that there is evidently a very good agreement in this respect if similar diagnostic investigations and procedures are considered in Central Europe.

Comparison between the course in patients with a single aneurysm and those with multiple aneurysms does not show any appreciable differences. In principle, this justifies application of the procedure in multiple aneurysms, i.e., unruptured aneurysms should and can also be dealt with. We have carried out a single-stage operation in all aneurysms which could be reached via one approach. In the cases with an aneurysm of the pericallosal artery and other locations, two approaches in the same session were chosen. As a rule, we waited for 6 months and longer before carrying out the second operation in aneurysms which were located on both sides, after improvement of the clinical symptoms and normalization of the findings. There were no demonstrable differences compared with the patients with a single aneurysm with regard to the results and the severity of the preoperative clinical picture. The large number of second operations which were refused indicates the severity of the rating of the cerebral hemorrhage and the postoperative course in many patients.

References

1. Fox JL (1983) Intracranial Aneurysma, vol I. Springer, New York, pp 290–291
2. Heiskanen O, Marttila I (1970) Risk of rupture of a second aneurysm in patients with multiple aneurysms. J Neurosurg 32:295–299

3. Hunt WE, Hess RM (1968) Surgical risk as related to time of intervention in the repair of intracranial aneurysms. J Neurosurg 28:14–20
4. Ianagawa T (1991) Surgical treatment of multiple intracranial aneurysms. Acta Neurochirurgia (Wien) 108:22–29
5. Jennett B, Bond M (1975) Assessment of outcome after severe brain damage. A practical scale. Lancet 1:480–484
6. Paterson A, Bond MR (1973) Treatment of multiple intracranial arterial aneurysms. Lancet 1:1302–1304
7. Reif J (1991) Personal communication

Circulatory Arrest and Hypothermia in the Treatment of Cerebral Aneurysms: Preliminary Results

A. Brawanski[1], O.-W. Ullrich[1], U. Hartung[2], P. Eigel[3], and I. Danhauser-Leistner[2]

Introduction

Some cerebrovascular lesions cannot be treated definitively by conventional means despite all advanced neurosurgical and anesthesiological techniques. Especially large or giant intracerebral aneurysms have a badly defined neck, and the size and location often impede anatomical intraoperative orientation and definitive clip placement.

In the last decade several neurosurgical centers have been using circulatory arrest to treat such complex lesions with encouraging postoperative results [3, 4, 7, 8]. We want to report our preliminary experience in the treatment of complicated intracranial aneurysms utilizing circulatory arrest and profund hypothermia.

Patients and Method

In 1990 we operated on three patients with a large intracranial aneurysm under hypothermia and cardiac arrest. The pertinent data are given in Table 1. Two of the patients (cases 1 and 2) had a subarachnoid hemorrhage, and one (Fig. 2) had a progredient loss of vision (case 3). One patient (case 1) had three additional aneurysms. One was clipped together with the giant aneurysm; the other two were treated in a second operation 3 months later. At the time of the operation the patients were in good clinical condition.

The diagnostic means comprised computer tomography (CT), magnetic resonance imaging (MRI), and digital subtraction angiography (DSA). Embolization or occlusion of the aneurysm by an endovascular approach was considered, but was not possible. Once the indication for the operation under cardiac arrest and hypothermia was set, each patient underwent medical assessment, extensive blood tests, and cardiological evaluation, which included electrocardiography (ECG), echocardiography, and coronary angiography in two patients.

[1] Neurochirurgische Klinik und Poliklinik der Universität Würzburg, Josef-Schneider-Str. 11, W–8700 Würzburg, FRG.
[2] Institut für Anästhesiologie der Universität Würzburg, Josef-Schneider-Str. 11, W–8700 Würzburg, FRG.
[3] Abteilung für Thorax-, Herz- und Thorakale Gefäßchirurgie der Universität Würzburg, Josef-Schneider-Str. 11, W–8700 Würzburg, FRG.

Advances in Neurosurgery, Vol. 20
K. Piscol, M. Klinger, M. Brock (Eds.)

Table. 1. Clinical data cases treated

Case	Name	Age (years)	Aneurysm location	Size
1	L.H.	38	Middle cerebral artery, right	Giant
2	K.K.	53	Anterior communicating artery	Giant
3	F.T.	65	Ophthalmic artery, left	Large

On the day of the operation several intravenous and arterial lines are introduced to allow intraoperative monitoring of blood pressure and cardiovascular parameters. Two temperature probes register the esophageal and rectal temperature.

After induction the neurosurgical team performs the craniotomy and exposes the aneurysm as far as possible. Then the cardiac surgeons implant a femorofemoral bypass. The patient is now fully heparinized; the heart-lung-circulation machine with a heat exchanger and exogenator is started to cool the patient. The heart starts to fibrillate at an approximate temperature of 28°C and eventually stops spontaneous activity completely. When the target temperature of 18°C is reached, the neurosurgical team continues the operation. If necessary the pump is stopped, and the patient's head is elevated to drain the patient's blood into the reservoir of the heart-lung-circulation machine. This maneuver causes the aneurysm to collapse and helps further dissection of the aneurysm and clip application. The maximum possible time for complete circulatory arrest amounts to 60 min. After clipping of the aneurysm the patient is rewarmed slowly at 0.4°–0.6°C/min. Overly rapid rewarming is dangerous because it can induce tissue acidosis and ischemia by a mismatch of energy supply and metabolism. If a spontaneous sinus rhythm of the heart does not start, cardioversion is necessary. In the case of persistent cardiac fibrillation, a thoracotomy would be necessary. When the cardiac output is sufficient and the core temperature is about 35°C, the femorofemoral bypass is removed by the thoracic surgeons, and the heparinization is antagonized with protamine sulfate. The craniotomy is closed after meticulous hemostasis. Then the patient is transferred to the ICU and sedated overnight. After an inconspicuous CT scan sedation is stopped.

Results

The three patients were treated according to the described protocol. All aneurysms were dissected via the pterional approach. The mean time of complete circulatory arrest was 13 min. All patients survived the operative procedure, two (cases 1 and 3) with excellent results, one with a good outcome (case 2). We observed no postoperative hemorrhage. Reangiography 3 months later showed a complete occlusion of the aneurysms (Figs. 1 and 2).

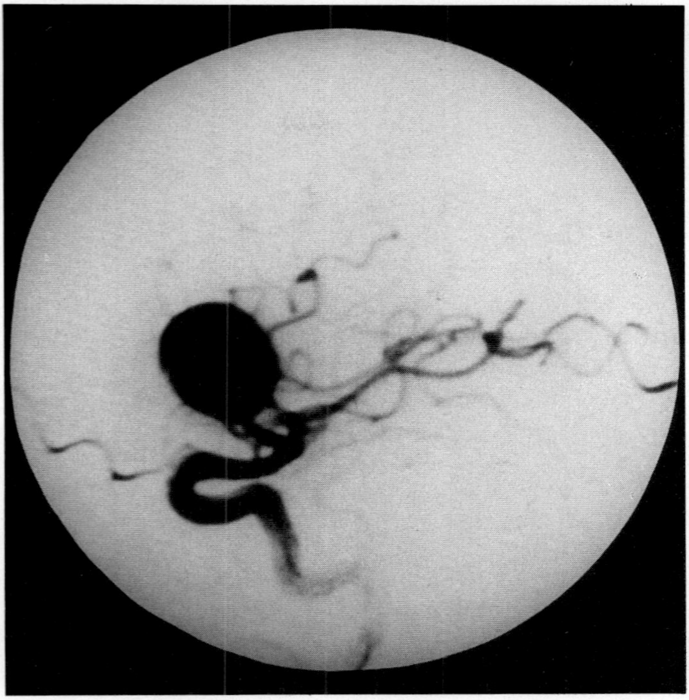

Fig. 1. Preoperative angiogram of case 2

Discussion

The introduction of cardiac arrest and deep hypothermia is a routine and safe procedure from an anesthesiological point of view [1, 5, 6]. It is utilized daily in cardiac surgery. The overall risk of this procedure is composed of several factors. The longer the circulatory arrest, the higher the risk is of ischemic damage to the brain. Thus, some neurosurgeons avoid total circulatory arrest and work with a very reduced circulation only [4].

The hypothermia has effects on blood viscosity, the partition coefficient of blood gases, and the glucose metabolism. These facts require corrresponding anesthesiological knowledge and experience. During the bypass normal coagulation is abandoned. Thus, all neurosurgeons report an increased risk of postoperative hemorrhage, which has significant influence on the outcome. The cannulation of the femoral vein increases the overall risk of postoperative embolism or deep venous thrombosis [2].

We did not see any of these complications in the small group of patients which we have treated so far. In general, the technique seems safe enough to offer it to a specific group of neurosurgical patients.

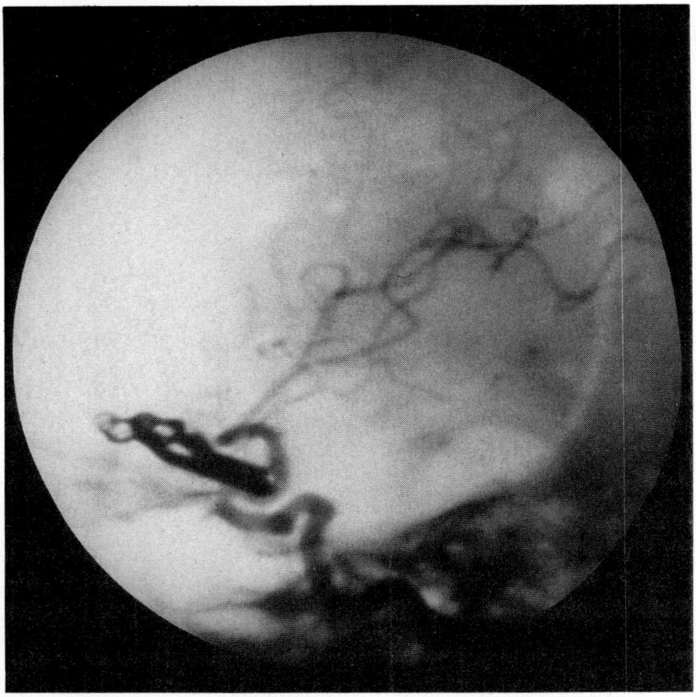

Fig. 2. Postoperative angiogram of case 2

We see the indication for circulatory arrest and deep hypothermia under the following conditions: The patient lacks specific cardiac risk factors. The aneurysm cannot be treated by any other means. Especially endovascular procedures are not possible. The anatomical situation allows no transient clipping for a longer time without the risk of ischemia, whereas the complexity and location of the aneurysm require a longer dissection time. We do not see the size of the aneurysm as sole indicator, but also consider anatomy and location.

References

1. Barrat-Boyes BG, Neutze JM, Seelye ER et al. (1972) Complete correction of cardiovascular malformations in the first year of life. Prog Cardiovasc Dis 15:229–253
2. Baumgartner WA, Silverberg GD, Ream AK et al. (1983) Reappraisal of cardiopulmonary bypass with deep hypothermia and circulatory arrest for complex neurosurgical operations. Surgery 94:242–249
3. Chyatte D, Elefteriades J, Kim B (1989) Profound hypothermia and circulatory arrest for aneurysm surgery. J Neurosurg 70:489–491
4. Keravel Y, Sindou M (1988) Giant intracranial aneurysms. Springer, Berlin Heidelberg New York Tokyo

5. Reitz BA, Ream AK (1982) Uses of hypothermia in cardiovascular surgery. In: Ream AK, Fogdall RP (eds) Acute cardiovascular management: anesthesia and intensive care. JB Lippincott, Philadelphia, pp 830–848
6. Ritterhouse EA, Mohri H, Dillard DH et al. (1974) Deep hypothermia in cardiovascular surgery. Ann Thorac Surg 17:63–98
7. Spetzler RF, Hadley MN, Rigamonti D, Carter LP et al. (1988) Aneurysms of the basilar artery treated with circulatory arrest, hypothermia, and barbiturate cerebral protection. J Neurosurg 68:868–879
8. Silverberg GD, Reitz BA, Ream AK (1981) Hypothermia and cardiac arrest in the treatment of giant aneurysms of the cerebral circulation and hemangioblastoma of the medulla. J Neurosurg 55:337–346

Principles of Aneurysm Surgery in the Acute Stage of Subarachnoid Hemorrhage

K. Sano[1]

We experienced 1646 cases of intracranial aneurysms up to the end of 1989; 1519 cases exhibited subarachnoid hemorrhage (SAH). Of these 1519 cases, 171 (11.3%) died of rebleeding while waiting for surgery mostly within 1 week after SAH. The fact has made us consider a possible advantage of early surgery for patients with ruptured aneurysms. However, if we compare the mortality (at 6 months following SAH) of early surgery (within 1 week after SAH) with that of surgery done later than the 1st week, the former was 14.5% (95/655) and the latter was 3.9% (26/674). Therefore, the latter seemed apparently better (Table 1). The latter became 15.2%, however, if the above 11.3% were added to it. Therefore, there was no marked difference in mortality between the two groups, or, one may say, early surgery was a little bit better.

Table 1. Timing of microsurgery of ruptured aneurysms

Location of aneurysms	Total	Within 1 week from the last SAH	Later than the 1st week	Death
ICPcom	284	124 (18)	160 (4)	22 (7.7%)
Ic-bif	31	13 (6)	18 (1)	7 (22.6%)
Ant. chor.	52	27 (5)	25 (2)	7 (13.5%)
Acom	380	192 (24)	188 (10)	34 (8.9%)
A_1, A_2	63	29 (4)	34 (1)	5 (7.9%)
MC	254	160 (25)	94 (1)	26 (10.2%)
V-B	80	18 (4)	62 (5)	9 (11.3%)
Multiple	185	92 (9)	93 (2)	11 (5.9%)
Total	1329	655 (95 = 14.5%)	674 (26 = 3.9%)	121 (9.1%)

ICPcom, internal carotid-posterior communicating (here including ophthalmic); IC-bif, internal carotid bifurcation; Ant. chor., anterior choroidal; Acom, anterior communicating; A_1, A_2, A_1 and A_2 portions of the anterior cerebral artery; MC, middle cerebral; V-B, vertebro-basillar; multiple, multiple aneurysms. ( ), deaths.

[1] Department of Neurosurgery, University of Tokyo, Teikyo University Hospital and Fuji Brain Institute, 2-11-1 Kaga, Itabashi-Ku, Tokyo 173, Japan.

Advances in Neurosurgery, Vol. 20
K. Piscol, M. Klinger, M. Brock (Eds.)

Table 2. Operative mortality and morbidity of cases with ruptured aneurysms according to grading

WFNS Grade	GCS	Cases	Death	GR	MD	SD, V
I	15	840	24 (2.9%)	732 (87.1%)	56 (6.7%)	28 (3.3%)
II, III	14-13	282	29 (10.3%)	177 (62.8%)	46 (16.3%)	30 (10.6%)
IV	12-7	153	36 (23.5%)	39 (25.5%)	39 (25.5%)	39 (25.5%)
V	6-3	54	32 (59.3%)	3 (5.6%)	5 (9.2%)	14 (25.9%)
Total		1329	121 (9.1%)	951 (71.6%)	146 (11.0%)	111 (8.3%)

GR, good recovery; MD, moderate disability; SD, severe disability; V, vegetative state (Glasgow Outcome Scale).

The three greatest causes of mortality and morbidity in aneurysmal subarachnoid hemorrhage are (a) rebleeding of ruptured aneurysms, (b) cerebral vasospasm causing delayed ischemic neurological deficits (DIND), and (c) direct effects of SAH or acute ischemic neurological deficits (AIND) [6–8, 13]. Rebleeding can be prevented by early (acute stage) surgery. Some factors of AINDs may be alleviated by early surgical interventions (e.g., acute hydrocephalus, intracerebral hematoma). In the acute stage (within 1 week after SAH), however, the surgeon most often encounters patients in poor condition or with serious grades due to AINDs. The fact inevitably constitutes a major cause of bad surgical results. Besides, contrary to our expectations, early surgery and removal of subarachnoid clots may often be too late or too incomplete to prevent development of delayed cerebral vasospasm or DINDs. When should surgery for patients with ruptured aneurysms be performed? To solve the problem of timing of surgery, our own series of 1329 cases of ruptured aneurysms submitted to microsurgery was analyzed. The patients were classified according to the state of consciousness just prior to surgery (not on admission), which was expressed by scores of the Glasgow Coma Scale (GCS) [5, 16] or the World Federation of Neurological Surgeons (WFNS) grading [1], namely, grade I (GCS 15), grades II and III (GCS 14-13), grade IV (GCS 12-7), and grade V (GCS 6-3). In Hunt's grading [3], which is still popular, grades I and II correspond to GCS 15; grades III, IV, and V roughly correspond to GCS 14 - 13, GCS 12-7, and GCS 6-3, respectively. The Glasgow Outcome Scale [4] is used for the classification of outcome at 6 months following SAH in patients submitted to surgery.

As far as the operative (postoperative) mortality (death at 6 months following SAH) is concerned, the χ^2 test shows that WFNS grade I cases (GCS 15) are superior to grades II and III (GCS 14-13) ($P < 1\%$), grade IV (GCS 12-7) ($P < 1\%$), or grade V (GCS 6-3) ($P < 1\%$) cases. Grade II and III cases are definitely better than grade IV cases or grade V cases ($P < 1\%$), and grade IV cases are superior to grade V ($P < 1\%$) (Table 2).

It is concluded that the grading of patients' conditions based on GCS just prior to surgery is the definitive factor which influences the (post)operative mortality and morbidity. Since cerebral vasospasm, at least angiographic vasospasm, appears first on day 4 and not before [10, 11], the 1st week after SAH was divided into two periods: from day 0 (the day of aneurysmal rupture) to day 2 (48 h after SAH) and from day 3 to day 7. In the 1st week, of 655 cases that underwent microsurgery, WFNS grade I cases comprised 345 (52.7%), grade II and III cases 162 (24.7%), grade IV cases 97 (14.8%), and grade V cases 51 (7.7%), i.e., grade II-V cases constituted 47.3% of the total. On days 0 through 2, however, grade I cases represented only 47.8% and grade II-V cases 52.2%.

The (post)operative mortality in 477 cases that underwent surgery on day 0 through day 2 (that is, within 48 h after SAH) and the mortality in 178 cases submitted to surgery on day 3 through day 7 were relatively high (15.9% and 10.7%, respectively) as compared with that in 155 cases submitted to surgery in the 2nd week after SAH (5.2%) and that in 519 cases operated on later than the 2nd week (3.5%), as seen in Table 3.

As far as the (post)operative mortality is concerned, the χ^2 test revealed that there was no statistically significant difference at any timing of surgery in each of WFNS grade I, IV, or V cases, except that grade I cases submitted to surgery on days 0 through 2 showed a slightly higher mortality (5.3%) as compared with those submitted to surgery later than the 2nd week (1.9%) ($P < 5\%$). In grade II and III cases (GCS 14-13), however, surgery on days 3–7 resulted in a higher (post)operative mortality as compared with surgery in the 2nd week ($P < 5\%$) or later than the 2nd week ($P < 1\%$) or even with surgery on days 0–2 ($P < 110\%$). On the other hand, the mortality of surgery on days 0–2 was not significantly different from that of surgery in the 2nd week or later in grade II and III cases (GCS 14-13).

Therefore, as for the (post)operative mortality, it can be said that for WFNS grade II and III cases with GCS 14-13, surgery on days 3–7 is best avoided, as was suggested by us years ago [10–12]. This mortality is mostly due to cerebral vasospasm. Surgery on days 0–2 in grade II and III cases, however, may be performed without significantly higher mortality as compared with surgery at a later timing. Grade I cases showed good results at any timing of surgery; therefore, early surgery is indicated for them. Grade IV and V cases exhibited poor results at any timing of surgery. Surgery, therefore, may better be postponed until they show better grades or better GCS.

For timing of surgery, age should also be considered. There was a singificant difference ($P < 1\%$) in the (post)operative mortality between the group younger than 60 years (5.4%) and the group 60 years and over (11.7%). In the former group, there was no significant difference by the χ^2 test in the (post)operative mortality (at 6 months following SAH) at any timing of surgery, except that the mortality in surgery on days 0–2 or days 3–7 was higher than that in surgery later than the 2nd week ($P < 1\%$). In the group 60 years and over, the (post)operative mortality in cases submitted to surgery on day 0 through day 2 (19.7%) was significantly higher than that later than the 2nd week ($P < 1\%$), but not significantly higher than that on day 3 through day 7 (11.1%). This high mortality in early surgery in the higher age group was probably partly because these mortality cases belonged to the higher grades (II or higher) and partly because in the higher age group the

Table 3. Microsurgery of ruptured aneurysms. Timing, grade at operation and follow-up results (1329 cases)

		1st week after SAH 0 (SAH day) – day 2					Day 3–7				
WFNS Grade	GCS	Cases	Death	GR	MD	SD, V	Cases	Death	GR	MD	SD, V
I	15	228	12	192	15	9	117	2	102	9	4
II, III	14-13	120	13	75	21	11	42	10	20	9	3
IV	12-7	82	26	17	20	19	15	3	4	5	3
V	6-3	47	25	3	5	14	4	4	0	0	0
Total		477	76	287	61	53	178	19	126	23	10
			15.9%	60.2%	12.8%	11.1%		10.7%	70.8%	12.9%	5.6%
		2nd week after SAH					Later than 2nd week				
WFNS Grade	GCS	Cases	Death	GR	MD	SD, V	Cases	Death	GR	MD	SD, V
I	15	80	2	75	2	1	415	8	363	30	14
II, III	14-13	54	3	42	6	3	66	3	40	10	13
IV	12-7	20	2	12	2	4	36	5	6	12	13
V	6-3	1	1	0	0	0	2	2	0	0	0
Total		155	8	129	10	8	519	18	409	52	40
			5.2%	83.2%	6.5%	5.2%		3.5%	78.8%	10.0%	7.7%

GR, good recovery; MD, moderate disability; SD, severe disability; V, vegetative state (Glasgow Outcome Scale).

ability to recover from pathological conditions due to direct effects of SAH may be lowered.

From these data, one may conclude that for patients 60 years of age or above, surgery may better be postponed to timing later than the 2nd week, especially when they are of WFNS grades II, III, or higher.

To evaluate the mortality and morbidity together, the *U* test (Mann-Whitney) may be suitable. WFNS grade I cases (GCS 15) had significantly less mortality and morbidity than grades II and III ($P < 1\%$), which were better than grade IV ($P < 1\%$), which was, in turn, significantly better than grade V ($P < 1\%$).

Grade I cases showed no statistically significant difference in the mortality and morbidity at different timing of surgery except that surgery done in the 2nd week showed better results than that on days 0–2 ($P < 5\%$). The results in WFNS grade II and III cases (GCS 14-13) were better in cases submitted to surgery in the 2nd week than on days 0–2 ($P < 5\%$) or days 3–7 ($P < 1\%$) or later than the 2nd week ($P < 5\%$). In the group younger than 60 years of age, cases that underwent surgery on days 0 through 2 and days 3 through 7 showed poorer results as compared with cases operated on at a later timing ($P < 1\%$), whereas in the group aged 60 years or above cases submitted to surgery on days 0 through 2 showed poorer results than the others ($P < 1\%$).

The borderline of 60 years of age was adopted here arbitrarily. We are not sure whether this borderline is valid or not. We are even more uncertain whether this borderline is valid for different gradings or not. Therefore, we checked the latter in 145 recent cases of aneurysmal SAH that were submitted to surgery. The results were not too different whether the borderline was 60 years or 65 years. And the younger age group (59 years and younger or 64 years and younger) showed good surgical results in grades I, II, and III. Considering the individual biological variability, the borderline can be set between the ages of 60 and 65 years.

In consideration of the results of the χ^2 test and the *U* test, the following conclusions may be drawn:

1. Grading according to GCS just prior to surgical intervention seems reasonable. Cases with GCS 15 (grade I of WFNS) showed better surgical results than cases with GCS 14-13 (grades II and III of WFNS) which were superior to cases with GCS 12-7 (grade IV of WFNS). Cases with GCS 12-7, in turn, showed better results than cases with GCS 6-3 (grade V of WFNS).
2. As for the (post)operative mortality (at 6 months following SAH), there was no significant difference at any timing of surgery in each of WFNS grade I, IV, or V cases (low mortality in I, higher mortality in IV and V).
3. For WFNS grade II and III cases with GCS 14-13, surgery on days 3–7 may better be avoided because of a higher (post)operative mortality than at another timing. However, surgery on days 0–2 may be performed without significantly higher mortality as compared with surgery in the 2nd week or a later timing (χ^2 test) (Fig. 1).
4. For patients 60 years or older (particularly in II or higher grades), surgery may better be postponed to the 2nd week or later.

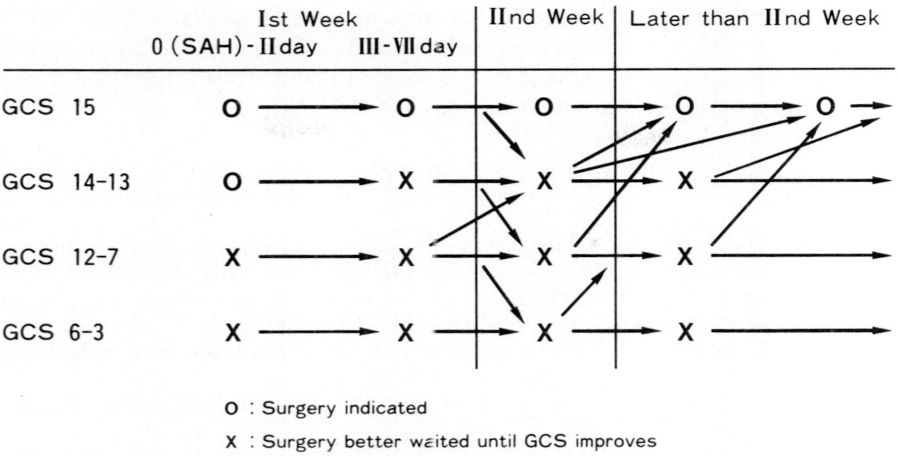

Figure 1

As seen from the statistics, the results of surgery are the same at any timing of operation in WFNS grade I patients with GCS 15. This means that in those patients AIND is minimal, and the effects of surgical intervention in the early stage of SAH are not different from those in the chronic stage of SAH. Therefore, these cases with GCS 15 should be submitted to surgery as soon as possible after SAH (Fig. 1). In cases of grade II, III, IV, or V patients who have already incurred a considerable degree of AIND, surgery in the early stage may exert a harmful influence on the brain. If the patient is relatively young, the brain may soon recover from the infliction. In elderly patients, however, the brain may not be able to fully tolerate surgical interventions and as a result, AINDs may become aggravated. This may be why the result of early surgery for elderly patients is rather poor.

In the 2nd week or later, if a patient develops cerebral vasospasm, the grading becomes worse, and surgery may have to be postponed. Because of this inadvertent selection, the results of delayed surgery may seem to be better than those of early surgery. This observation is shared by other authors [2, 14].

One of the reasons why we are inclined to be in favor of early surgery is that the mortality in rebleeding cases is very high. The Japanese part [9] of the International Cooperative Study [7, 8], which consists of 1131 cases, shows that 64.4% of rebleeding cases in that series were fatal. If we clip aneurysms in the very early stage, we can concentrate our efforts on prevention and treatment of cerebral vasospasm by using calcium blockers, free radical scavengers, hypervolemia, hypertension, etc. Recently, our Japanese group devised a simple and most effective means to remove subarachnoid and intraventricular blood clots after aneurysm clipping [15]. This is the head shaker by which the patient's head is intermittently shaken (amplitude 4 cm, frequency 1–1.4 c/s) in the horizontal plane while ventriculocisternal irrigation with 500 ml of lactate Ringer with or without urokinase (6000 IU) is carried out for 24–48 h so that clots can be extensively removed. This procedure has remarkably decreased the incidence of cerebral vasospasm and may be a strong tool to prevent delayed cerebral vasospasm and DIND.

References

1. Drake CG (1988) Report of World Federation of Neurological Surgeons Committee on a Universal Subarachnoid Hemorrhage Grading Scale. J Neurosurg 68:985–986
2. Hugenholtz H, Elgie RG (1982) Considerations in early surgery on good-risk patients with ruptured intracranial aneurysms. J Neurosurg 56:180–185
3. Hunt WE, Hess RM (1968) Surgical risk as related to time of intervention in the repair of intracranial aneurysms. J Neurosurg 28:14–26
4. Jennett B, Bond M (1975) Assessment of outcome after severe brain damage. A practical scale. Lancet I:480–484
5. Jenett B, Teasdale G (1977) Aspects of coma after severe head injury. Lancet I:878–881
6. Kassell NF, Torner JC (1984) The International Cooperative Study on timing of aneurysm surgery: An update. Stroke 15:566–570
7. Kassell NF, Torner JC et al. (1990) The International Cooperative Study on the timing of aneurysm surgery: Part 1: Overall management results. J Neurosurg 73:18–36
8. Kassell NF, Torner JC et al. (1990) The International Cooperative Study on the timing of aneurysm surgery: Part 2: Surgical results. J Neurosurg 73:37–47
9. Kitamura K, Kassell NF, Torner JC et al. (1987) The Japanese results in the International Cooperative Study on timing of aneurysm surgery. Neurol Surg 15:1155–1166
10. Saito I, Udea Y, Sano K (1977) Significance of vasospasm in the treatment of ruptured intracranial aneurysms. J Neurosurg 47:412–429
11. Sano K (1983) Cerebral vasospasm and aneurysm surgery. Clin Neurosurg 30:13–58
12. Sano K, Saito I (1978) Timing and indication of surgery for ruptured intracranial aneurysms with regards to cerebral vasospasm. Acta Neurochir 41:49–60
13. Sano K, Asano T, Tamura A (1987) Acute aneurysm surgery: pathophysiology and managment. Springer, Wien New York
14. Suzuki J, Onuma T, Yoshimoto T (1979) Results of early operation on cerebral aneurysms. Surg Neurol 11:407–412
15. Suzuki I, Shimizu H, Takahashi H, Ishijima B (1990) Effect of head shaking method on clot removal in cisternal irrigation. In: Sano K et al. (eds) Cerebral vasospasm. Univ of Tokyo Press, Tokyo, pp 314–316
16. Teasdale G, Jennett B (1974) Assessment of coma and impaired consciousness. A practical scale. Lancet II:81–84

Prognosis of Aneurysmal Subarachnoid Hemorrhage: Prospective Study on 543 Patients

N. Freckmann, H.-D. Herrmann, and D. Winkler[1]

Introduction

Prevention of rebleeding and cerebral vasospasm is essential for the prognosis of aneurysmal subarachnoid hemorrhage (SAH). Only early elimination of the rebleeding risk permits appropriate management of SAH and its sequelae due to cerebral vasospasm [2, 3]. Since March 1984 we therefore use a more aggressive management strategy [5, 7]: As soon as the diagnosis of SAH is made, i.v. administration of nimodipine is started. Earliest operation follows except for patients grade IV/V (according to Hunt and Hess) without relevant intracranial hematoma [12] and those harboring aneurysms of the proximal basilar artery. The morbidity of early surgery will be reduced by:

1. Use of external ventricular drainage [6] for preoperative lowering of intracranial pressure (ICP), increase of intraoperative space, and reduction of surgical trauma. It is further advantageous for postoperative ICP monitoring and clearing of bloody CSF.
2. Use of intraoperative "brain protection" (isoflurane/Brevimytal) [8]
3. Liberal temporary clipping [11]
4. Induction of hypertonia/hypervolemia immediately after definitive clipping [4]
5. Intravenous and cisternal administration of nimodipine
6. Controlled hypotension in basilar aneurysm only

The postoperative therapy of SAH is directed toward safeguarding a sufficient cerebral perfusion to minimize the risk of permanent neurological deficits due to cerebral ischemia:

1. Prevention of vasospasm: Nimodipine i.v. (0.5–0.7 mg/kg, 7–14 days), monitoring by transcranial Doppler sonography [9]
2. Lowering of ICP: dexamethasone, ventricular drainage
3. Increase in mean arterial pressure (MAP): hypertension (catecholamine), hypervolemia [4]
4. Improvement of rheology and microcirculation (high molecular weight dextrans)

[1] Neurochirurgische Abteilung, Universitätskrankenhaus Eppendorf, Martinistr. 52, W-2000 Hambnurg 20, FRG.

Advances in Neurosurgery, Vol. 20
K. Piscol, M. Klinger, M. Brock (Eds.)

Table 1. Selected characteristics

	Series A (n = 135)		B (n = 408)	
Preop. re. SAH	34	(25%)	77	(19%)
Preop. vasospasm	30	(22%)	65	(16%)
Preop. mortality	25	(18%)	55	(14%)
Surgery	103	(76%)	343	(84%)
Early surg.	35	(35%)	249	(73%)
Delayed surg.	67	(65%)	94	(27%)
Postop. vasospasm	11	(9%)	55	(13%)
Postop. mortality	12	(12%)	37	(11%)
Early surg.	8	(22%)	34	(14%)
Delayed surg.	4	(6%)	3	(3%)
Overall mortality	37	(27%)	92	(23%)
Mean age of death (years)	52.8		51.3	

Patients

From January 1981 to March 1991, 543 patients who suffered aneurysmal SAH were admitted and prospectively documented. Patients with vertebrobasilar, multiple, or giant aneurysms were not excluded from this study. In accordance with the modification of our therapeutic strategy we built two series: series A (1/81–2/84; $n = 135$) and series B (3/84–3/91; $n = 408$).

In series A early surgery was aimed at only in grade I/II patients [7]. Before surgery these patients generally were treated by sedation and lowering the blood pressure. In most cases induced hypotension was used during aneurysm clipping [3].

The series did not differ in their age and sex distribution. The mean age was 49 years. The ratio between male and female patients was 1 : 1.7.

The distribution of clinical grading on admission, however, was significantly different between patients in series A and B. The amount of poor-grade patients (i.e., presenting in grade III–V) increased from 29% in series A to 46% in series B; 11% of the patients in series A but 22% of the patients in series B were classified as grade IV and V.

Results

The most relevant clinical data and results are summarized in Tables 1–4. Further, we observed the development of permanent ischemic neurological deficits due to delayed-onset cerebral vasospasms in 4 of 29 (14%) "good-risk patients" of series A operated on early. In 208 patients of series B permanent lesions occurred in only 10 cases (5%). The incidence of transitory neurological deficits was about the

Table 2. Admission grade/mortality (%)

Series A	*n*	%	Preop.	Postop.	Total
I	58	43	3	3	6
II	39	29	5	8	13
III	23	17	25	13	39
IV	12	9	58	25	83
V	3	2	33	67	100
Series B					
I	143	35	2	6	8
II	77	19	4	5	9
III	99	24	9	11	20
IV	53	13	23	19	42
V	36	9	81	8	89

Table 3. Outcome (Glasgow Outcome Scale, GOS) after early surgery

		GOS					
Preop. grade		1	2	3	4	5	Death
Series A	(*n* = 36)						
I	(*n* = 17)	7	5	2	2		1
II	(*n* = 9)	3	2	3			1
III	(*n* = 3)		1		1		1
IV	(*n* = 2)			1		1	3
V	(*n* = 2)						2
Series B	(*n* = 249)						
I	(*n* = 104)	25	42	24	6		7
II	(*n* = 43)	5	17	11	5	1	4
III	(*n* = 60)	5	19	24	6	2	4
IV	(*n* = 33)		2	7	9	3	12
V	(*n* = 9)				1	1	7

same: 3 cases among the patients of series A (10%) and 18 cases (9%) among those of series B. An excellent or favorable outcome was achieved by 181 (73%) patients of series B operated on early.

Discussion

The evaluation of our clinical data shows that our present management regime has had a positive impact on the prognosis of SAH. At 12 months after SAH, 73% of our patients had achieved an excellent or good outcome [10].

Table 4. Age/mortality (%)

Age (years)	*n*	Preop.	Postop.	Total
< 20	10	20		20
20–29	27		11	11
30–39	64	9	12	20
40–49	113	11	7	17
50–59	95	19	13	28
60–69	71	17	14	28
> 70	28	18	16	28

Especially the improvement of the outcome in grade III patients (Table 3), a substantial group making up 24% of our population, is particularly striking. The outcome of grade III patients in whom surgery was planned after an interval of 8–14 days showed particularly unsatisfactory results: 50% of them had a drastic deterioration of their state and died before surgery from rebleeding or the sequelae of cerebral vasospasm without any chance of being helped. Now the total mortality in this group is reduced to 20%. Therefore, in spite of the drawback of a higher postoperative mortality and morbidity, the tendency to early surgery prevailed. It is indeed this group of patients which should undergo diagnosis and surgery as soon as possible.

Accordingly, advanced age should not represent a criterion for exclusion from early surgery because there is no difference in the overall mortality of patients above 50 years (Table 4). After all, particularly elderly patients are in danger because of the inherent risks after SAH. These are mainly related to cerebral ischemia, but also apply to general pulmonary and cardiovascular complications [3].

On the other hand, we do not presently see any possibility of improving prognosis and outcome in patients in grade IV and especially grade V without space-occupying hematomas.

The subgroup of patients presenting in poor neurological condition on admission increased during the last 2–3 years. There was consequently an increase of the mortality rate from 19% to 23% (Tables 1 and 2). As some patients died prior to or shortly after admission without being included in our series, we assume that a fairly realistic mortality rate should be estimated at least 10% higher. These data indicate that aneurysmal SAH still is associated with a high mortality rate and it is difficult to improve its prognosis further.

In accordance with the results recently reported in the literature, we can state that our present strategy for the treatment of SAH, the overall catalogue of measures for safeguarding sufficient cerebral perfusion, including treatment with the calcium antagonist nimodipine and surgery at the earliest possible moment, eliminates the rebleeding risk, reduces the complications due to cerebral vasospasm, and thus allows a reduction in mortality and morbidity.

References

1. Ammerer HP, Perneczky G, Böck F (1985) Appearance of cerebral vasospasm after break of Nimotop-prophylaxis and their treatment. In: Auer LM (ed) Timing of aneurysm surgery. de Gruyter, Berlin New York
2. Auer LM (ed) (1985) Timing of aneurysm surgery. de Gruyter, Berlin New York
3. Ausman JI, Diaz FG, Malik GM et al. (1985) Current management of cerebral aneurysms: Is it based on facts or myths? Surg Neurol 24:625–635
4. Baumann H, Samii M, Ramina R et al. (1985) Experience with Nimodipine in combination with postoperative hypertensive, hypervolemic treatment in the management of ruptured intracranial aneurysms. In: Auer LM (ed) Timing of aneurysm surgery. de Gruyter, Berlin New York
5. Cristante L, Freckmann N, Winkler D, Herrmann H-D (1990) Nimodipine in the treatment of subarachnoid hemorrhage secondary to aneurysm rupture: Five years experience. In: Bushe KA, Brock M, Klinger M (eds) Advances in neurosurgery. Springer, Berlin Heidelberg New York Tokyo
6. Dolenc VV (1985) The value of CSF drainage during aneurysm surgery and prevention of the development of hydrocephalus. In: Auer LM (ed) (1985) Timing of aneurysm surgery. de Gruyter, Berlin New York
7. Freckmann N, Noll M, Winkler D et al. (1987) Does the timing of aneurysm surgery neglect the real problems of subarachnoid haemorrhage? Acta Neurochir 89:91–99
8. Freckmann N, Renz D, Müchler H-Ch, Rehn H (1985) Hirnprotektive Maßnahmen aus der Sicht des Neurochirurgen. In: Heuser D, Freckmann N, Renz D, Schoeppner H, Wiedemann K (eds) Indikation und Praxis cerebroprotektiver Maßnahmen in der Neurochirurgie. Springer, Berlin Heidelberg New York Tokyo
9. Harders A, Gilsbach J (1985) Timecourse of cerebrovascular spasm in early aneurysm operation: transcranial Doppler findings. In: Auer LM (ed) Timing of aneurysm surgery. de Gruyter, Berlin New York
10. Stegen G, Freckmann N (1991) Outcome and rehabilitation after aneurysmal subarachnoid haemorrhage. Zentralbl Neurochir 52:37–39
11. Symon L (1985) Thresholds of ischaemia applied to aneurysm surgery. Acta Neurochir 77:1–7
12. Weelock B, Weir B, Watts R et al (1983) Timing of surgery for intracerebral haematomas due to aneurysm

Early Versus Delayed Aneurysm Surgery in Subarachnoid Hemorrhage in Clinical Grade Hunt–Hess III

K. Lukow, W. Köning, and J. Menzel[1]

Introduction

Timing of aneurysm surgery in patients in grade III (according to Hunt and Hess) is still being discussed controversially, even reviewing last year's literature. The main argument for early surgery [1, 2, 5, 7, 10] is recurrent hemorrhage. Its frequency is reported ranging from 9% to 22% during the first 2 weeks. Opponents of early surgery [4, 8, 9] list difficult intraoperative conditions, which include brain edema and the risk of vasospasm. Other authors do not see any essential difference between the results of early or delayed surgery [3, 6, 11]. They decide upon timing according to circumstances [12].

Material and Methods

During the period of 1983–1989, 110 patients in grades I–III with subarachnoid hemorrhage (SAH) after ruptured aneurysm underwent surgery in the neurosurgical department of the municipal hospital in Cologne-Merheim. The patients' ages ranged from 12 to 78 years (average 47.0 years): 47 of the patients were male and 63 female (Table 1).

In 58 cases the aneurysms were located at the anterior circulation, in 28 at the site of the middle cerebral artery, in 8 at the internal carotid artery, and in 6 in the area of the vertebrobasilar artery.

On the day of surgery 70 patients were classified as grade I/II and 40 patients as grade III. Sixty patients underwent early surgery within 3 days after SAH; 50 patients were operated on day 4 or later. The causes for delayed surgery were late admission to the neurosurgical department, logistic reasons, and grades IV or V at admission.

To determine the operative conditions the following findings of grade III patients were evaluated retrospectively:

1. Brain swelling
2. Vasospasm observed intraoperatively
3. Intracerebral hemorrhage

[1] Neurochirurgische Klinik der Städtischen Krankenanstalten Köln-Merheim, Ostmerheimer Str. 200, W–5000 Köln 91, FRG.

Advances in Neurosurgery, Vol. 20
K. Piscol, M. Klinger, M. Brock (Eds.)

Table 1. Characteristics of patients grade I–III (1983–1989)

Total cases		110
Sex		
	Male	47 (43%)
	Female	63 (57%)
Age		
	Range	12–78 years
	Average	47.0 years
Clinical grade		
	I/II	70
	III	40

Table 2. Operative conditions of grade III patients ($n = 40$)

Conditions	Acute surgery ($n = 16$)		Delayed surgery ($n = 24$)	
	n	%	n	%
Brain swelling	8	50	2	8
Spasm	6	38	1	4
Hematoma	5	31	8	33
Difficult dissection[a]	9	56	4	17

[a] Premature rupture, temporary clipping, multiple clipping.

4. Difficult dissection such as early rupture of the aneurysm, temporary or multiple clipping (Table 2).

Regarding the Glasgow Outcome Scale (GOS), the results 6 months after surgery were evaluated as follows: GOS 1/2 = favorable, GOS 3/4 = unfavorable, and GOS 5 = dead.

Results

Early surgery for grade III patients showed a remarkable increase in brain swelling and therefore in two cases the operation had to be interrupted. A similar rate occurred for vasospasm and operative dissection.

The grade I and II patients showed the known recovery rate of 95% and 85%, respectively, and low mortality of 2.5% and 3.8%, respectively, independent of the time of surgery (Table 3). The recovery rate of the grade III patients with early surgery was within 75%, whereas only 33.3% with delayed surgery recovered well (Table 4).

Table 3. Six-month outcome of grade I/II patients ($n = 70$)

Timing of surgery	Favorable		Unfavorable		Dead		Total cases
	n	%	*n*	%	*n*	%	*n*
Acute (0–3 days post SAH)	42	(95.0)	1	(2.5)	1	(2.5)	44
Delayed (≥ 4 days post SAH)	22	(84.6)	3	(11.5)	1	(3.8)	26

Table 4. Six-month outcome of grade III patients ($n = 40$)

Timing of surgery	Favorable		Unfavorable		Dead		Total cases
	n	%	*n*	%	*n*	%	*n*
Acute (0–3 days post SAH)	12	(75.0)	2	(12.5)	2	(12.5)	16
Delayed (≥ 4 days post SAH)	7	(29.2)	8	(33.3)	9	(37.5)	24

The total mortality of the grade III patients was 27.5%, essentially higher than in grade I/II patients. The highest mortality rate was 37% for the grade III patients treated by delayed surgery. Two of them died because of medical problems (endocarditis and pulmonary embolism), and a further two patients because of intraoperative complications.

The remaining five patients died as a consequence of a delayed neurological deficit. They were operated on day 11 after SAH or later and without nimodipine treatment. Three of these five patients were admitted late, four of them were grade IV or V and improved before surgery, and one patient had two rebleedings.

Discussion

As expected, the frequency of intraoperative findings such as brain swelling, vasospasm, and difficult dissection in grade III patients was much higher in early than in delayed surgery. Nevertheless, the mortality rate was quite lower in early surgery than in delayed surgery. Similar rates resulted for morbidity and good recovery. We suggest that the differences are not related to intraoperative conditions in early surgery, but are due to the late admittance to the neurosurgical department and to the fact that the surgery was delayed because the patients were in a worse clinical grade before.

This study leads to the conclusion that grade III patients with delayed admission to the neurosurgical department have a relatively poor outcome, whereas grade III patients admitted early are not disadvantaged because of the early surgery.

References

1. Adams HP Jr, Kassell NF, Torner JC et al. (1981) Early management of aneurysmal subarachnoid hemorrhage. A report of the cooperative aneurysma study. J Neurosurg 54:141–145
2. Gilsbach JM, Reulen HJ, Ljunggren B, Brandt L, v Holst H, Mokrey M, v Essen C, Conzen M (1990) Early aneurysm surgery and preventive therapy with intravenously administered nimodipine: a multicenter, double-blind, dose-comparison study. Neurosurgery 26:458–464
3. Kassel NF, Torner JC, Jane JA, Haley EC Jr, Adams HP et al. (1990) The international cooperative study on the timing of aneurysm surgery. J Neurosurg 73:37–47
4. Ljunggren B, Säveland H, Brandt L (1983) Causes of unfavorable outcome after early aneurysm operation. Neurosurgery 13:629–633
5. Öhman J, Heiskanen O (1989) Timing of operation for ruptured supratentorial aneurysms: a prospective randomized study. J Neurosurg 70:55–60
6. Samson DS, Hodosh RM, Reid WR et al. (1979) Risk of intracranial aneurysm surgery in the good grade patient: early versus late operation. Neurosurgery 5:422–426
7. Sano K, Saito I (1978) Timing and indication of surgery for ruptured intracranial aneurysms with regard to cerebral vasospasm. Acta Neurochir 41:49–60
8. Sundt TM (1977) Cerebral vasospasm following subarachnoidal hemorrhage: evolution, management, and relationship to timing of surgery. Clin Neurosurg 56:228–239
9. Sundt TM, Kobayashi S, Fode NC, Whisnant JP (1982) Results and complications of surgical management of 809 intracranial aneurysms in 722 cases. J Neurosurg 56:753–765
10. Suzuki J, Onuma T, Yoshimoto T (1979) Results of early operations on cerebral aneurysms. Surg Neurol 11:407–412
11. Weir B, Aronyk K (1981) Management mortality and the timing of surgery for supratentorial aneurysms. J Neurosurg 54:146–150
12. Yasargil MG (1984) Microneurosurgery II. Thieme, Stuttgart, pp 10–11

Poor-Grade Patients with Aneurysmal Subarachnoid Hemorrhage: Early or Late Operation?

H. A. Trost[1], V. Seifert[2], C. Goetz[2], and H. Dietz[2]

Introduction

Early surgery in low-risk aneurysm patients (Hunt and Hess I–III) has led to a considerable improvement of the perioperative management morbidity and mortality and is now an almost generally accepted regimen of treatment. Except for those patients with a space-occupying intracerebral hematoma, patients in grades IV and V (according to Hunt and Hess) are often not considered to be surgical candidates. Thus, surgery is delayed, hoping that with improvement of the clinical condition the patient will be later amenable to aneurysm clipping. However, with this form of treatment many of these patients will finally die from recurrent hemorrhage or from the effect of delayed ischemic deficits. The following study was performed to examine the clinical management of a population of grade IV and V patients with the aim to clarify whether certain variables of treatment, including early surgery, could be defined that might help to improve the so far almost hopeless outlook for the stuporous or comatose patient after aneurysm rupture.

Material and Methods

Between January 1983 and December 1990, 755 patients who had suffered from subarachnoid hemorrhage (SAH) were admitted to the Neurosurgical Clinic, Hannover Medical School, Germany. After neurological examination and grading of the patients according to the Hunt and Hess scale [2], diagnosis of SAH was confirmed by computerized tomography. Of the SAH patients, 191 (25.3%) were poor-risk patients: 114 (15.1%) grade IV and 77 (10.2%) grade V. In case of acute hydrocephalus, an immediate ventriculostomy and continuous external CSF drainage was performed. Four-vessel angiography was undertaken in 137 of these 191 patients (71.7%), who were considered to be potential surgical candidates. The strategy of surgical or nonsurgical treatment in each patient was left to the decision of the surgeon responsible for the individual patient. Surgery was performed under neuroleptic anesthesia using standard microsurgical techniques including washout

[1] Neurochirurgische Klinik, Universität – GHS – Essen, Hufelandstr. 55, W-4300 Essen, FRG.
[2] Neurochirurgische Klinik, Medizinische Hochschule Hannover, Konstanty-Gutschow-Str. 8, W-3000 Hannover 61, FRG.

Advances in Neurosurgery, Vol. 20
K. Piscol, M. Klinger, M. Brock (Eds.)

of the basal cisterns from subarachnoid blood collections. Postoperatively induced hypertension and hypervolemia were installed. All surviving patients were reexamined 6–12 months postsurgery and graded according to the criteria of the Glasgow Outcome Scale [3].

Results

Of the 191 poor-risk patients, 131 (68.5%) suffered from aneurysmal SAH: 14 patients (7.3%) had bled from an arteriovenous malformation, 23 patients (12.0%) had SAH of unknown origin assumed by "negative angiography" or proved by autopsy, and in a further 23 patients (12.0%) the origin of SAH remained unclear because neither angiography nor autopsy was undertaken. Of our patients 58% were admitted within 24 h after SAH and 87% were admitted within the first 72 h after SAH. No differences could be found between the surgical and nonsurgical groups concerning age, sex, and admission pattern. The ruptured aneurysm was located at the anterior communicating artery complex in 54 patients (41.2%), in 39 patients (29.8%) at the middle cerebral artery, at the internal carotid artery in 22 patients (16.8%), and at the vertebrobasilar artery complex in 16 patients (12.2%). Fourteen patients had multiple aneurysms (11 times two aneurysms, 3 times three aneurysms). Seventy-seven patients (58.8%) were operated on: 52 patients (39.7%) were operated on early; 25 patients (19.1%) had delayed surgery. Thirteen patients (10.0%) died within a few hours after admission, not allowing enough time for diagnostic procedures and operation. Four patients (3.1%) had false negative angiography, 18 (13.7%) patients were not considered to be surgical candidates because of age, poor clinical condition, or otherwise poor prognosis, and 38 (27.5%) of the 52 early operated patients had been operated on schedule. The remaining 16 (12.2%) patients had emergency operations for space-occupying hemorrhage (12 patients) or rebleeding (4 patients). Forty-four (33.6%) patients were scheduled for delayed surgery; 19 (14.5%) of them died while waiting for the operation, 8 (6.1%) patients as a result of fatal rebleeding, 11 (8.4%) from sequelae of the initial hemorrhage, of vasospasm, or medical complications, and 25 patients (19.1%) managed to live long enough for delayed surgery (Table 1).

In grade V patients mortality was 54%. In the nonsurgical group only 1 of 16 patients survived severely disabled (4%). In the surgical group we had excellent outcome in one patient (7%), who recovered well after drainage of acute hydrocephalus and had delayed surgery. Another 7 patients (47%) survived severely disabled. The 69 grade IV patients did somewhat better. Mortality in the early surgery group was 48%, 50% in emergency operations, and 47% in operation on schedule, respectively. An excellent or good outcome was reached by 32% of the early surgery group. Decision for delayed surgery in 25 patients led to 40% mortality: 7 patients (28%) died while waiting for operation; 18 patients finally operated on late had 17% mortality and 44% excellent or good outcome (Table 2).

Table 1. Management of poor-risk aneurysmal subarachnoid hemorrhage

Nonsurgical treatment	54 patients	(41.2%)	
19	died before scheduled late operation	(14.5%)	
	8 died from lethal rebleeding		(6.1%)
	11 died from sequelae of initial hemorrhage, vasospasm, or medical complications		(8.4%)
18	decided against operation	(13.7%)	
13	died before angiography/surgery	(9.9%)	
4	aneurysms not detected by anigography	(3.0%)	
Surgical treatment	77 patients	(58.8%)	
52	early operations	(39.7%)	
	36 early operations on schedule		(27.5%)
	12 emergency operations (space-occupying hemorrhage)		(9.2%)
	4 emergency operations (rebleeding)		(3.0%)
25	late operations on schedule	(19.1%)	

Discussion

Despite the fact that poor-risk patients after aneurysmal SAH represent between 15% and 30% of all aneurysm patients reported in larger series, detailed analyses of the management morbidity and mortality are surprisingly scarce and recommendations for treatment are vague, based mostly on personal experience and intuition [1, 4, 5]. Our data demonstrate that patients subjected to aneurysm clipping had a far better outcome (mortality 42%) as compared with those who were treated nonoperatively (mortality 98%). The timing of poor-risk aneurysm surgery is still under discussion. In 1990 we recommended early diagnosis and operation in grade IV patients and a wait-and-see policy in grade V patients based on our results during 1983 to 1987 [7]. The more aggressive treatment in grade IV patients in 1988 to 1990 led to a rise in operative mortality (34% vs 39%) and fall in good surgical outcome (GOS 1+2) (49% vs 35%). This changed the relation between severely disabled (10% vs 18%) and good outcome (31% vs 24%); the overall mortality in these patients, however, remained stable (58%). In grade V patients we had another 3 severely disabled and 11 fatal outcomes; overall mortality remained at about 80%, the rest being severely disabled (15% vs 18%) and one lucky excellent outcome survivor. Treatment of grade V patients remains disappointing. Mortality in nonsurgical treatment is almost 100%; a decision for early surgery leads to 75% mortality as well as a decision for delayed surgery. A wait-and-see policy in these patients seems to be justified since the only excellent outcome was achieved after secondary improvement after ventriculostomy followed by delayed surgery. In

Table 2. Outcome of poor-grade aneurysmal subarachnoid hemorrhage

		Outcome (GOS)							
		1		2		3		5	
Surgical treatment									
IV	62	12	(19%)	10	(16%)	16	(26%)	24	(39%)
V	15	1	(7%)			6	(40%)	8	(53%)
IV+V	77	13	(17%)	10	(13%)	22	(29%)	32	(42%)
(Early operation on schedule)									
IV	32	6	(19%)	4	(13%)	7	(22%)	15	(47%)
V	4					1	(25%)	3	(75%)
IV+V	36	6	(17%)	4	(11%)	8	(22%)	18	(50%)
(Emergency operation)									
IV	12			4	(33%)	2	(17%)	6	(50%)
V	4					1	(25%)	3	(75%)
IV+V	16			4	(25%)	3	(19%)	9	(56%)
(Late operation on schedule)									
IV	18	6	(33%)	2	(11%)	7	(39%)	3	(17%)
V	7	1	(14%)			4	(57%)	2	(29%)
IV+V	25	7	(28%)	2	(8%)	11	(44%)	5	(20%)
Nonsurgical treatment									
IV	29							29	(100%)
V	25					1	(4%)	24	(96%)
IV+V	54					1	(2%)	53	(98%)
Overall outcome poor-risk group									
IV	91	12	(13%)	10	(11%)	16	(18%)	53	(58%)
V	40	1	(3%)			7	(18%)	32	(80%)
IV+V	131	13	(10%)	10	(8%)	23	(18%)	85	(65%)

grade IV patients we still advocate early diagnosis and operative treatment since aneurysm clipping facilitates treatment of delayed ischemic deficits by administration of hypervolemic hypertension, tissue plasminogen activator, or nimodipine [6] and prevents rebleeding.

References

1. Bailes JE, Spetzler RF, Hadley MN, Baldwin HZ (1990) Management morbidity and mortality of poor-grade aneurysm patients. J Neurosurg 72:559–566
2. Hunt WE, Hess RM (1968) Surgical risk as related to time of intervention in repair of intracranial aneurysm. J Neurosurg 28:14–19
3. Jennet B, Bond M (1975) Assessment of outcome after severe brain damage. Lancet I:480–484
4. Kassell NF, Torner JC, Haley EC et al. (1990) The International Cooperative Study on the Timing of Aneurysm Surgery. Part 1: Overall management results, Part 2: Surgical results. J Neurosurg 73:18–36, 37–47

5. Petruk KC, West M, Mohr G et al. (1988) Nimodipine in poor grade aneurysm patients. Results of a multicenter double-blind placebo-controlled trial. J Neurosurg
6. Seifert V, Eisert WG, Stolke D, Goetz C (1989) Efficacy of single intracisternal injection of recombinant tissue plasminogen activator to prevent delayed cerebral vasospasm after experimental subarachnoid hemorrhage. Neurosurg 25:590–598
7. Seifert V, Trost HA, Stolke D (1990) Management morbidity and mortality in grade IV and V patients with aneurysmal subarachnoid haemorrhage. Acta Neurochir (Wien) 103:5–10

Timing and Grading: Problems in Poor-Grade Subarachnoid Hemorrhage

R. Laumer, R. Naraghi, C. Nimsky, R. Fahlbusch, and U. Machera[1]

Introduction

The management of aneurysmal subarachnoid hemorrhage (SAH) is mainly based on timing and grading. Meanwhile these problems seem to be solved for Hunt and Hess grades I, II, and III. The early operation within 48 h after SAH is the most adequate therapy to prevent rebleeding before onset of vasospasm.

However, for grades IV and V there is no generally accepted guideline at all. As in most other neurosurgical departments, these poor-grade aneurysm patients were excluded from surgery, and especially comatose grade V patients were sent back to peripheral hospitals without receiving any active treatment.

In a recent study [1], good results were obtained by early operative intervention, including immediate ventriculostomy placement, early surgery, and aggressive postoperative hypervolemic, hypertensive, hemodilutional therapy. The indication for craniotomy and aneurysm clipping was seen in relationship to the intracranial pressure (ICP). If this parameter was controllable (< 30 cm H_2O without an intracranial clot or > 50 cm H_2O in the presence of a clot) the active treatment was started.

In view of this regime and the good results, the following questions were investigated and discussed in our own material:

1. Was there really no change in neurological status between the initial and the preoperative examination?
2. Is the ICP really the most appropriate parameter for early aneurysm surgery in grades IV and V?
3. Does the Hunt and Hess classification allow a comparison between different studies at all [3]?

Clinical Material and Methods

In the period between 1987 and 1990, 232 patients with SAH were treated in the neurosurgical department of the Unviersity of Erlangen. In all cases a ruptured aneurysm was responsible for the hemorrhage, documented by angiography, au-

[1] Neurochirurgische Klinik der Universität Erlangen-Nürnberg, Schwabachanlage 6, W–8520 Erlangen, FRG.

Advances in Neurosurgery, Vol. 20
K. Piscol, M. Klinger, M. Brock (Eds.)

topsy, or intraoperative findings. In this period, the management, clinical course, and outcome of 84 patients presenting with grades IV and V were investigated.

Based on previous experiences, a management protocol was established and applied to all poor-grade aneurysm patients. This regime consisted of immediate implantation of a ventriculostomy, ICP monitoring, CSF drainage, and close neurological examinations documented as the Hunt and Hess grade and the additional Glasgow Coma Scale (GCS). In contrast to Bailes and Spetzler [1], the indication for angiography and surgery was seen in relationship to the clinical reaction to ventriculostomy and CSF drainage. If there was a shade of improvement at least, angiography and clipping were performed. If there was no clinical improvement at all, the patients were excluded from further treatment.

Results

According to the modified regime, an increase in operations performed on grade IV and V patients from 12% in 1987 to 40% in 1990 could be documented (Fig. 1). Investigations revealed a notable clinical improvement due to CSF drainage. Generally, this improvement consisted of an increase in GCS, but in many cases there was even a change from one Hunt and Hess grade to another. This improvement proceeded in a very short time: within 12 h in more than 25% and within 24 h already in 50%.

After ventriculostomy and CSF drainage, the neurological status improved in 38 of 84 patients, initially graded IV and V. This was documented in 32 of 60 grade IV and 6 out of 24 grade V patients. From these 60 grade IV patients, 7 improved to grade II, 19 to grade III, 32 patients remained grade IV, and 2 deteriorated to grade V. From those remaining grade IV, 6 improved in GCS, however.

Of 24 patients initially presenting in grade V, 2 improved to grade IV and 4 to grade III.

All patients improving to grade II or III were operated on for the aneurysm, whereas of 34 grade IV patients only in 8 cases was the indication for surgery seen. Two of these eight patients were initially graded V; the other six cases remained

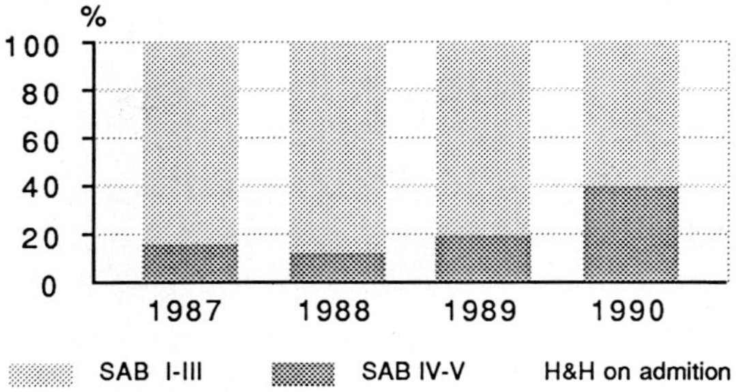

Fig. 1. Aneurysm clipping operations performed on grade IV and V SAH patients ($n = 232$) between 1987 and 1990 in the neurosurgical department of the University of Erlangen

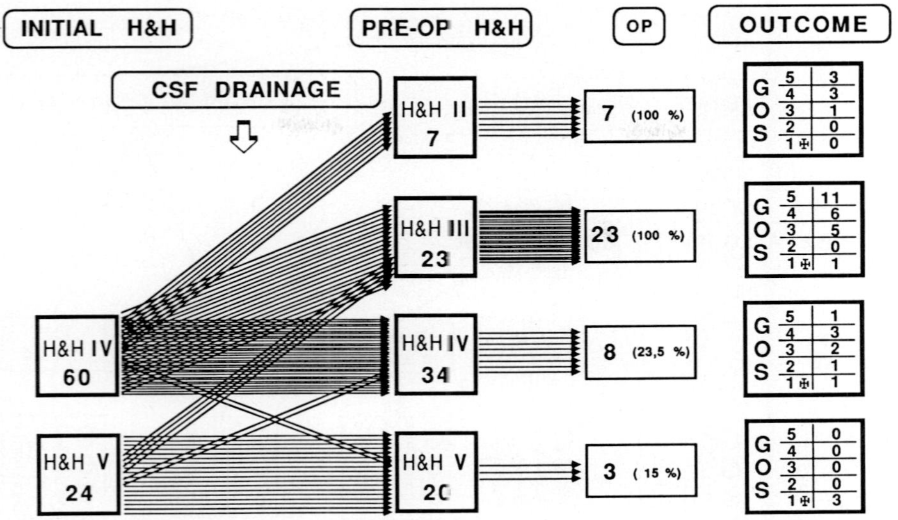

Fig. 2. *Left*, clinical improvement in 84 patients presenting with Hunt and Hess grades IV and V at admission due to CSF drainage (each *arrow* indicates one patient). *Right*, outcome in 41 patients undergoing aneurysm clipping according to preoperative Hunt and Hess grading (classification according to original Glasgow Outcome Scale, GOS)

GOS	H&H II	H&H III	H&H IV	H&H V
5	3	11	1	0
4	3	6	3	0
3	1	5	2	0
2	0	0	1	0
1 ✠	0	1	1	3

grade IV, but they showed an improvement in GCS. Of 20 cases remaining grade V, only 3 were operated on due to a large hematoma (Fig. 2).

Of these 30 patients, preoperatively graded II or III, 23 achieved good results: scores of 5 and 4, respectively, according to the Glasgow Outcome Scale (GOS) [4].

Four of eight operated grade IV patients also had good results, whereas all grade V patients died. In view of initial ICP, two groups of patients resulted after ventriculostomy:

1. In 41 patients ICP was elevated
2. In 43 patients ICP was normal

Due to CSF drainage, ICP could be reduced in 12 of 41 patients. Of these 12 patients 10 were operated with good results in 6 cases. Two patients with GCS 3 were excluded from further active treatment because of a lack of clinical improvement despite reduced ICP. Vice versa, seven patients were operated on due to a clinical improvement despite elevated ICP (Fig. 3).

Of 43 patients with normal ICP, 24 were operated with good results in 19 cases; 19 patients had no clinical improvement at all and thus no operation.

All patients who were excluded from further active treatment because of a lack of clinical improvement died. These 43 cases never had a score better than 5 points on the GCS. Almost 50% had the lowest possible score of 3 points at admission

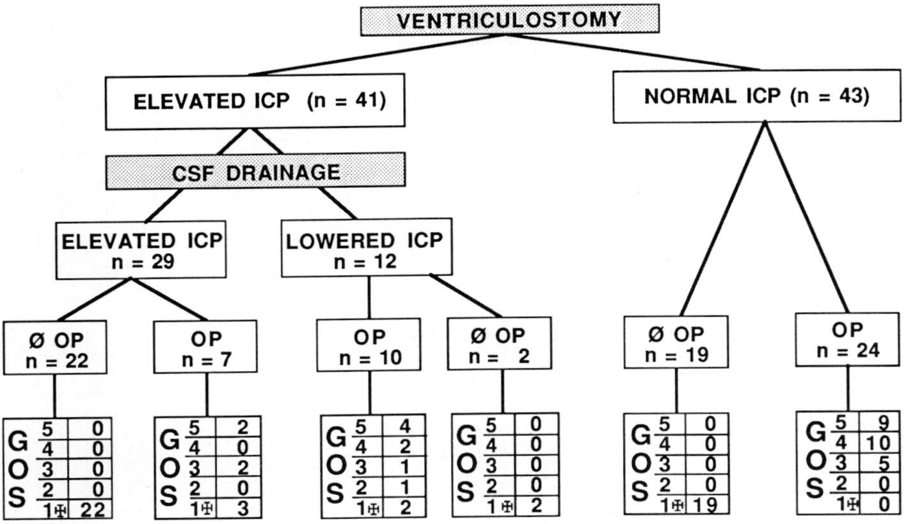

Fig. 3. Management and outcome in grade IV and V patients according to the behavior of ICP after ventriculostomy and CSF drainage. If there was no clinical improvement, the patients were excluded from further operative treatment (ø *OP*)

Table 1. Problems of Hunt and Hess classification due to a variety of possible Glasgow coma scores, especially in grade IV

Grade	Glasgow Coma Scale
III	15–10
IV	15– 5
V	4– 3

and remained in this extremely unfavorable condition without any improvement (Fig. 4).

In view of the Hunt and Hess classification, there is a lack of accuracy which could enable a comparison between different studies. In the Hunt and Hess grade IV, completely awake patients with hemiparesis and unconscious patients with decerebrate rigidity and vegetative disturbances are mixed, according to scores 15 and 5, respectively, on the GCS (Table 1).

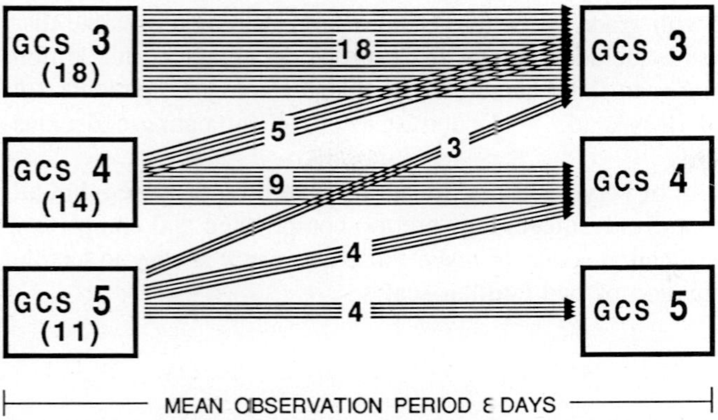

Fig. 4. Level of consciousness according to Glasgow Coma Scale (GCS) of 43 patients who were excluded from further operative treatment due to a lack of clinical improvement after ventriculostomy and CSF drainage

Discussion

In view of the good results of this series, in all unconscious grade IV and V patients a ventriculostomy placement should be performed immediately after admission. The ICP may be a parameter for further treatment, but as a single guideline it is not sufficient. The prognostic value of clinical reaction to CSF drainage should also be drawn into consideration. Under this regime in two cases a very good outcome could be achieved despite constantly elevated ICP. On the other side, in many cases unnecessary operations could be avoided because it makes no sense to perform aneurysm clipping in patients with GCS 3 with no clinical improvement after CSF drainage for several days.

Furthermore, it is hard to believe that in those cases an aggressive treatment would be able to avoid an unfavorable outcome, whereas it is possible in cases with a clinical improvement as a reaction to CSF drainage.

However, in many cases there was an improvement not only in GCS but also in Hunt and Hess grades. This means that many patients, initially graded IV and V, were immediately preoperatively grade III or still better. Generally, this happened within a few hours.

Furthermore, the Hunt and Hess classification enables a comparison between different studies only exceptionally. Apart from observer variabilities, reported by Teasedale et al. [5], especially in Hunt and Hess grade IV, so many possibilities from awake to comatose patients are mixed that no general statement is possible.

The WFNS SAH scale, proposed by the World Federation of Neurological Surgeons in 1988 [2], is better than the Hunt and Hess classification without doubt, but it is accepted only exceptionally by a few neurosurgeons. The reason may be that now nearly all neurosurgeons are familiar with the Hunt and Hess classification and it will take a lot of time to become familiar with a completely new classification.

Therefore, beginning with grade III, where besides mild deficits a possible disturbance of consciousness is included, the GCS should be documented, in addition to the Hunt and Hess grade. In this manner, IV/5 indicates comatose patients not far away from Hunt and Hess grade V in contrast to IV/14, indicating conscious patients with a hemiparesis.

In the last 10 years, a lot of very good classifications have been proposed, but all of them have an important disadvantage: they are too complicated and completely new. This proposed classification seems to make sense because it is easy to handle due to the simple combination of two familiar scales.

References

1. Bailes JE, Spetzler RF, Hadley MN, Baldwin HZ (1990) Management morbidity and mortality of poor-grade aneurysm patients. J Neurosurg 72:559–566
2. Drake CG (1988) Report of World Federation of Neurological Surgeons Committee on a Universal Subarachnoid Hemorrhage Grading Scale. J Neurosurg 68:985–986
3. Hunt WE, Hess RM (1968) Surgical risk as related to time of intervention in the repair of intracranial aneurysms. J Neurosurg 28:14–20
4. Jennett B, Bond M (1975) Assessment of outcome after severe brain damage. A practical scale. Lancet I:480–484
5. Lindsay KW, Teasdale G, Knill-Jones R et al. (1982) Observer variability in grading patients with SAH. J Neurosurg 56:628–633

Early Operation in the Elderly?

A. Laun, C. Eulgem, and O. Hoffmann[1]

Introduction

Since the report presented by Ljunggren et al. (1981) and later studies confirming these findings [17], it has become standard practice in neurosurgery to perform early operation – within 72 h – for aneurysmatic subarachnoid hemorrhage on patients in Hunt and Hess grade I and II, and to a limited extent also on those in grade III. Some less recent studies are also available concerning aneurysm operation in the elderly [4, 6–9, 18], as well as individual observations about the influence of internal disorders, for example, hypertension [5, 10]. In view of some unfavorable developments in individual elderly patients after early operation, we decided to perform this retrospective study on the basis of the patient group in the Neurosurgical Department of the University of Giessen.

Material and Methods

Since 1978 all data on patients with subarachnoid hemorrhage, with or without aneurysm as well as all patients with paralytic aneurysms, plus data on their complete neuroradiological findings and outcome have been registered. Between 1 January 1978 and 30 June 1990 there was a total of 795 patients.

When classifying them according to age (borderline 65 years) and sex (Table 1), it becomes obvious that there is an overproportional percentage of females in the 65 and over age group. At the end of 1986/beginning of 1987 the early operation was introduced, i.e., the timing and the strategy of the operation were completely changed, giving rise to a rapid increase in the number of elderly patients from 5%–10% up to 1986 to 20%–25% after 1987 (Fig. 1). The admission findings, classified in Hunt and Hess grades, have shown a significant improvement since 1987 ($P < 0.0001$). If a further differentiation is made on the basis of age, taking 65 as the borderline, then it becomes apparent that the improvement in the admission findings relates primarily to those patients under 65 years.

The treatment outcome for all aneurysmatic subarachnoid hemorrhage patients did not differ very much after changing the operation timing. Using another classification – this time showing the different age groups – reveals a gradual improve-

[1] Neurochirurgische Klinik, Justus-Liebig-Universität Gießen, Klinikstr. 29, W–6300 Gießen, FRG.

Advances in Neurosurgery, Vol. 20
K. Piscol, M. Klinger, M. Brock (Eds.)

Table 1. Distribution of age and sex

	$\leq$ 65 years	> 65 years
Male	330 (47.2%)	22 (22.9%)
Female	396 (52.8%)	74 (77.1%)

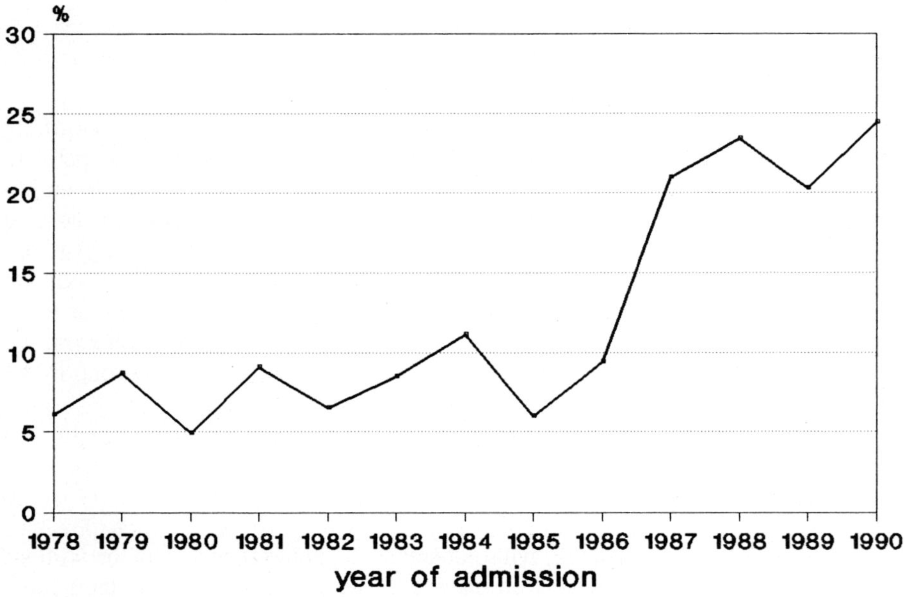

Fig. 1. Proportion of elderly patients in the years of admission since 1978

ment in the result of young patients, but a much worse one for elderly patients ($P = 0.0004$). The special outcome for all aneurysm patients over 65 years who had been classified in Hunt and Hess I and II on admission is much less favorable after early operation than after late operation. These figures are not significant ($P = 0.088$) on account of the small number of cases.

Results

The following points could account for a worse result in the higher age group:

1. In the higher age group the proportion of aneurysms on the internal carotid artery at the junction of the posterior communicating artery was 22.9% compared with 9.2% among those under 65.
2. In the higher age group multiple aneurysms constituted 16.7%, in the younger ones 11.7%.

3. An intraventricular hemorrhage could be observed in 42.2% of those over 65, in only 23.2% of the younger patients.

An identical or better outcome in those over 65 might be achieved by the following means:

1. Spasms shown in transcranial Doppler sonography are much less frequent in the higher age group.
2. An intraoperative rupture occurred in 26.5% of the younger patients and in 11.1% of the older ones.
3. The development of a hydrocephalus aresorptivus was observed with equal frequency in both age groups.
4. The frequency of seizures is the same in both age groups, though focal seizures predominated in the younger patients and generalized seizures predominated in the older ones.

Thus, the reason for the less successful outcome must be sought in other factors, e.g., internal ones.

Diabetes Mellitus

In the whole population of the Federal Republic of Germany there is a 3% expected incidence of diabetes mellitus. The proportion of diabetic patients among those with subarachnoid hemorrhage is, however, 4.3%. In the group under 65 years the incidence is 2.9%, within the range that would be expected for the whole population. In those over 65, the figure is 14.6% which is more than four times as high. No connection between admission findings and treatment outcome could be established.

Manifest Hypertension

The patients who were administered antihypertensive medication before the onset of the subarachnoid hemorrhage were classed as manifest hypertensive patients.

The influence of manifest hypertension on admission findings and operation outcome was studied, comparing those patients suffering manifest hypertension with all those not affected by it (Fig. 2). Furthermore, three groups were formed on the basis of the admission findings for Hunt and Hess grades I and II, grade III, and grades IV and V. These three groups were juxtaposed to the operation outcome graded as per the Glasgow Outcome Scale. The Hunt and Hess I and II groups for the manifest hypertensive patients revealed a significantly worse outcome ($P = 0.0014$) than the group without this disorder. The tendencies in groups 2 and 3 were identical, but not significant ($P = 0.1032$; $P = 0.601$).

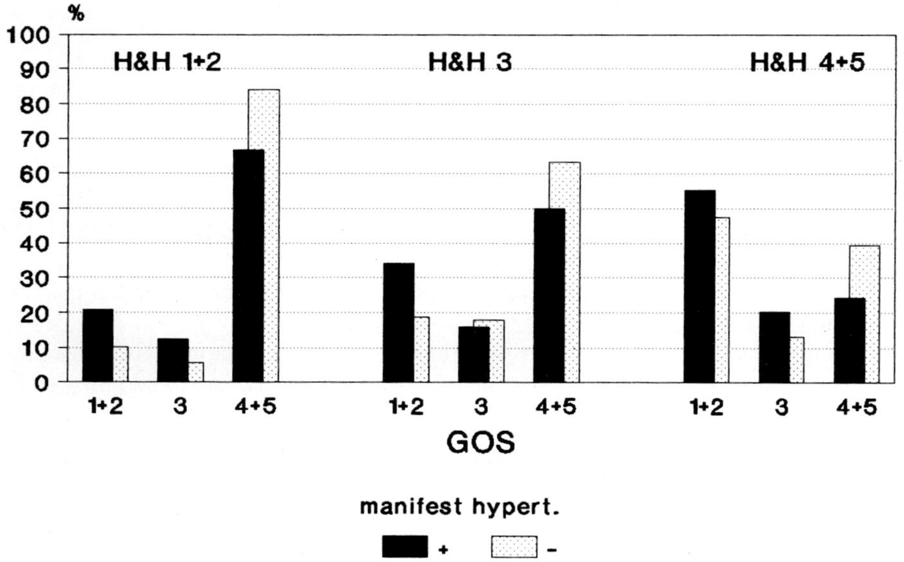

Fig. 2. Influence of manifest hypertension on outcome

Coronary Heart Disease

The groups were classified in an identical way to the manifest hypertension groups (Fig. 3). A very significant negative influence on the outcome was established in group 1, classified as Hunt and Hess grades I and II on admission, when a coronary heart disorder was present ($P = 0.0001$). Groups 2 and 3 tended in a similar direction, but were not significant ($P = 0.0652$; $P = 0.0227$).

Discussion

After evaluating the patients grouped into categories spanning 5 years each, the age limit of 65 was arrived at, which corresponds to the literature [19]. The view that elderly patients would not benefit from neurosurgical treatment [17] or should not undergo operation at all [7] due to a possibly less successful outcome is, in our opinion, not ethically tenable in regard to the natural course [19]; on the other hand, some favorable observations have been reported [6, 8, 18, 20, 21], and it is known that the less successful outcome possibly only applies to posterior circulation aneurysm [2, 3]. The reasons for a poorer outcome cannot only be "neurosurgical" ones; they must reside in the combination of subarachnoid hemorrhage and internal disorders in the elderly [10]. An additional factor is the decreasing CBF as the patient ages and the impaired autoregulation [15, 24]. An internally impaired brain may possibly tolerate the reduced perfusion pressure from brain retraction less

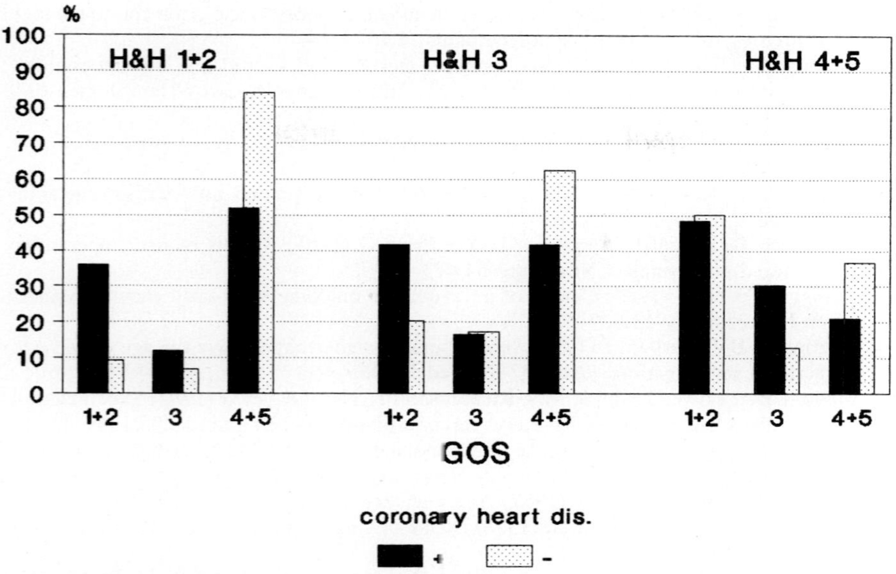

Fig. 3. Influence of coronary heart disease on outcome

well. The influence exercised by calcium channel blockers [1] and the question of whether they have actually even improved these present results must be examined in a more detailed study on a larger number of patients. The precise reasons and correlations of the less favorable outcome in those over 65 after early operation are still unknown. Including all anamnestic data and internal disorders we would like to endorse what Ljunggren [13] stated: "... that it is principally the patient's condition during the acute stage that determines the outcome."

References

1. Allen GS, Ahn HS et al. (1983) Cerebral arterial spasm – A controlled trial of nimedipine in patients with subarachnoid hemorrhage. N Engl J Med 308:619–624
2. Amacher AL (1980) Aneurysm surgery in the elderly. Neurosurgery 6:612, letter
3. Amacher AL, Ferguson GG, Drake CG et al. (1977) How old people tolerate intracranial surgery for aneurysm. Neurosurgery 1:242–244
4. Drake CG (1980) Viewpoint: Senior citizen with ruptured aneurysm. Neurosurgery 6:605–606
5. Erkesen V, Rosenorn J, Schmidt K, Ronde F (1987) Preexisting arterial hypertension in subarachnoid haemorrhage: an unfavourable prognostic factor. Brit J Neurosurg 1:455–461
6. Fein JM (1982) Aneurysms in geriatric patients. In: Hopkins LN, Long DM (eds) Clinical management of intracranial aneurysms. Raven Press, New York, pp 183–191
7. Giammusso V, Vassallo A (1975) Medical treatment of subarachnoid hemorrhage due to cerebral aneurysm in old patients. J Neurosurg Sci 19:70–71

8. Hogusson R (1973) Intracranial arterial aneurysms: Considerations on the upper age limit for surgical treatment. Acta Neurochir 28:157–164
9. Hornig CR, Tonn JC, Agnoli AL, Laun A, Dorndorf W (1988) Die Subarachnoidalblutung im höheren Lebensalter. Poster. 61. Jahrestagung Dt Ges f Neurologie, 20.–24.9.88, Frankfurt
10. Keller AZ (1970) Hypertension age and residence in the survival with SAH. Am J Epid 91:139–147
11. Langfitt TW, Kassell NF, Weinstein JD (1965) Cerebral blood flow with intracranial hypertension. Neurology 15:761–773
12. Ljunggren B, Brandt L, Kagström E, Sundborg G (1981) Results of early operations for ruptured aneurysms. J Neurosurg 54:473–479
13. Ljunggren B et al. (1983) Causes of unfavourable outcome after early aneurysm operation. Neurosurgery 13:629–633
14. Martindale BV, Garfield J (1978) Subarachnoid haemorrhage above the age of 59: Are intracranial investigations justified? Br Med J 1:465–466
15. Meyer CHA, Lowe D, Meyer MN, Richardson PL, Neil-Dwyer G (1982) Subarachnoid haemorrhage: older patients have low cerebral blood flow. Br Med J 285:1149–1153
16. Muizelaar JP et al. (1988) Outcome of aneurysmal subarachnoid hemorrhage in patients 66 years of age and older. Clin Neurol Neurosurg 90:203–207
17. Sano K, Asano T, Tamura A (1987) Acute aneurysm surgery. Springer, Wien
18. Sengupta RP, Lassman JP et al. (1978) Scope of surgery for intracranial aneurysms in the elderly. Br Med J 2:246–247
19. Sengupta RP, McAllister VL (1986) Subarachnoid haemorrhage. Springer, Berlin Heidelberg New York Tokyo
20. Shephard RH (1978) Subarachnoid haemorrhage in patients over 59. Br Med J 1:921, letter
21. Shephard RH (1983) Ruptured cerebral aneurysms: early and late prognosis with surgical treatment. J Neurosurg 59:6–15
22. Steward J, Shephard RH, Millac P (1975) Neurosurgery in the old patient. Postgrad Med J 51:453–456
23. Tonn JC, Hornig CR, Laun A, Büttner C, Hoffmann O (1989) Subarachnoidalblutung im höheren Lebensalter unter besonderer Berücksichtigung des Einsatzes von Calciumantagonisten. Poster. 40. Jahrestagung Dt Ges Neurochirurgie, 7.–10.5.1989, Würzburg
24. Yasni N, Ito Z, Ohta H, Suzuki A (1982) Surgical problems and pathophysiology in severe cases with ruptured aneurysm in the acute stage. Acta Neurochir 63:163–174

Management Results of a Series of Predominantly Delayed Operations on Ruptured Aneurysms

W. Krupp, W. Heienbrok, and R. Müke[1]

Introduction

Using a comprehensive statistical analysis, Kassell and Drake [9] were able to illustrate the fatal consequences of aneurysmal rupture. Many authors have advocated an early operation to reduce both the rebleeding and vasospasm rates [2, 4, 11–13, 21]. Nevertheless, the results of early operations have been varied and, in their interpretation, are not uncontroversial. Discussion centered mainly on the range of criteria for an early operation in terms of aneurysm site and grade at the time of admission [1, 5, 7, 9, 10, 15, 20]. A comparison of the various treatment strategies reveals methodological problems due to differences in selection when the patients are allocated to the clinics and due to the choice of outcome parameters [13, 16]. Generally recognized as comparison values are the definitions of management mortality and management morbidity, which were coined by Lougheed [14]. In this paper, we present the management results of a series of predominantly delayed operations on ruptured aneurysms.

Patients and Methods

The criteria for an early operation were kept restricted. Only those patients with an admission grade of I or II on the Hunt and Hess scale or those with very severe intracerebral hematoma underwent an early operation. Exceptions to this rule were patients with vertebrobasilar or giant aneurysms, those with signs of an incipient vasospasm, those over the age of 65, or with serious accompanying diseases. The patients were administered nimodipine intravenously from the day of admission.

The grade at the time of admission was classified according to Hunt and Hess, while the results were categorized according to the Glasgow Outcome Scale (GOS) 4 weeks after operation. On an average of 3 years (38 ± 16 months) after the operation, 90% ($n = 88$) of the patients belonging to GOS categories 1 and 2 were interviewed as to their subjective assessment vis-à-vis their ability to take stress both in their everyday life and at work.

[1] Neurochirurgische Klinik, Alfried-Krupp-Krankenhaus, Alfried-Krupp-Str. 21, W-4300 Essen, FRG.

Advances in Neurosurgery, Vol. 20
K. Piscol, M. Klinger, M. Brock (Eds.)

Table 1. Grade on admission (Hunt and Hess) and location of aneurysm ($n = 131$)

	I	II	III	IV	V	Total cases (%)
Anterior cerebral artery	9	14	21	7	4	42
Internal carotid artery	10	13	7	2	1	25
Middle cerebral artery	8	9	8	2	8	27
Vertebrobasilar system	0	4	1	2	1	6
Total cases (%)	21	31	28	10	11	100

Results

During the period covering 1985 to 1990, a total of 131 patients with subarachnoid hemorrhage (SAH) due to aneurysmal rupture were diagnosed. Eleven patients with SAH could not – owing to their extremely poor condition – be prescribed an angiography and are not included in this series.

Grades on admission and aneurysm sites are laid out in Table 1. Seventy-four percent (97) of the patients were admitted within the first 72 h after SAH, whereas 26% (34) were admitted at a later point in time, i.e., only after 7 days at the earliest were they operated on.

Eight percent (11) of the patients diagnosed with an aneurysm died before the chance of operation: 3.1% (4) died of initial hemorrhage consequences; 3.8% (5) of rebleeding; and 1.5% (2) of the effects of a vasospasm.

Operative Mortality

Ninety-two percent (120) of the patients were operated on; 15% (20) of the patients received an early operation. Operation mortality amounted to 5% altogether and to 2.5% for admission grades I–III ($n = 99$). Following early operation, 15% of the patients died and 6% for admission grades I–III ($n = 16$).

Management Mortality

Table 2 shows management mortality. The overall mortality rate was 13.0%. Of grade I–III patients 7.7% (8) died, 4.8% (5) preoperatively and 2.9% (3) postoperatively. There was rebleeding with 2.9% (3) of these "good-risk" patients and vasospasm with 1.9% (2). Vasospasm combined with cerebral edema led to death in the case of 1.9% (2) patients. One patient (1.0%) succumbed to embolism relapse with mitral insufficiency.

No patient classified as grade I on admission died, whereas 2.9% (3) grade II and 4.8% (5) grade III died. Of grade IV/V patients 33% died.

Table 2. Management mortality in patients with aneurysmal subarachnoid hemorrhage (SAH)

	Total cases (*n* = 131)	Admission within 72 h after SAH (*n* = 97)
Management mortality	13.0%	14.4%
Management mortality/admission grade I–III	7.7%	7.1%

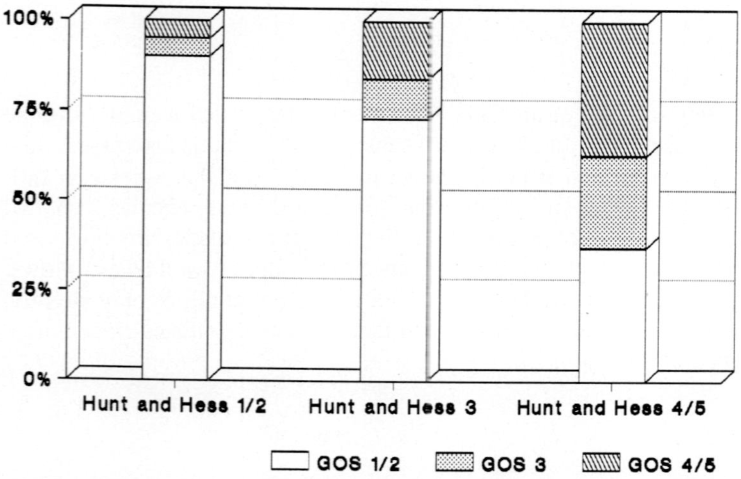

Fig. 1. Grade on admission (Hunt and Hess) and management results (Glasgow Outcome Scale) of patients who were admitted within 72 h after subarachnoid hemorrhage (*n* = 97)

Management Outcome

Figure 1 illustrates the relationship between admission grades and management outcome for the patients admitted within 72 h. In the overall sample (*n* = 131) 75% of the patients and 85% of the patients with admission grades I–III (*n* = 104) were designated as GOS categories 1 or 2.

Twenty-seven patients were admitted at grades IV or V. Owing to very severe intracerebral hematoma, three of these were sent for early surgery. Of the remaining 24 patients, 17 – due to the decision to wait – were operated on at grades I–III and 53% of these obtained satisfactory results (GOS 1/2): 88% of the 17 patients were designated to the GOS categories 1–3; the corresponding management value including all grade IV or V patients lay at 63%.

Table 3. Subjective assessment of ability to withstand stress during the daily routine. Survey of GOS 1/2 patients on an average of 3 years (38 ± 16 months) after operation

	n	%
No, or slight, inhibition	73	83
Considerable inhibition	15	17
Great inhibition	0	

Follow-up Results

Prior to their operations, 59% of the GOS 1/2 patients interviewed were in full-time work, 24% were housewives, and 17% were pensioners. The subjective assessment as to their ability to withstand stress is shown in Table 3. Of the patients in full-time employment, 60% were still in the same job after 3 years whereas 21% had changed. Nineteen percent were pensioners. If the interview statistics are transposed to the overall number of patients, then the management values would be as follows: 62% of the patients claimed that their daily routine was not at all, or only slightly, inhibited; 58% of the respondents claimed that there was no significant impediment to the performance of their job.

Discussion

The proportion of rebleeding and fatal vasospasm in our series was less than that sometimes described for delayed operations [17, 23]. Similarly, the chances of stabilization and delayed operation results for admission grade IV/V patients are remarkable and demonstrate the need for a discussion about the treatment strategies concerning "poor-grade" patients.

Criteria for recommending an early operation have broadened owing to the deployment of calcium antagonists and owing to enhanced possibilities of procedure control such as rCBF measurements and transcranial Doppler sonography [3, 8, 18, 22].

However, the results discussed here confirm that strict criteria for an early operation continue to be justified; in other words, poor management results are not necessarily the outcome of predominantly delayed operations on patients.

References

1. Adams HP (1986) Early management of the patient with recent aneurysmal subarachnoid hemorrhage. Stroke 17:1068–1070
2. Auer LM (1983) Acute surgery of cerebral aneurysms and prevention of symptomatic vasospasm. Acta Neurochir (Wien) 69:273–281

3. Auer LM, Brandt L, Ebeling U, Gilsbach J, Groeger U, Harders A, Ljunggren B, Oppel F, Reulen HJ, Saeveland H (1986) Nimodipine and early aneurysm operation in good condition SAH patients. Acta Neurochir 82:7–13
4. Ausman JI, Diaz FG, Malik GM, Fielding AS, Son CS (1985) Current management of cerebral aneurysms: Is it based on facts or myths? Surg Neurol 24:625–635
5. Chyatte D, Fode NC, Sundt TM (1988) Early versus late intracranial aneurysm surgery in subarachnoid hemorrhage. J Neurosurg 69:326–331
6. Disney L, Weir B, Petruk K (1987) Effect on management mortality of deliberate policy of early operation on supratentorial aneurysms. Neurosurgery 20:695–701
7. Flamm ES (1986) The timing of aneurysm surgery 1985. Clin Neurosurg 33:147–158
8. Gilsbach JM, Harders AG (1989) Morbidity and mortality after early aneurysm surgery – a prospective study with nimodipine prevention. Acta Neurochir 96:1–7
9. Kassell NF, Drake CG (1982) Timing of aneurysm surgery. Neurosurgery 10:514–519
10. Kassell NF, Kongable GL, Torner JC, Adams HP, Mazuz H (1985) Delay in referral of patients with ruptured aneurysms to neurosurgical attention. Stroke 16:587–590
11. Ljunggren B, Brandt L, Kagström E, Sundbärg G (1981) Results of early operations for ruptured aneurysms. J Neurosurg 54:473–479
12. Ljunggren B, Brandt L, Säveland H, Nilson PE, Cronqvist S, Andersson KE, Vinge E (1984) Outcome in 60 consecutive patients treated with early aneurysm operation and intravenous nimodipine. J Neurosurg 61:864–873
13. Ljunggren B, Säveland H, Brandt L, Zygmunt S (1985) Early operation and overall outcome in aneurysmal subarachnoid hemorrhage. J Neurosurg 62:547–551
14. Lougheed WM (1969) Selection, timing, and technique of aneurysm surgery of the anterior circle of Willis. Clin Neurosurg 16:95–113
15. Marsh H, Maurice-Williams RS, Lindsay KW (1987) Differences in the management of ruptured intracranial aneurysms: a survey of practice amongst British neurosurgeons. J Neurol Neurosurg Psychiatry 50:965–970
16. Maurice-Williams RS, Marsh H (1985) Ruptured intracranial aneurysms: the overall effect of treatment and the influence of patient selection and data presentation on the reported outcome. J Neurol Neurosurg Psychiatry 48:1208–1212
17. Milhorat TH, Krautheim M (1985) Results of early and delayed operation for ruptured intracranial aneurysms in two series of 100 consecutive patients. Surg Neurol 26:123–128
18. Öhman J, Heiskanen O (1988) Effect of nimodipine on the outcome of patients after aneurysmal subarachnoidal hemorrhage and surgery. J Neurosurg 69:683–686
19. Ropper AH, Zervas NT (1984) Outcome 1 year after SAH from cerebral aneurysm. Management morbidity, mortality, and functional status in 112 consecutive good-risk patients. J Neurosurg 60:909–915
20. Säveland H, Ljunggren B, Brandt L, Messeter K (1986) Delayed ischemic deterioration in patients with early aneurysm operation and intravenous nimodipine. Neurosurgery 18:146–150
21. Sakaki S, Ohta S, Kuwabara H, Shiraishi M (1987) The role of ventricular and cisternal drainage in the early operation for ruptured intracranial aneurysms. Acta Neurochir 88:87–94
22. Seiler RW, Reulen HJ, Huber P, Grolimund P, Ebeling U, Steiger HJ (1988) Outcome of aneurysmal subarachnoid hemorrhage in a hospital population: a prospective study including early operation, intravenous nimodipine, and transcranial Doppler ultrasound. Neurosurgery 23:598–604
23. Taneda M (1982) The significance of early operation in the management of ruptured intracranial aneurysms – an analysis of 251 cases hospitalized within 24 hours after subarachnoid haemorrhage. Acta Neurochir (Wien) 63:201–208

Analysis of Relevant Intervals Between Subarachnoid Hemorrhage and Surgery on Patients with Aneurysm and Its Influence on the Decision for Early or Delayed Surgery

W. Pinz, J. Meissner, G. Bertram, J. Janus, P. Assimakopoulos, M. Pusfurosh-Tehrani, and K. Piscol[1]

The decision for early versus late surgery often is affected by factors not related to the neurological field. These factors especially occur in the period prior to admission of the patient to the neurosurgical unit and immediately thereafter.

In regard to the recommendation for early surgery after the World Congress in Munich and the following Symposium in Graz in 1981, a computer-assisted analysis was carried out in our clinic to evaluate the timing of surgery in dependence on relevant intervals between subarachnoid hemorrhage and the earliest point of time patients could be subjected to surgical intervention. The consideration of these intervals also includes the analysis of the time of admission to any clinic and the time of transfer to the neurosurgical unit thereafter.

Our investigation comprises a total of 402 fully evaluated patients with aneurysms operated on between 1972 and 1990. These patients were operated on in two different periods, which we called eras: in era 1 (1972–1981; before the World Congress in Munich) delayed surgery was favored. Unconscious or severely impaired patients were admitted only after they had survived the unstable interval. In era 2 (1982–1990; the period after the World Congress in Munich) decision for early surgery was propagated.

The number of admissions and surgical treatments have more than doubled in era 2 and, therefore, for ease of comparison we present our data as percentages. The group of patients with early surgical intervention increased from 3.7% in the first era to 31.5% in the second era. Nevertheless we still had 48.7% delayed surgical treatments in era 2 and 19.8% of patients who were subjected to surgical intervention in the interval between the 3rd and the 14th day after subarachnoid hemorrhage.

Analyzing the reasons for the delayed surgery in era 2, we see that one of the major factors is the time of arrival of the patients in the neurosurgical department. Between 95% (era 1) and 85% (era 2) of patients were transferred from other hospitals, mainly from neurological or medical units.

Comparing era 1 (1972–1981) and era 2 (1982–1990), there is a slight change toward direct admission, from 5.2% to 15%, in the recent past. Nevertheless, it was disappointing to realize that within this group the number of early admissions has decreased from 85% to 72%. On the other hand, even though the overall number of

[1] Neurochirurgische Klinik, Zentralkrankenhaus St.-Jürgen-Str., W–2800 Bremen 1, FRG.

Advances in Neurosurgery, Vol. 20
K. Piscol, M. Klinger, M. Brock (Eds.)

Table 1. Time of admission to the neurosurgical department in relation to SAH, divided into different periods (early = 0–3 days; interval = 4–10 days; late = 11 days)

	Early	Interval	Late
Era 1 (1972–1981)	17.0%	24.5%	58.5%
Era 2a (1982–1985)	37.3%	22.5%	40.2%
Era 2b (1986–1990)	67.9%	18.2%	13.9%

transfers from other hospitals has decreased slightly, the number of early transfers from these medical centers has quadrupled from 13.3% to 53.2%, which is even more significant as these are by far the larger total figures. Therefore, the decisive change has occurred in the nonsurgical specialities. The positive view of them toward early surgery and our modified admission policy account for this alteration.

In accordance with the previous findings, the average time of stay in the other hospitals has decreased from 15 days in era 1 to 12 days in 1982–1985, and finally to 3 days in 1986–1990. Within era 2 there was a distinctive development that permits a further division of era 2 into era 2a and era 2b.

Table 1 shows the increase in the early admissions from 17% in era 1 to 37.3% in era 2a and 67.9% in era 2b. This increase can be traced to a reduction of the length of stay in other hospitals prior to the patient's transfer to our facility.

Looking at era 2 representing the last decennium, there were only 56.2% of patients available for early surgery (Fig. 1). Within this group there were 10.5% grade IV and V patients, reducing the percentage of suitable candidates for surgery. In fact, an early surgery was performed in only 31.5% of patients. Figure 2 shows the situation of early admitted patients with the above-explained division of era 2 to demonstrate the present state of patient care.

Even though there was a marked increase of patients for whom early surgical treatment was feasible, from 21.8% in era 1 to 62.5% in era 2, the portion of early admitted patients who were not operated on initially remained remarkably high: 37.5%.

Our analysis revealed the following reasons that led to their exclusions from early surgical intervention:

1. Initial angiography revealed no evidence of aneurysm in 14%
2. The time spent on diagnostic evaluation exceeded the time frame allowed for early intervention in 7.5%
3. Serious accompanying illnesses, worsening of patients' condition, and initial refusal to be operated on in 16%

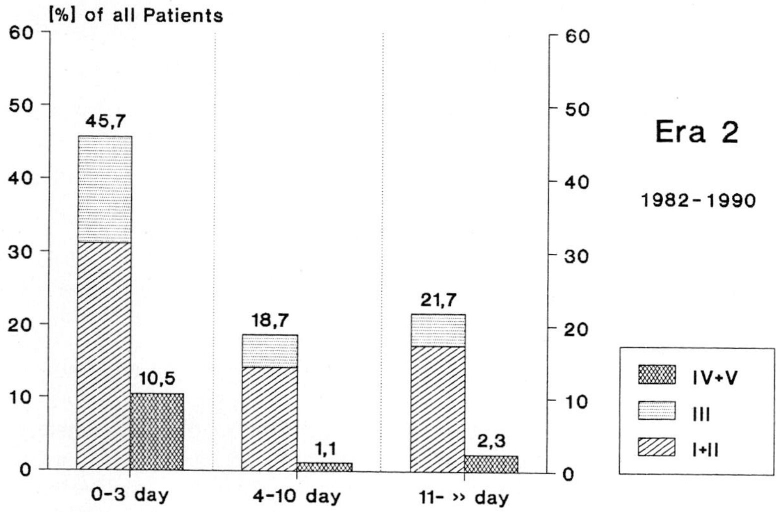

Fig. 1. Interval between SAH and admission to the neurosurgical department in relation to the patients' neurological grades according to Botterell in era 2

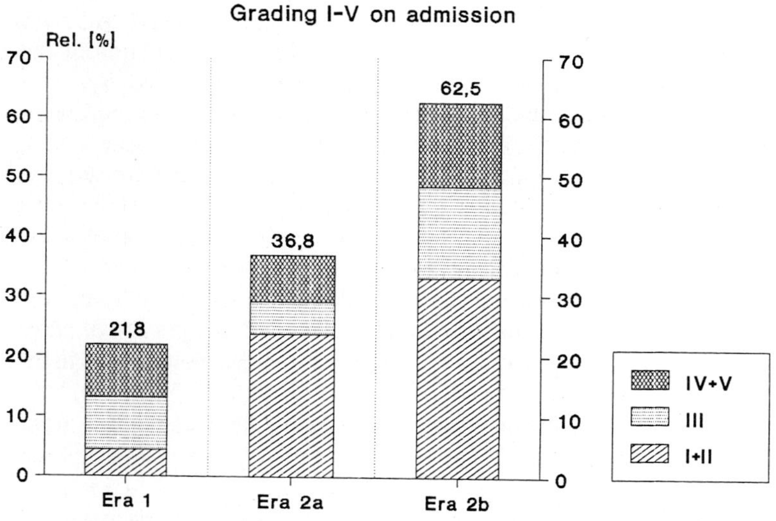

Fig. 2. A comparison between the different eras in regard to the percentage fraction of all early admitted patients who were subjected to early surgical intervention; the fractions are divided into the patients' neurological stages according to Boterell

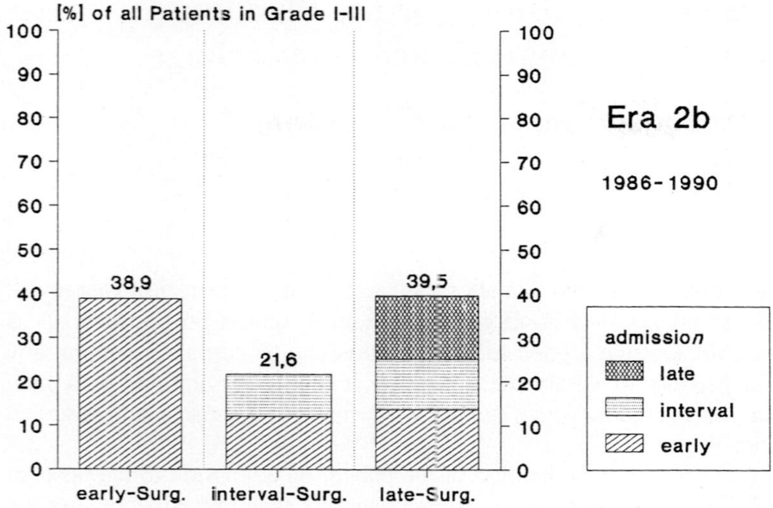

Fig. 3. Point of time when patients were subjected to surgical intervention in relation to their time of admission to the neurosurgical department

All of the early operated patients in poor condition (12.5%) had acute cerebral hematomas. The outcome in grade IV patients was astonishingly good (84.2% in GOS 1–3), worse in grade V patients (only 25% in GOS 1–3).

Lastly, the current state of surgical candidates in grades I–III is shown in Fig. 3: about 40% of these patients can be treated early, 32% reach the neurosurgical department in more than 72 h after the subarachnoid hemorrhage, and the final 28% are excluded because of the above-stated criteria. That is the reason why 21.6% of patients could only be treated in the interval, and 39.5% were only candicates for delayed surgery without the neurosurgeon's ability to influence this.

The main findings of our analysis were: In regard to the World Congress in 1981 the number of patients who were subjected to early surgical intervention after SAH had distinctly increased in era 2. This increased number particularly resulted from a trend toward early transfer to the neurosurgical unit from other hospitals and obviously from our own policy toward early intervention, if possible.

A further increase of early surgery can only be achieved through a decrease of the number of patients with delayed admission. Since this is commonly known and already practiced by the colleagues transferring from nonsurgical departments, it is necessary to emphasize this point with the general practitioners and people in general.

Significance of the History for the Planning of Therapy After Subarachnoid Hemorrhage

C. Woertgen[1], M. Schirmer[1], and M. Bettag[2]

There is relative clear agreement that after a subarachnoid hemorrhage an aneurysm demonstrated in patients in a good general condition should be operated on as rapidly as possible. Despite a good initial condition and an operation without any complications, patients in whom there are appreciable deteriorations or a fatal outcome after the operation which cannot be explained at present are observed time and again.

Assuming that it is not the condition of the patient on admission to the hospital which is crucial for the further course, but the patient's state immediately after the subarachnoid hemorrhage, 255 patients with proved intracranial aneurysm were investigated catamnestically. All these patients were admitted and treated in the Neurosurgical Department of Düsseldorf University Hospital between 1983 and 1987.

Of the patients, 38% were admitted to the neurosurgical department on the day of the subarachnoid hemorrhage, and 30% in the next 3 days. At the *time of the hemorrhage,* the most pronounced symptoms were headache (77.2%), clouding of consciousness (61.6%), as well as nausea and vomiting (49%); meningism was detected in 37.5%. *On admission to the hospital,* meningism was the symptom which was found most frequently (51.8%); only 44.3% of the patients then showed a clouding of consciousness, and headache was only present in 11.9%. Substantial changes in the symptoms which affect the appraisal are thus shown. These are further underscored by the neurological deficits detected.

The evaluation of the results after aneurysm operation does indeed reflect these differences: of the 79 patients in whom the postoperative result could be rated as good ($n = 18$) or excellent ($n = 61$), 42% were in the stages I and II according to Hunt and Hess [1] at the time of the hemorrhage, 21% in stage III, and 37% in stages IV and V; of these patients with excellent or good postoperative results, 65% were in stages I and II and 32% in stage III, but only 3% in stages IV and V at the time of admission to the hospital. In 57 patients, we rated the postoperative result as disappointing; 75 patients died. Of these 132 patients, only 20% were in stages I and II according to Hunt and Hess at the time of the hemorrhage; likewise, 20% in stage III, but 60% in stages IV and V. At the time of admission to the

[1] Neurochirurgische Klinik, Städtisches Krankenhaus Solingen, Gotenstr. 1, W–5650 Solingen, FRG.
[2] Neurochirurgische Universitätsklinik, Moorenstr. 5, W–4000 Düsseldorf 1, FRG.

Advances in Neurosurgery, Vol. 20
K. Piscol, M. Klinger, M. Brock (Eds.)

hospital, 27% of these 132 patients were in stages I and II, 37% in stage III, but only 43% in the poorer stages IV and V.

Our investigations [2] show unequivocally that it is not the condition of the patient on admission to the neurosurgical departments, but his/her condition immediately after subarachnoid hemorrhage which is of crucial importance for the planning of further therapy.

References

1. Hunt WE, Hess RM (1968) Surgical risk as related to time of intervention in the repair of intracranial aneurysms. J Neurosurg 28:14
2. Woertgen C (1990) Die therapeutische und prognostische Bedeutung der Anamnese bei Subarachnoidalblutungen. Dissertation, Universität Düsseldorf

Microsurgical Strategy and Surgical Results in Carotid Ophthalmic Artery Aneurysms

A. G. Harders, J. M. Gilsbach, and G. Laborde[1]

Introduction

Carotid ophthalmic artery aneurysms are of special interest because the direct microsurgical clipping procedure requires a special surgical strategy and technique. Worthy of mention are temporary internal carotid artery (ICA) occlusion in the neck, temporary clipping of the carotid artery near the cavernous sinus, retrograde or direct evacuation of the aneurysm, special (fenestrated) clips, removal of the clinoid process and the roof of the optic canal, and precise knowledge of the anatomy in the cavernous sinus and the relationship of the clinoid process to the internal carotid artery.

This article describes the special characteristics of carotid ophthalmic aneurysms, our indication for operation, and the different operative strategies based on the author's experience with this type of aneurysm.

Patients

Between 1979 and 1990, 21 patients with carotid ophthalmic artery aneurysms were surgically treated by the authors (17 patients at the Department of Neurosurgery of the University of Freiburg and 4 at the RWTH Aachen). According to Yasargil's aneurysm classification [18] there were 4 (19%) patients with small aneurysms, 9 (43%) were medium size, 5 (24%) large, and 3 (14%) giant aneurysms. In 15 (17%) of the patients the aneurysm originated from the left ICA, in 6 (29%) from the right ICA. The typical characteristics of ophthalmic artery aneurysms, multiplicity and symmetry, are reflected by the figures: in 12 (57%) of the patients the aneurysms were multiple and in 2 (9%) symmetrically located; 67% (14) of the patients were female and 33% (7) were male; the average age was 48 years.

Clinical symptoms of the carotid ophthalmic aneurysm consisted in most cases of subarachnoid hemorrhage (SAH) in 11 (52%), followed by visual deficits in 6 (28%) of the patients. Eight (38%) of the ophthalmic artery aneurysms were incidental, and in four (19%) the source of an acute SAH was an aneurysm of a different location.

[1] Neurochirurgische Klinik der RWTH Aachen, Pauwelsstr. 30, W-5100 Aachen, FRG.

Advances in Neurosurgery, Vol. 20
K. Piscol, M. Klinger, M. Brock (Eds.)

Table 1. Timing of the operation in the 15 patients who suffered SAH of the total of 21 patients

Delay	No.	%
1–3 days	5	34
4–7 days	2	13
1–2 weeks	2	13
2–4 weeks	3	20
1–3 months	1	7
> 3 months	2	13

Table 2. Incidence of special surgical strategies

Operative strategy	No.	%
Removal of clinoid process and unroof optic canal	15	71
Temporary occlusion of ICA neck	15	71
Temporary clip of ICA	4	20
Fundus resection	8	38
Bipolar coagulation	21	100

Surgical Strategy

Of the 15 patients presenting with SAH, 5 (34%) were operated early and 9 (60%) of them within the first 2 weeks (Table 1).

In every patient suffering from acute SAH, a lumbar drainage was placed perioperatively to reduce intracranial volume. A dissection of the cervical ICA was carried out in large and giant aneurysms so that temporary occlusion could be performed to reduce intra-aneurysmal pressure and/or to control bleeding due to aneurysm rupture. After carrying out the classic pterional transsylvian approach [18], the carotid cistern was opened laterally from the carotid artery because the dome of the aneurysm is mainly directed infero-medial-subchiasmatically [18]. In all cases the lamina terminalis was additionally opened to release CSF. Resection of the anterior clinoid process and unroofing of the optic canal were necessary in 15 (71%) of the patients. In all of them a temporary occlusion of the cervical ICA was performed (Table 2). The techniques most often used for occlusion of the aneurysm were coagulation of the aneurysm neck, followed by clipping with fenestrated clips in combination with multiple clips in cases where the aneurysm neck was calcified or very thick. Applying this operative strategy the relationship of aneurysm neck to the ophthalmic artery was identified in every single case and kept patent. Figure 1 shows the pre- and postoperative angiogram of an ophthalmic aneurysm. Intraoperative microvascular Doppler sonography [6] was a very useful monitor-

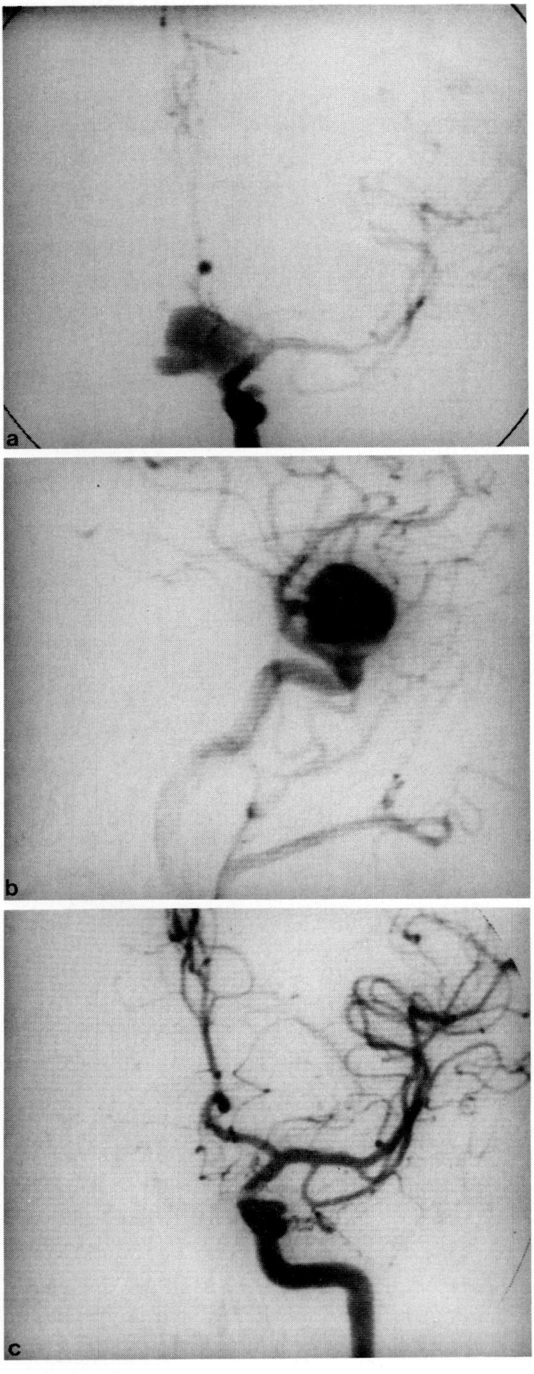
a
b
c

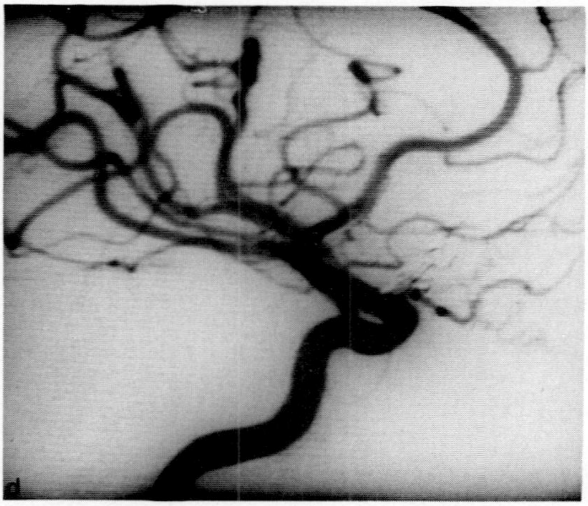

Fig. 1a–d. A 20-year-old male with a large carotid ophthalmic aneurysm on the left side **a, b** and clinical symptoms of SAH 7 days before operation, small intracavernous ICA aneurysm on the right side, preoperative clinical condition grade I (Hunt and Hess) **c, d.** The control angiography shows exclusion of the aneurysm. The clinical result was graded as good; the patient had no postoperative neurological deficits

ing device especially during the clipping maneuver in large and giant aneurysms because the clip sometimes severely stenosed or occluded the parent artery. Intraoperative Doppler sonography may prevent permanent neurological deficits by an intraoperative repositioning of the clip based on the Doppler findings.

Results

One patient of 21 died due to intraoperative ischemia caused by prolonged temporary clipping with inadvertent intraoperative hypotension in acute aneurysm surgery with severely raised intracranial pressure. This patient was preoperatively classified as grade IV according to Hunt and Hess (Table 3). In one patient with preoperative Hunt and Hess grade II, the aneurysm was incompletely clipped and rebled. The remaining 19 (90%) patients had a good clinical outcome.

Discussion

Regarding the well-described anatomical details and operative techniques [10–12, 18] concerning the pterional-transsylvian approach, temporary proximal and/or distal ICA clipping, and the resection of the clinoid process and the unroofing of the optic canal, direct microsurgical clipping of the aneurysms is presently the best method of treatment.

Table 3. Clinical outcome of the patients in relation to the preoperative condition according to Hunt and Hess

Outcome	Grade I–III	Grade IV–V
Good	19	–
Fair	–	–
Poor	1 rebleeding	–
Dead	–	1 ischemia

To reduce intra-aneurysmal pressure, intradural temporary ICA occlusion, the so-called trapping evacuation technique [17] and the retrograde suction decompression of giant paraclinoidal aneurysms has been described [2]. Direct suction decompression of aneurysms has been described by Flamm [5].

The anatomical structures and the surgical approaches to the cavernous sinus by the extradural approach have been described by Dolence in detail [4]. A clearly illustrated intradural approach to the sinus cavernous and the carotid cistern, applied in five cases of large and giant carotid ophthalmic aneurysms and in two cases of intracavernous aneurysms that arose from the anterior siphon knee, has been described [13].

The special location of proximal intra- and/or extradural aneurysms and the operative technique have been described [1–3, 8, 9, 11, 13, 16, 17]. For large and giant aneurysms special clips have been developed, ultralong clips [14], booster clips [15], so that the technical problem of clipping large or giant aneurysms has been solved from this point of view. Especially in giant aneurysms with a calcified wall the possibility of performing an extracranial-intracranial bypass should be kept in mind already while planning the skin incision [7, 15]. The typical multiplicity of aneurysms in patients with a carotid ophthalmic artery aneurysm [18] not only implies a complete four-vessel angiography but should also influence the choice of the operative approach. As many aneurysms as possible should be clipped in one session and one approach. Taking into consideration the literature of the last 7 years [3, 8, 9, 11–13, 17], morbidity is very low and mortality of the surgical results in ophthalmic artery aneurysm ranges between 0 and 5%. These findings are comparable to our results.

Except for the one patient who died postoperatively, all the other six who were operated within the first 7 days after SAH showed a good postoperative clinical course. Patients in a preoperative clinical condition rates III or less according to Hunt and Hess and carotid ophthalmic artery aneurysms should also be operated early because in those patients a good clinical result can be obtained.

References

1. Aldrich F (1991) Anterior (dorsal) paraclinoid aneurysm: Case report. Surg Neurol 35:374–376
2. Batjer H, Samson D (1990) Retrograde suction decompression of giant paraclinoidal aneurysms. J Neurosurg 73:305–306
3. Bather H, Frankfurt A, Purdy P, Smith S, Samson D (1988) Use of etomidate, temporary arterial occlusion, and intraoperative angiography in surgical treatment of large and giant cerebral aneurysms. J Neurosurg 68:234–240
4. Dolenc V (1989) Anatomy and surgery of the cavernous sinus. Springer, Wien New York
5. Flamm E (1981) Suction decompression of aneurysms. J Neurosurg 54:275–276
6. Gilsbach JM (1983) Intraoperative Doppler sonography in neurosurgery. Springer, Wien New York
7. Hosobuchi Y (1979) Direct surgical treatment of giant intracranial aneurysms. J Neurosurg 51:743–756
8. Kobayashi S, Kyoshima K, Gibo H, Hedge S, Takemae T, Sugita K (1989) Carotid cave aneurysms of the internal carotid artery. J Neurosurg 70:216–221
9. Nishioka T, Kondo A, Aoyama I, Nin K, Takahashi J (1990) Subarachnoid hemorrhage possibly caused a saccular carotid artery aneurysm within the cavernous sinus. J Neurosurg 73:301–304
10. Nutik St (1978) Carotid paraclinoid aneurysms with intradural origin and intracavernous location. J Neurosurg 48:526–533
11. Nutik St (1978) Ventral paraclinoid carotid aneurysms. J Neurosurg 69:340–344
12. Nutik St (1988) Removal of the anterior clinoid process for exposure of the proximal intracranial carotid artery. J Neurosurg 69:529–534
13. Ohmoto T, Nagao S, Mino S, Ito T, Homme Y, Fujiwara T (1991) Exposure of the intracavernous carotid artery in aneurysm surgery. J Neurosurg 28:317–324
14. Sugita K, Shigeaki K, Inoue T, Takemae T (1984) Characteristics and use of ultra-long aneurysm clips. J Neurosurg 60:145–150
15. Sundt TM, Piepgras DG (1979) Surgical approach to giant intracranial aneurysms. J Neurosurg 51:731–742
16. Sundt T, Piepgras D, Marsh R (1984) Booster clips for giant and thick-based aneurysms. J Neurosurg 60:751–762
17. Tamaki N, Shigekuni K, Kazumasa E, Masahiro A, Katsuzo F, Katsushi T, Satoshi M (1991) Giant carotid-ophthalmic artery aneurysms: direct clipping utilizing the "trapping-evacuation" technique. J Neurosurg 74:567–572
18. Yasargil M (1984) Microneurosurgery, vol I, II. Thieme, Stuttgart New York

Surgery in Cases of Subarachnoid Hemorrhage Without Definite Angiographic Evidence of Vascular Malformation

A. Perneczky[1], J. C Mäurer[1], and W. Müller-Forell[2]

Introduction

In 20% of cases with subarachnoid hemorrhage (SAH) the source remains unknown in the initial angiography. Suspicious angiographic findings of vascular malformations raise the question of the indication to perform explorative surgery. Based on experiences with seven cases, we would like to discuss the indication for surgery in cases of SAH without definite angiographic evidence of vascular malformation.

Material

Case 1

A 34-year-old male with SAH (Hunt and Hess grade III) was admitted to our department. The CT scan revealed an SAH (Fisher grade II) with accumulation of clots in the fossa interpeduncularis. Angiography showed an irregularity in the caliber of the right P1 segment but no evidence of vascular malformation. Explorative surgery was performed 1 day after the initial bleeding. Intraoperatively we found a microangioma on the surface of the right pedunculus cerebri which could be coagulated. The postoperative course was uncomplicated. Vasospasm did not occur and the patient recovered completely.

Case 2

A 63-year-old female with SAH (Hunt and Hess grade II) was admitted. The CT scan showed blood clots mainly in the pentagon cistern (Fisher grade II). Angiography was negative except for a suspicious finding concerning the left posterior communicating artery (PCoA). Two days after the initial bleeding surgery was performed. A large blood clot at the left PCoA was the only pathological finding. The patient recovered completely.

[1] Neurochirurgische Universitätsklinik und Poliklinik, Langenbeckstr. 1, W–6500 Mainz, FRG.
[2] Abteilung Neuroradiologie der Universitätsklinik, Langenbeckstr. 1, W–6500 Mainz, FRG.

Advances in Neurosurgery, Vol. 20
K. Piscol, M. Klinger, M. Brock (Eds.)

Case 3

A 44-year-old male, classified on admission as Hunt and Hess grade I, deteriorated and suffered a tonic-clonic seizure. He had to be classified as grade IV right after the presumable rebleeding. The CT showed blood clots in all basal cisterns (Fisher grade III) and hydrocephalic configuration. The angiography revealed a suspicious area concerning the anterior communicating artery (ACoA). Surgery was performed on the same day. We found intraoperatively a large blood clot around the ACoA, but no vascular malformation. The postoperative course showed delayed recovery with extreme vasospasm. The patient still does not have a satisfactory outcome, although no neurological deficits are present.

Case 4

A 51-year-old female with left hemiparesis and third nerve palsy was admitted to our department. The CT scan showed an SAH with largest blood clot accumulation in the basal cisterns. Angiography showed a suspicious finding in the course of the right PCoA. Explorative surgery was performed on the same day. No vascular malformation was seen. The recovery was delayed by vasospasm, but the patient did finally recover completely.

Case 5

A 60-year-old male was admitted with CT scan confirmed SAH and hydrocephalus. The clinical picture was consistent with Hunt and Hess grade II. The history of the present illness was unknown. Angiography showed a suspicious finding at the right ACoA. Surgery was performed on the same day. Again no evidence of vascular malformation was seen. The postoperative course was delayed. The patient turned out to suffer from a symptomatic epilepsy induced by chronic alcohol abuse and had severe generalized arteriosclerosis. The patient still needs nursing care.

Case 6

A 58-year-old male presented with a right hemiparesis. The CT scan showed blood clots mainly in the left fissure of Sylvius. Irregularities in diameter of the left middle cerebral artery (MCA) were seen on angiography. TCD revealed the presence of critical vasospasm. For that reason surgery was performed on day 16 after the initial bleeding. Arteriosclerotic alteration of the left MCA but no vascular malformation was found. The patient recovered completely.

Case 7

A 56-year-old female was admitted with a right hemiparesis. The CT scan showed the blood mainly in the left side of the pentagon cistern. The findings on angiography were irregularities in the diameter of the left anterior choroid artery. Because of vasospasm surgery was performed on day 14 after the initial bleeding. Intraoperatively a small aneurysm of the anterior choroid artery was found and coagulated. The patient recovered completely.

Discussion

According to 350 operations in cases of intracranial aneurysms performed by the authors the seven cases without definite angiographic evidence of vascular malformation comprise a minor group (2%). Of the seven cases presented, three showed a vascular malformation without definite corresponding angiographic findings.

What are the arguments which lead to the decision to perform surgery without clear angiographic evidence of vascular malformation?

1. All cases presented had a diagnosed SAH and all angiographies showed suspicious findings. Irregularities seen on the angiographic films were topographically correlated to the maximal accumulation of blood clots on CT or MRI or correlated to the neurological deficits. Two cases needed to be operated on because of hydrocephalus.
2. Surgery in SAH has the following advantages [4]:
   a) Elimination of the bleeding source (i.e., angiomas, aneurysms)
   b) Reduction of the amount of subarachnoid blood clots
   c) Treatment of posthemorrhagic hydrocephalus
3. The risk of rebleeding while waiting for the second angiography seems to be higher than the surgical risk, based on our own experiences

The last 290 angiograms performed at the Department of Neuroradiology at the University of Mainz were analyzed.

In 90 cases the initial angiography showed no vascular malformation, meaning that in 31% of the cases the source of the SAH could not be documented. These findings correlate to the data in the literature (20%–30%) [1, 2, 5, 6]. By repeated angiography 4–8 weeks after the initial bleeding, vascular malformation was seen in nine cases (10%). According to the literature 38.8% of patients with SAH and diagnosed aneurysm died in the first 3 months; of this group 78% were due to proved or suspected rebleeding [3]. This implies an incidence of fatal rebleeding of 30%. The morbidity of explorative surgery with special regard to rebleeding, infection, or parenchymatous damage was 1% in our department, meaning that the risk of explorative surgery is much smaller than the risk of rebleeding by a missed vascular malformation.

Conclusion

We see the indication for explorative surgery in cases of SAH without definite angiographic evidence of vascular malformation under the following conditions:

1. Confirmed SAH
2. Suspicious finding in angiography
3. Topographic correlation between suspicious finding in angiography to CT or MRI
4. Occasionally additional correlation between suspicious location in angiography and clinical symptoms, for example, third nerve palsy.

The decision to perform surgery is forced by the fact that the risk of surgery is much smaller than the risk of rebleeding in cases of a false negative angiography.

References

1. Brismar J, Sundbärg G (1985) Subarachnoid hemorrhage of unknown origin: prognosis and prognostic factors. J Neurosurg 63:349–354
2. Forster DMC, Steiner L, Hakanson S, Bergvall U (1978) The value of repeat panangiography in cases of unexplained subarachnoid hemorrhage and negative cerebral panangiography. J Neurosurg 48:712–716
3. Graf CJ, Torner JC, Perret GE, Nibbelink DW (1981) Cooperative aneurysm study. Long-term follow-up evaluation of randomized study. In: Sahs AL, Nibbelink DW, Torner JC (eds) Aneurysmal subarachnoid hemorrhage. Urban & Schwarzenberg, Baltimore Munich, pp 203–248
4. Ljunggren B, Brandt L, Säveland H, Nilsson RE, Cronqvist S, Andersson KE, Vinge E (1984) Outcome in 60 consecutive patients treated with early aneurysm operation and intravenous nimodipine. J Neurosurg 61:864–873
5. Nishioka H, Torner JC, Graf CJ, Kassell NF, Sahs AL, Goettler LC (1984) Cooperative study of intracranial aneurysm and subarachnoid hemorrhage: a long-term prognostic study. III. Subarachnoid hemorrhage of undetermined etiology. Arch Neurol 41:1147–1151
6. Redfern RM, Zygmunt S, Pickard JD, Foy PM, Shaw MDM (1988) The natural history of subarachnoid haemorrhage with negative angiography: a prospective study and 3-year follow-up. Br J Neurosurg 2:33–41

Differential Diagnostic Problems and Treatment of Thrombosed Giant Intracranial Aneurysms

C. B. Lumenta, J. Kiwit, and M. Sabel[1]

Introduction

Although modern neuroradiological equipment for diagnostic procedures of cerebrovascular disease is available, it is not always possible to reveal an aneurysm by these methods preoperatively.

In patients with thrombosed giant aneurysms, we may have an additional problem in that they do not have an intracranial hemorrhage but show neurological symptoms due to the intracranial mass lesion.

Among 162 patients who were operated on by the authors in the last 3.5 years, there were 20 patients with giant aneurysms. In this patient group the diagnosis of an aneurysm, however, could only be established preoperatively in 16 patients.

In this paper we report on the findings and our surgical management of the other four patients in whom the diagnosis was made during surgery (Table 1).

Case 1 (Pat. M.H.)

This 27-year-old man complained of cervicocephalalgia. The orthopedic surgeon did not find any pathological alterations of the cervical spinal column. Because of that he consulted a neurologist, who arranged an MRI scan examination. The neurological finding was normal; the MRI scan showed a roundish mass lesion anterior to the brainstem on the left, suspected to be a clival meningioma. The left vertebral angiography revealed an avascular mass. The patient was operated on through a lateral suboccipital approach on the left. The surgical finding was a thrombosed giant aneurysm of the vertebral artery just proximal to the proximal internal carotid artery (PICA) junction. The vertebral artery was trapped. The postoperative clinical finding was excellent. A control angiography was refused by the patient.

[1] Neurochirurgische Universitätsklinik, Moorenstr. 5, W-4000 Düsseldorf 1, FRG.

Advances in Neurosurgery, Vol. 20
K. Piscol, M. Klinger, M. Brock (Eds.)

Table 1. Clinical, neuroradiological, and surgical findings as well as outcome of four patients with thrombosed giant aneurysm

No.	Inititals	CT/MRI	Clinic	Localization	Outcome
1.	M.H.	Clival tumor	Cephalgia	V1 lt trapping	Excellent
2.	D.K.	Sphenoid wing tumor	Seizures	M1 rt trapping	Excellent
3.	G.S.	Suprasellar tumor	Seizures	ACoA clipping	(POS)
4.	S.D.	Clival tumor	Seizures	P1 lt trapping	(Hemianopia)

ACoA, anterior communicating artery; M1, medial cerebral artery; P1, posterior cerebral artery; POS, psycho-organic syndrome; V1, vertebral artery; (-), transient.

Case 2 (Pat. D.K.)

This 41-year-old man had a history of focal seizures on the left 2 months before admission to the hospital. The clinical and neuroradiological diagnostic procedures were performed at the Department of Neurology of our University Hospital. His neurological finding was normal. The patient was transferred to our service for surgery because of the results of a CT scan and right brachial angiography with a suspected large meningioma of the medial sphenoid wing on the right (Figs. 1 and 2). The patient was operated on through a subtemporal approach on the right. The intraoperative finding was a giant, completely thrombosed aneurysm of the M1 on the right, which had to be trapped. The postoperative clinical finding was excellent. The angiography after surgery showed a rarefaction of the M1 area, but good collateral perfusion by the posterior cerebral aretery on the right (Fig. 3).

Case 3 (Pat. G.S.)

After a general seizure, this 57-year-old man was admitted to our service. Postictal he merely showed a psycho-organic syndrome, but no focal neurological deficit. CT and MRI scans revealed a large suprasellar mass lesion, suggesting a craniopharyngioma. The cerebral panangiography showed a suprasellar mass lesion with a moderate spasm of both anterior cerebral arteries. Because of the close proximity to the circle of Willis and the previous experience with the other two patients, we took into consideration the differential diagnosis of a thrombosed giant aneurysm of the anterior circulation. The patient was operated on through a pterional approach on the right. Indeed, we found a thrombosed giant aneurysm which could be clipped and resected. The postoperative neurological finding was unchanged, although the angiography revealed increased spasm of both anterior cerebral arteries.

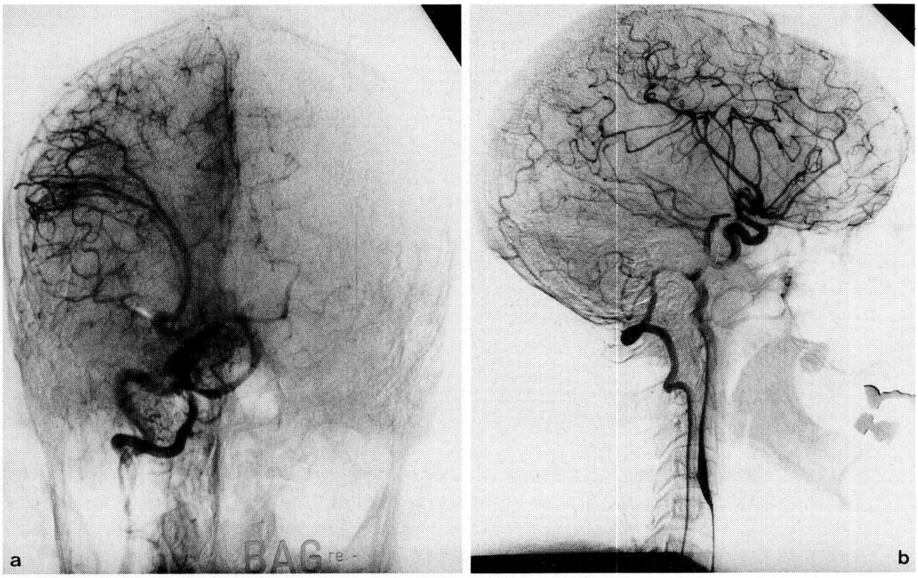

Fig. 1a, b. Right brachial angiogram of patient D.K. (case 2) with thrombosed giant aneurysm of the M1 segment. **a** AP view; **b** lateral view

Case 4 (Pat. S.D.)

The history of this 27-year-old man included general seizures with postictal homonymous hemianopia to the right. On admission to our service the neurological finding was normal. CT and MRI scans showed a large mass lesion at the clival edge on the left, simulating a meningioma. Cerebral panangiography revealed a vascular malformation of the posterior cerebral artery on the left, but an exact diagnosis for a giant aneurysm or a cavernoma could not be made. The patient was operated on through a subtemporal approach. The intraoperative finding was a serpentine giant aneurysm, which was not completely thrombosed. The P1 segment was trapped. After surgery the patient showed a transient oculomotor palsy and a homonymous hemianopia to the right for 6 months. The angiographic control 6 months after surgery showed the P1 segment up to the area of clipping without aneurysm. On CT and MRI there was no infarct zone.

Discussion

Completely thrombosed giant aneurysms can sometimes not be identified in either CT or MRI scans or the angiogram so that the diagnosis is not made until surgery [1]. The clinical findings with signs of intracranial space-occupying lesions were

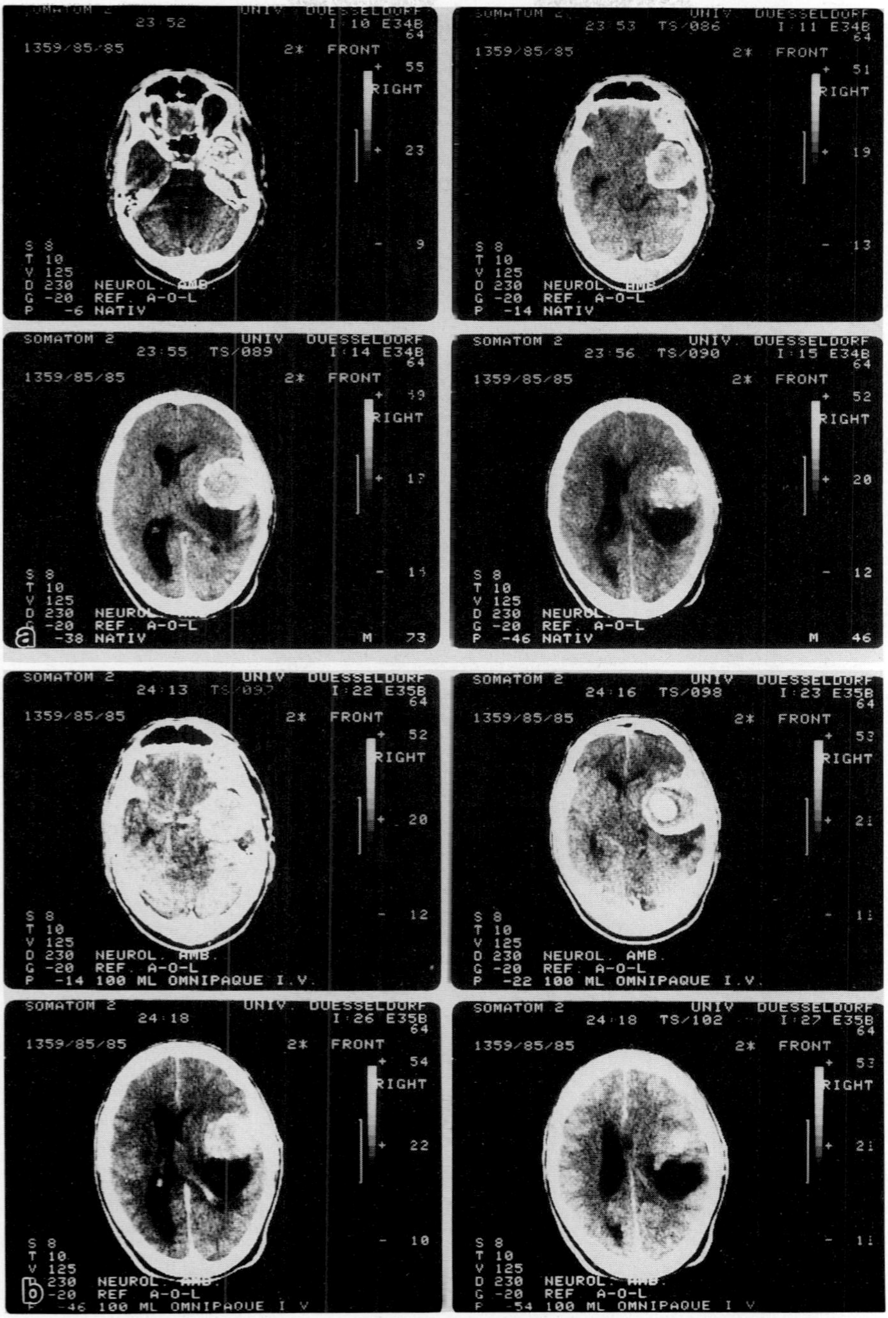

Fig. 2a, b. The same patient as in Fig. 1. CT scan **a** before and **b** after contrast enhancement

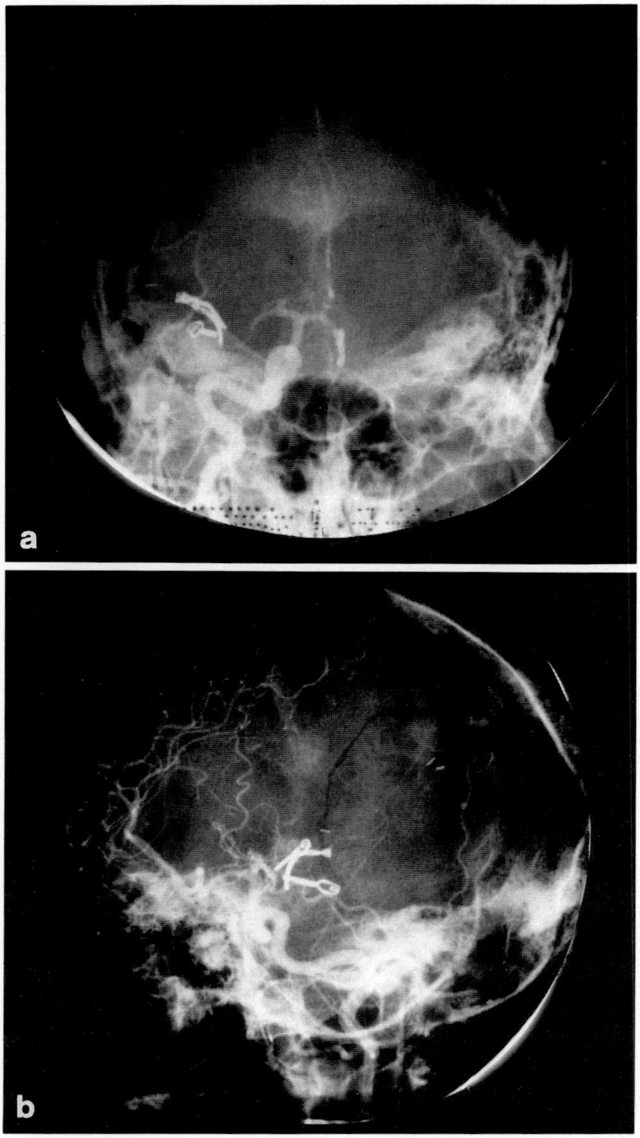

Fig. 3a, b. The same patient as in Fig. 2. Right carotid angiogram after surgery. **a** AP view; **b** lateral view diagnostically misleading as they suggested an intracranial tumor [3, 5, 6] or an arteriovenous malformation [2].

Our experience with aneurysm surgery showed that 12% of surgically treated aneurysms were giant and 2% completely thrombosed so the diagnosis could not be made preoperatively. This fact caused difficulty in surgical planning and strategy. In cases in which the intracranial mass lesion is localized close to cerebral vessels and the diagnosis of aneurysm could not be excluded, we prefer a large craniotomy so that an intensive inspection is always possible and the parent vessel can be identified.

Three of our patients were treated with trapping procedures because the clips could not be put over the neck of the aneurysm due to the thick wall. Nevertheless, the outcome of these patients was excellent. We supposed that due to the chronic mass lesion blood flow in the parent vessel was reduced so that the perfusion was maintained by spontaneously developed collateral circulation. Moret [4] also prefers the trapping procedure in patients with giant aneurysm by endovascular treatment with excellent results. In conclusion our cases demonstrate again that although modern neuroradiological procedures are available, the diagnosis of thrombosed giant aneurysm cannot always be made preoperatively.

References

1. Bien S, Schumacher M, Thron A, Klein HJ, Hassler W (1986) Neuroradiologische Diagnostik und Klinik intrakranieller Riesenaneurysmen. Radiologe 26 (11):515–519
2. Camras LR, Reicher MA, Bentson JR, Wilson GH (1987) Partially thrombosed giant aneurysm simulating an arteriovenous malformation on MR imaging. J Comp Assist Tomogr 11 (2):326–328
3. Dolenc V (1983) A tumor-simulating giant aneurysm of the vertebral artery. Case report. Zentralbl Neurochir 44 (3):215–220
4. Moret J (1991) Endovascular treatment of giant aneurysm. Presented at the meeting of American Association of Neurological Surgery in New Orleans
5. Nitta T, Makajima K, Maeda M, Ishii S (1987) Completely thrombosed giant aneurysm of the pericallosal artery: case report. J Comp Assist Tomogr 11 (2):140–143
6. Rusegger L, Grunert V (1983) Ein teilthrombosiertes Basilarisaneurysma als Tumor des 3. Ventrikels imponierend. Neurochirurgia 26 (2):59–62

Cerebral Artery Aneurysm in Childhood: Surgical Indications and Results

S. Vogel, R. Saballus, and A. Heinitz[1]

Introduction

The incidence of cerebral artery aneurysm in childhood has been quoted to be 0.6 to 100 000 individuals aged below 20 years and, consequently, is three times lower than in adult age. Twenty-five cases of aneurysms in patients below 15 years of age were compiled from the literature by Shapiro [4] who underlined the rare occurrence of aneurysm in childhood. Yasargil [7] mentioned seven patients below 20 years of age in a series of 355 patients. Only 8 children in a group of 1080 patients with cerebroarterial aneurysm were reported by Suzuki [5]. That group, nevertheless, is of particular interest, as it might be helpful to us in obtaining some information on the pathogenesis of cerebroarterial aneurysm and peculiarities of its clinical manifestation.

If Forbus' [3] assumption of the origin of congenital aneurysm in instability of walls or defects in the wall structure of developing and ramifying cerebral arteries has retained its validity, predetermination of an aneurysm should be timed in intrauterine human life, while manifestation could be verified only in postnatal life on the basis of hemodynamic development. With equal emphasis on the congenital wall defect, consequences most likely should occur at an earlier point in time from microvessels and high flow resistance. On the other hand, these distal vascular segments are directly located in between extracerebral and intracerebral structures. Hence, their rupture should be immediately covered by parenchymatous tissue.

Amacher [1], Becher [2], and Vincent [6] have actually emphasized that manifest aneurysm in childhood is preferably localized in the distal segment of the artery or at the connection of smaller arteries from larger vessels, such as the A1 or M2 segments of the rami perforantes, rami ad pontem of the vasilar artery, and at ramifications of the anterior and posterior choidal arteries. The dysplastic nature of cerebroarterial aneurysm, with its localization in concomitance with manifest hemorrhage being a timing criterion for the action of hemodynamic factors, is likely to be substantiated by incomplete connection of embryonically laid out arteries to mature vascular segments.

[1] Neurochirurgische Abteilung, Charité der Humboldt-Universität, Schumannstr. 20/21, O–1040 Berlin, FRG.

Advances in Neurosurgery, Vol. 20
K. Piscol, M. Klinger, M. Brock (Eds.)

Material

Surgical treatment was performed on 55 children up to 14 years of age for malformations of brain vessels at the neurosurgical department of the Berlin Charité Hospital over the past 10 years. Included were 3 cases of so-called aneurysm of the galenic vein, 41 with arteriovenous malformations of the brain, and 11 children with congenital aneurysm of the cerebral artery.

Aneurysms were recorded from the following sites in the distal arterial segment, more or less even distributed among age levels between 6 months and 14 years in these 11 patients:

Median cerebral artery, M2	2 patients
Posterior cerebral artery, P2	2 patients
Pericallosal artery, A2	2 patients
Anterior choroid artery	2 patients
Posterior choroid artery	1 patient
Rami ad pontem of the basilar artery	1 patient
Inferoposterior cerebellar artery	1 patient

No aneurysms were recorded by the authors from the internal carotid artery, vertebral artery, from the A1 or M1 segments. In all patients, symptoms were found to begin with disorders in cerebral functionality which, however, did not entail immediate diagnosis in any of them. In most cases, neuroradiological examination was performed only along with aggravating impairment of cerebral function and was accompanied in 8 of the above 11 children by lumbar puncture with evidence of subarachnoid hemorrhage. The latter was not recordable by lumbar puncture in three children. Cerebral vasospasm was clinically and neuroradiologically established in only two children, both of them 14 years of age. All children stayed at stage I–II or III according to Hunt and Hess.

Surgical indications for all children were not established until 2 weeks had passed from the first bleeding. The reasons were not related to our inability to perform an operation during the acute phase, but were attributable to delays by pediatric neurologists or pediatricians who had failed to establish early diagnoses so that all children were admitted with delay to our department.

Selected Case Reports

A 6-month-old infant suddenly turned pale in his mother's arm and exhibited hypotonia in the neck and extremity muscles together with somnolence for 1 h. The child was examined the same day, and an ultrasonographic checkup was scheduled for the next day. A hematoma in the frontal position on the right was ultrasonographically detected. The hemorrhage was verified by lumbar puncture. Computed tomography of the skull, after another 2 days, confirmed a mediobasal hematoma on the right (Fig. 1). In the meantime, flaccid hemiparesis had developed on the left. Cerebral angiography was performed only 3 weeks later, with evidence point-

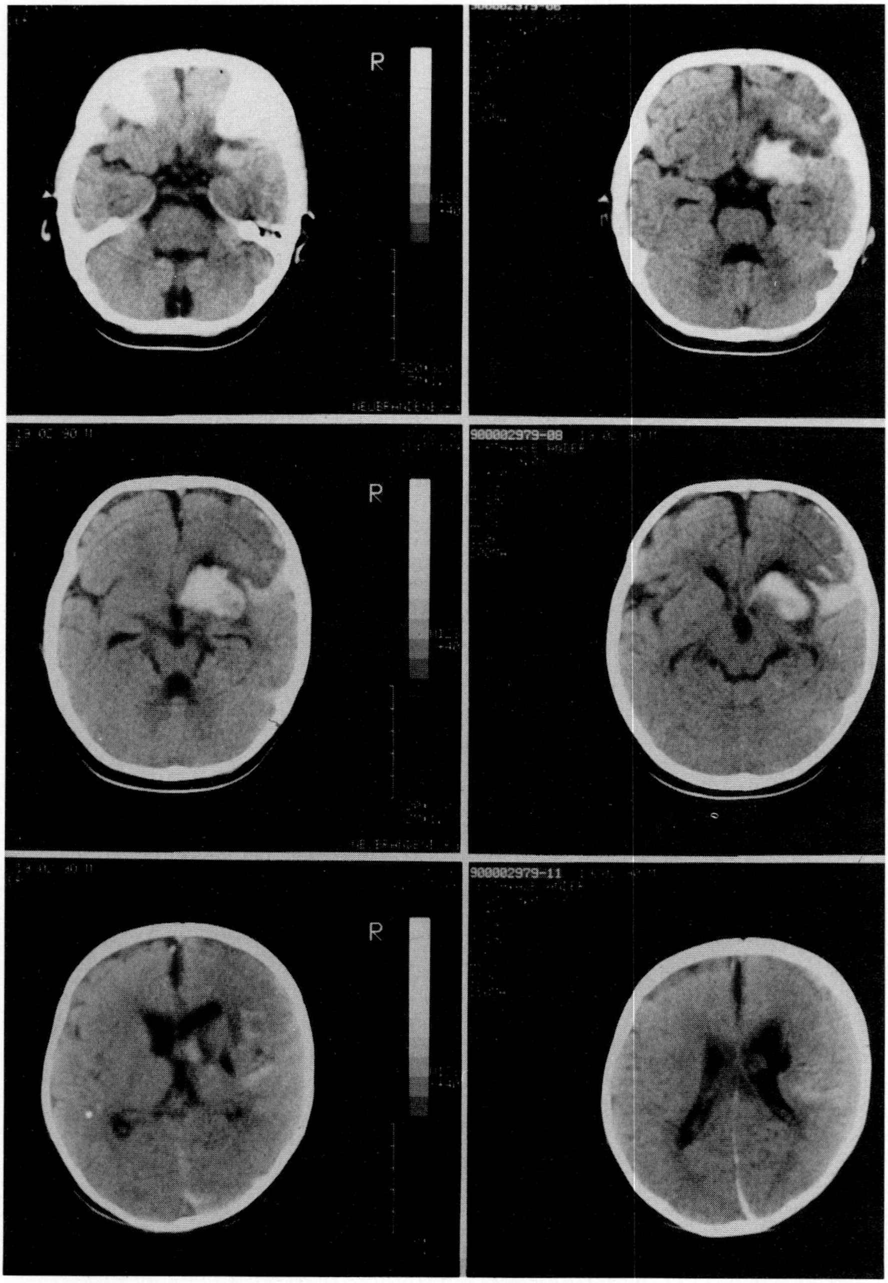

Fig. 1. This CT scan shows subarachnoid and intracerebral hemorrhage in a 6-month-old infant. This girl had a hemiparesis on the left

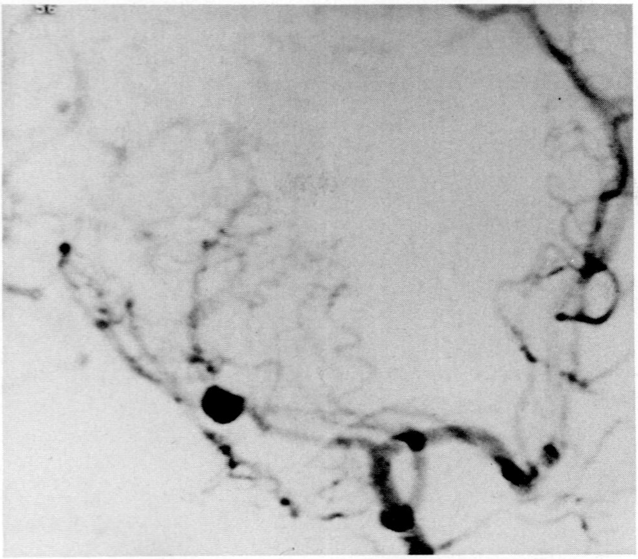

Fig. 2. This anterior-posterior projection of the carotid angiogram shows an aneurysm of the middle cerebral artery without vasospasm in a 6-month-old infant

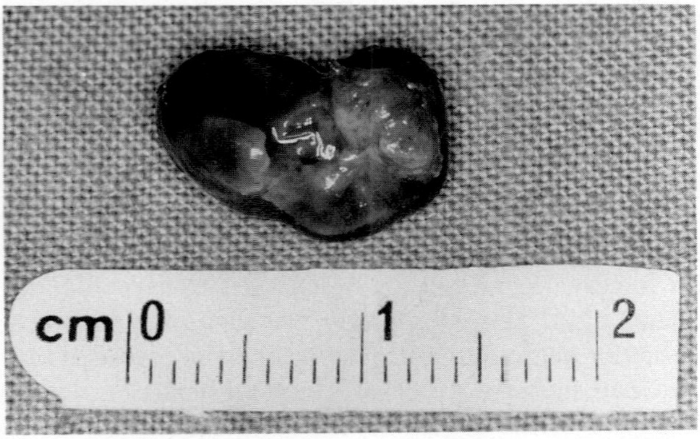

Fig. 3. This photograph shows the aneurysm from the middle cerebral artery after clip application and resection

ing to an aneurysm of the median cerebral artery on the right (Fig. 2). The child was then transferred for surgical intervention. The hematoma was removed and the aneurysm closed by a clip immediately (Fig. 3). On histological investigation, the extirpated aneurysm exhibited intraaneurysmal wall defect filled with granulation tissue (Fig. 4). Elastic fiber components were totally absent from the wall. The

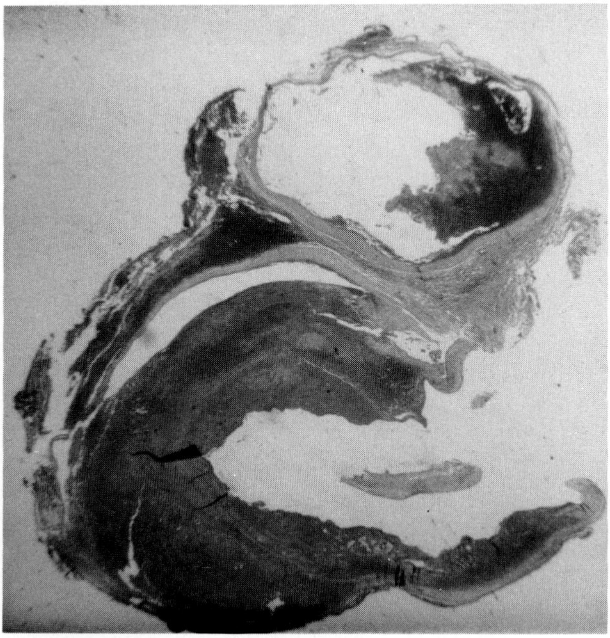

Fig. 4. The histological examination of the aneurysm demonstrated the defects in the muscle and elastic tissue of the artery will. H & E, 17 μm, $\times$12.5

lumen was filled with thrombi and fresh blood. Postoperative regression of the hemiparesis was satisfactory. Some problems relating to diagnosis and adequate decision making on therapeutic action may be seen from the following two cases.

A 2-year-old girl was struck by sudden hemiparesis on the playground of a kindergarten. The girl was immediately taken to a pediatrician, but cranial computed tomography was conducted only a week later. The child, suspected of having a tumor, was then referred for surgery. Representation of left-sided transventricular findings followed after another 2 days. This surprisingly revealed three mutually adherent aneurysms in the posterior choroid artery. The histological investigation provided evidence of defective wall structure with absence of elastic fibers. Hemiparesis has continued unchanged over the 2 years that have passed since those primary findings.

A boy aged 10 years suddenly noticed impairment of sensitivity in his left knee, "as if lukewarm water ran down his leg." The same phenomenon recurred 2 years later associated with visual disorders. Severe headache and vomiting occurred after another 2 days. Only then was a pediatrician called in for clinical consultation. He found incipient hemiparesis on the left and established subarachnoid hemorrhage on the left by lumbar puncture. Cranial computed tomography revealed a hyperdense, stratified growth, 3 cm in diameter, in the right thalamic pulvinar. The thrombotic and blood-filled part of the aneurysm was visualized by subsequent magnetic resonance imaging. The aneurysm was approached subtemporally and closed by application of a clip to the posterior choroid artery and removed within 24 h. A stratified dysontogenetic aneurysm with signs of repetitive thrombosis was histologically confirmed. Hemiparesis subsided rapidly, with only slight dysdiadochokinesia remaining in the left arm and leg.

Discussion

None of the 11 children died. All aneurysms were directly tackled by means of a clip and were removed. Postoperative courses were without problems. Some persistent neurologicofunctional disorders were attributable to major and lasting intracerebral bleedings. Spasms of cerebral arteries were recordable in only two of the above children, two boys aged 14 years. Newborns and infants obviously were not as strongly threatened by vascular spasms as adults were. The real problem associated with infantile cerebroarterial aneurysm has something to do with nontargeted diagnosis which may lead to delay of neurosurgical therapy.

References

1. Amacher AL, Drake CG (1975) Cerebral artery aneurysms in infancy, childhood and adolescence. Child's Brain 1:72–80
2. Becker DH, Silverberg GD, Nelson DH, Hanbery JW (1978) Saccular aneurysm of infancy and early childhood. Neurosurgery 2:1–7
3. Forbus WD (1930) Origin of miliary aneurysms of superficial cerebral arteries. Bull Johns Hopkins Hosp 47:239–284
4. Shapiro K (1985) Subarachnoid hemorrhage in children. In: Fein JM, Flamm ES (eds) Cerebrovascular surgery, vol 3. Springer, Berlin Heidelberg New York Tokyo, pp 941–965
5. Suzuki J, Miusma T (1979) Intracranial aneurysms associated with arteriovenous malformations. J Neurosurg 50:742–746
6. Vincent FM (1980) Intracranial aneurysms. Arch Neurol 37:602–608
7. Vasargil MG, Smith RD, Gasser JG (1978) Microsurgery of the aneurysms of the internal carotid artery and its branches Prog Surg 9:58–121

Multiple Intracranial Aneurysms: Considerations in Planning Surgical Management

M. Fylaktakis, P. Sakellariou, K. Polyzoidis, N. Baskinis, and J. Magras[1]

Introduction

Despite the rapid developments in the diagnosis of intracranial aneurysmal disease, with the advent of the CT scan, MRI scan, and selective cerebral angiography, and the remarkable experience with microneurosurgery during the last decades, the surgical treatment of multiple intracranial aneurysms in the same patient raises significant questions [8, 9].

Two main questions that the managing surgeon has to take into consideration are: (1) whether the second aneurysm, which has not bled, has caused no clinical symptoms and was detected entirely accidentally, has to be surgically treated and (b) which would be the optimal timing for the surgical management of this aneurysm [1, 2, 6, 7, 14, 15, 17].

The particular features of these aneurysms, the technical aspects, the results, and the complications of their management are described by reviewing the international literature and our material.

Material

During the last 5 years (1985–1990), 120 intracranial aneurysms were surgically treated in our department. Among them 11 multiple aneurysms were found, which comprise 9.2% of the total number. Seven patients were male and four female, most in their 5th decade of life. The youngest patient was 26 years old and the oldest 60.

The multiple aneurysms were located ipsilaterally in seven cases and contralaterally in four. In the last group, three patients were harboring aneurysms of the contralateral middle cerebral artery (MCA), while a 45-year-old woman had an aneurysm of the anterior communicating artery (ACoA) and a second one at the trunk of the basilar artery. Among the ipsilaterally located multiple aneurysms, three were originating from the internal carotid artery (ICA) in coexistence with aneurysms of the MCA, three of the ACoA in coexistence with MCA aneurysms, and one aneurysm of the ICA was paired with one of the ACoA (Table 1).

[1] Department of Neurosurgery, George Papanicolaou General Hospital, GR–Thessaloniki, Greece.

Advances in Neurosurgery, Vol. 20
K. Piscol, M. Klinger, M. Brock (Eds.)

Table 1. Location of the multiple aneurysm

Location	No.
Unilateral	7
Only ICA	0
Only MCA	0
Only ACA	0
ICA + MCA	3
ACA + ICA	1
MCA + ACA	3
Bilateral	4
Symmetrical (MCA)	3
Asymmetrical (ACA + BA)	1

In all of our patients the unruptured aneurysm was also operated apart from the one originating from the basilar artery. After the successful clipping of the ruptured aneurysm of the ACoA, the patient refused to have another operation for the second aneurysm.

The surgical procedure in eight cases was the unilateral pterional craniotomy, and in three cases the bilateral pterional approach in two stages for aneurysms of the contralateral MCA. The technical difficulties are considerable. In a 43-year-old patient of ours with bilateral MCA aneurysms, a recraniotomy was necessary for the definite clipping of a giant aneurysm that eventually required the application of five clips in total. Another 26-year-old patient, also with symmetrical aneurysms of the MCA had to be operated on an emergency basis because the ruptured aneurysm had produced a large intratemporal hematoma with clinical signs of tentorial herniation.

The results from the surgical treatment of our series of patients ranged from good to excellent. None of our patients died. The patient with the aneurysm of the basilar artery lives and works normally without neurological deficit 2 years after her operation (Figs. 1–3).

Discussion

The incidence of multiple intracranial aneurysms ranges between 12.9% and 22.7% in autopsy studies [5, 12]. In a large series reported by Winn et al. (1983) in collaboration with the University of Virginia, a comparison was made of the treatment of multiple aneurysms with that of single lesions. The incidence of rebleeding during the 1st decade after the hemorrhage was the same in both groups of aneurysms, which were treated conservatively [3, 4, 14, 15]. The risk of rebleeding in patients with surgical treatment of only the ruptured aneurysm was similar to that in patients harboring an incidental aneurysm [10, 13–15].

The location of the lesion, the surgical approach, and the treatment priorities must be taken into account to achieve the optimal planning of the operation [11,

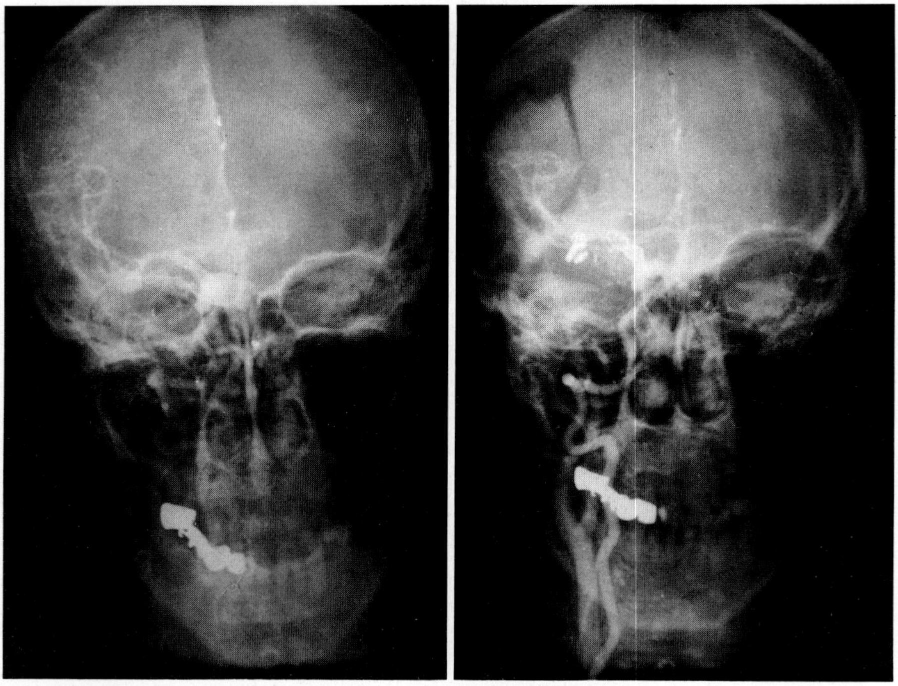

Fig. 1. Aneurysms of the right ICA and right MCA. Pre- and postoperative angiography (AP view)

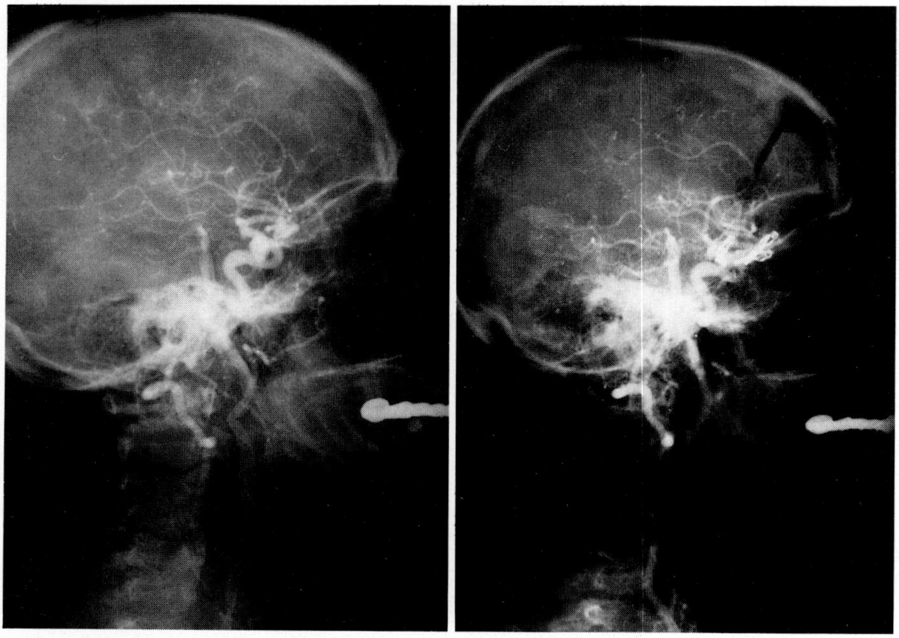

Fig. 2. Aneurysms of the right ICA and right MCA. Pre- and postoperative angiography (lateral view)

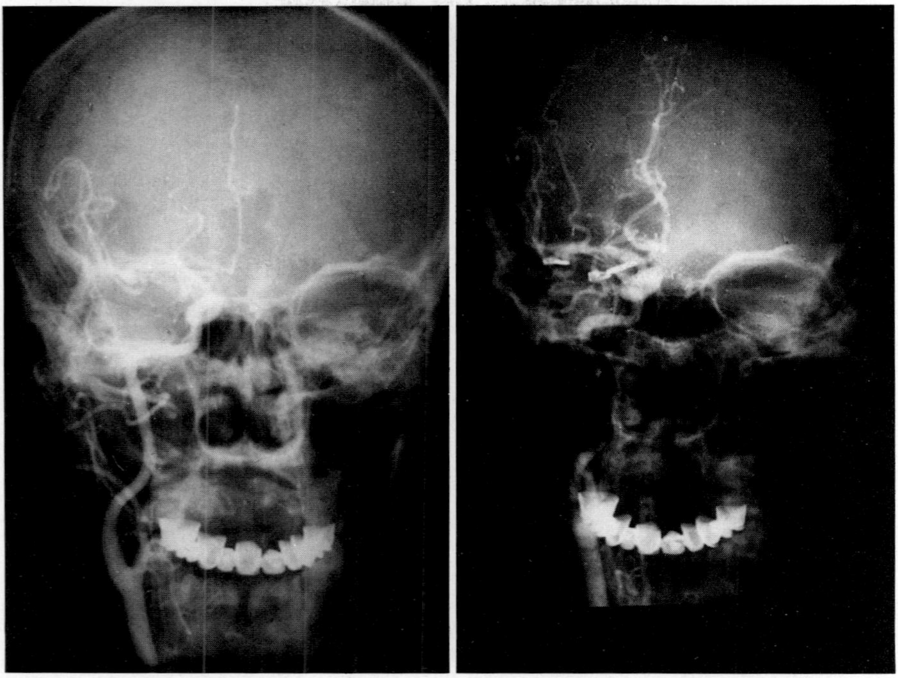

Fig. 3. Aneurysms of the ICA-PCoA and MCA. Pre- and postoperative angiography (AP view)

16, 17]. Through a pterional craniotomy, all ipsilaterally located aneurysms can be treated in one stage. With a single approach, aneurysms of the ICA, MCA, ACoA, basilar tip, as well as contralateral aneurysms of the ICA and the A1 segment of the ACA can be handled. The bilateral craniotomy is necessary for symmetrical aneurysms of the MCA and the other locations. The ruptured aneurysm should always be treated first [11, 12, 15–17].

In conclusion, a diagnosed aneurysm, if left untreated, is a cause of continuous, remaining risk for the patient's life. All aneurysms should be managed surgically, especially the ones that are located on the same side. A second craniotomy, if needed, should be performed as early as possible.

References

1. Drake CG, Girvin JP (1976) The surgical treatment of subarachnoid hemorrhage with multiple aneurysms. In: Morley TP (ed) Current controversies in neurosurgery. Saunders, Philadelphia, pp 274–278
2. Hamby WB (1959) Multiple intracranial aneurysms. Aspects of treatment. J Neurosurg 16:558–563

3. Heiskansen O (1981) Risk of bleeding from unruptured aneurysms in cases with multiple intracranial aneurysms. J Neurosurg 55:524–526
4. Jain KK (1974) Surgery of intact intracranial aneurysms. J Neurosurg 40:495–498
5. McKissok W, Richardson A, Walsh L et al. (1964) Multiple intracranial aneurysms. Lancet I:623–626
6. Maunt LA, Brisman R (1974) Treatment of multiple intracranial aneurysms – symptomatic and asymptomatic. Clin Neurosurg 24:166–170
7. Moyes PD (1971) Surgical treatment of multiple aneurysms and of incidentally-discovered unruptured aneurysms. J Neurosurg 35:291–295
8. Pappen JL, Fager CA (1959) Multiple intracranial aneurysms. J Neurosurg 16:581–589
9. Paterson A, Bond MR (1973) Treatment of multiple intracranial arterial aneurysms. Lancet I:1302–1304
10. Samson DS, Hodosh RM, Clark WK (1977) Surgical management of unruptured asymptomatic aneurysms. J Neurosurg 46:731–734
11. Suzuki J, Sakurai Y (1979) The treatment of intracranial multiple aneurysms. In: Suzuki J (ed) Cerebral aneurysm. Neuron, Tokyo, pp 293–307
12. Suzuki J, Yoshimoto T (1980) Distribution of cerebral aneurysms. In: Pia HW, Langmaid JC, Zierski C (eds) Spontaneous intracerebral haematomas. Advances in diagnosis and therapy. Springer, Berlin Heidelberg New York, pp 127–133
13. Wiebers DO, Whisnant JP, O'Fallon WM (1981) The natural history of unruptured intracranial aneurysms. N Engl J Med 304:696–698
14. Winn HR, Richardson AE, Jane JA (1977) The long-term prognosis in untreated cerebral aneurysms: I. The incidence of late hemorrhage in cerebral aneurysm: a 10-year evaluation of 364 patients. Ann Neurol 1:358–370
15. Winn HR, Almanii SW, Berga LS, Jane JA, Richardson AE (1983) The long-term outcome in patients with multiple aneurysms. J Neurosurg 59:642–651
16. Yasargil MG (1984) Microneurosurgery, vol I. Thieme, Stuttgart New York, pp 267–268
17. Yasargil MG (1984) Microneurosurgery, vol II. Thieme, Stuttgart New York, pp 305–328

Psychological Stress During Operations of Aneurysms: A Factor in the Surgical Treatment of Aneurysms. Cardiac Output and Blood Pressure of the Surgeon

B. Panning[1], M. R. Gaab[2], and H. Dietz[2]

It is usually the main task of an anesthesiologist in the operating theater to take care of the patient during surgery. Publications on cardiac stress reactions of physicians during work reporting on tachycardia [2–5] and occasionally ventricular arrhythmia [5] stimulated us to undertake similar investigations in neurosurgeons during clipping of aneurysms. This seemed interesting because there is a very unique combination of very high psychological stress and very low physical activity.

All measurements were done by the same anesthesiologist (B.P.), who was not charged with anesthesiological duties during the crucial period.

An oscillometric automatic blood pressure cuff (Dinamap, Johnson and Johnson, Norderstedt) and a thoracic bioimpedance cardiac output monitor (NCCOM 3, BoMed Medical Manufacturing, Irvine, Fig. 1) were used to measure the hemodynamic parameters. Both devices are used in our routine monitoring during anesthesia. Heart rate, stroke volume, and cardiac output were obtained from the BoMed, which measures the pulsatile changes of thoracic bioimpedance. The principles of this method have been described by Bernstein [1]. Eight ECG electrodes were

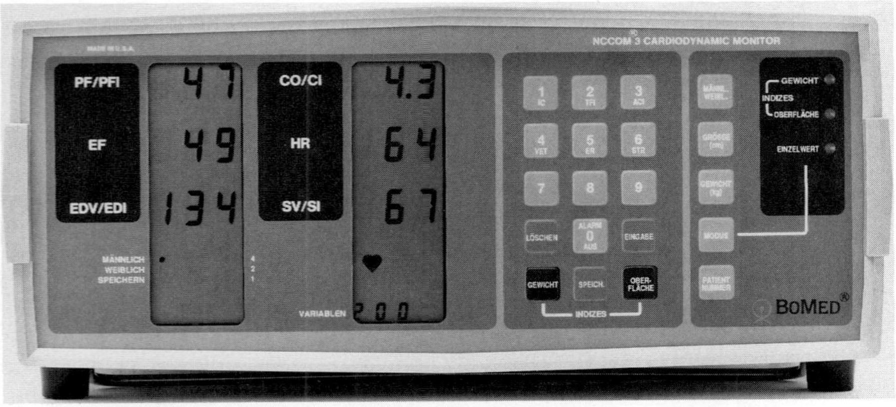

Fig. 1. The BoMed NCCOM 3 cardiovascular monitor

[1] Abteilung Anaesthesiologie II, Medizinische Hochschule Hannover, Konstanty-Gutschow-Str. 8, W–3000 Hannover 61, FRG.
[2] Neurochirurgische Klinik, Medizinische Hochschule Hannover, Konstanty-Gutschow-Str. 8, W–3000 Hannover 61, FRG.

Advances in Neurosurgery, Vol. 20
K. Piscol, M. Klinger, M. Brock (Eds.)

Table 1. Details of six cases of cardiovascular monitoring of a surgeon during operation of cerebral aneurysms

Localization and size	Therapy, special circumstances, complications
ACA 1 cm Ø	Bleeding, trapping, clipping
ACI l. 2 cm Ø	Thin-walled aneurysm, perforation (neck), clipping
MCA r. giant	Trapping (scheduled), neuromonitoring, clipping
MCA l. 1 cm Ø	135 kg BW, severe brain edema, clipping without problems
ACA 1 cm Ø	Bleeding (expected), clipping
ACI r. infraclinoidal giant	Temporary clipping, neuromonitoring, evacuation of clots, muscle filling

placed at the neck and the chest of the surgeon. The connecting cables were long enough to place the BoMed at an appropriate distance from the surgical field. Blood pressure measurements were taken at the lower leg occasionally; 70 mmHg were subtracted for height correction.

After having gathered some technical experience during other operations such as hypophysectomy or cervical spine surgery which even habituated the surgeon, six measurements during aneurysm clipping could be performed. Details concerning location of aneurysm, complications, and surgery are given in Table 1.

In general, we found two types of reactions which should be demonstrated. The first diagram (Fig. 2) shows an initially elevated heart rate which rises during the course of surgery to a maximum of approximately 140 bpm. The cardiac index shows the same tendency. An interesting finding was the decrease of heart rate from 120 to 98 bpm during the performance of the temporary occlusion of the carotid artery which was tolerated well. This seemed to calm the surgeon. On the contrary a sudden disturbance caused by EEG deterioration raised the heart rate from 100 to 130 bpm. During the manipulation of the aneurysm, the heart rate and cardiac index increased distinctly and declined slightly after successful clipping. The second example was recorded during an operation of a large aneurysm of the anterior cerebral artery (Fig. 3). This particular case was complicated by bleeding. In contrast to the first diagram, a cardiac hyperdynamic reaction could only be observed during the manipulation of the aneurysm. Similar circumstances were found during the four other measurements.

The blood pressure recordings were not very useful because during the periods of high stress this disturbance of the surgeon seemed not to be advisable. This measurement could only be used to demonstrate normal basic values. The bioimpedance electrodes did not disturb the surgeon.

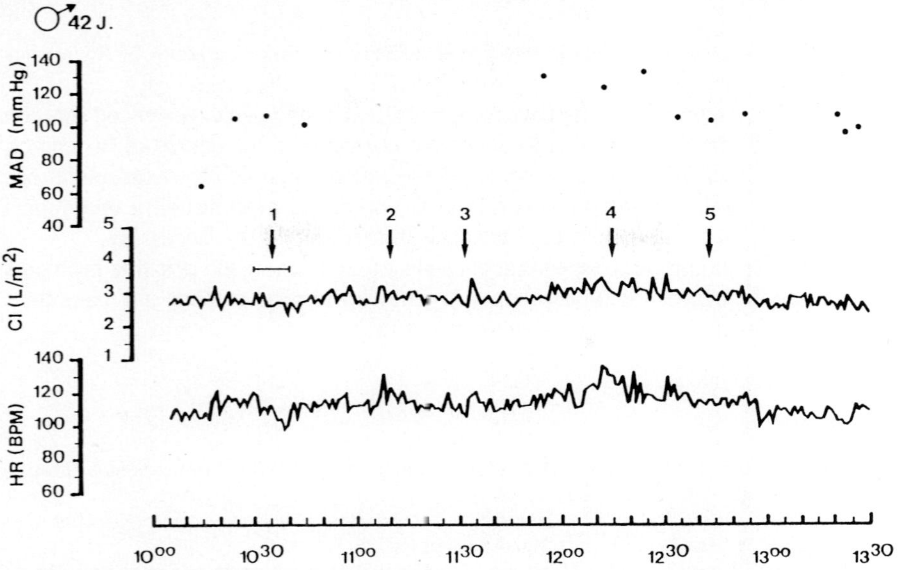

Fig. 2. Heart rate (HR), CI (cardiac index), and a mean arterial blood pressure (MAD) in a surgeon during operation of an infraclinoidal giant aneurysm of the internal carotid artery. The *numbered arrows* mark special events. *1*, temporary carotid occlusion (10 min) followed by decrease of heart rate; *2*, increase of heart rate possibly caused by announcement of suspicious EEG alterations (artifact); *3*, beginning of manipulation near aneurysm; *4*, incision of the aneurysm, removal of clots; *5*, distal carotid clip open

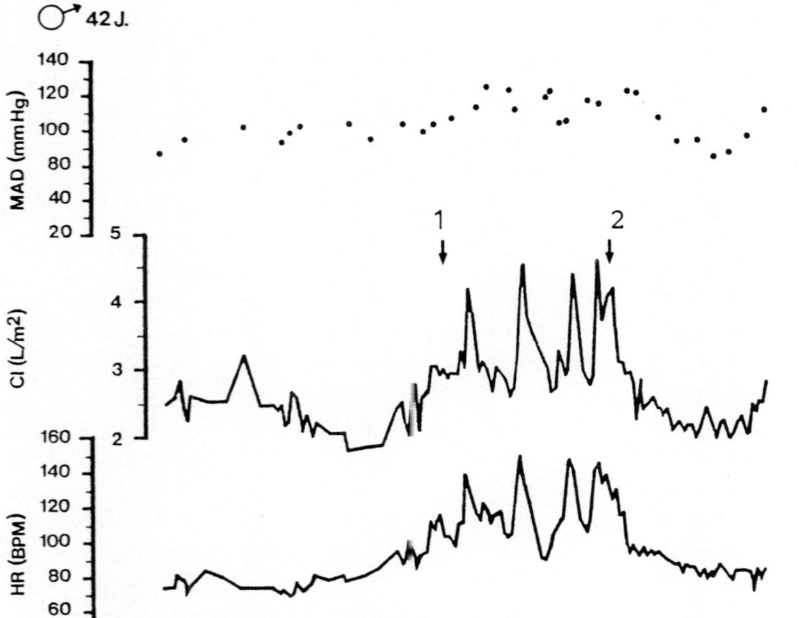

Fig. 3. Hemodynamics of a surgeon during operation of a bleeding anterior communicating aneurysm with trapping (abbreviations see Fig. 2). *Arrow 1* indicates the beginning of manipulation near the aneurysm; *Arrow 2*, final clipping

Our findings demonstrate the psychological stress even in an experienced surgeon who had performed more than 100 aneurysm clippings in the course of his career. Compared with the results from other studies which found much lower accelerations of heart rate, surgery of aneurysms might be one of the most stressful operations. More should not be discussed here because further studies are necessary.

However, it should be stressed that anesthesiologists know the possible problems confronting the neurosurgeon and hopefully they try to respect them and make their task as easy as possible by considerate behavior.

References

1. Bernstein DP (1986) A new stroke volume equation for thoracic bioimpedance. Theory and rationale. Crit Care Med 14:904–909
2. Lazarus G, Weis KH (1977) Herzfrequenz von Anaesthesisten unter physischer und psychischer beruflicher Belastung. Anaesthesist 26:375–380
3. Payne RL, Rick JT (1986) Heart rate as an indicator of stress in surgeons and anaesthetists. J Psychosom 30:411–419
4. Woitowitz HJ, Obersteiner A, Kindermann G, Roitowitz R (1972) Radiotelemetrische Untersuchungen von Herzschlagfrequenz, Elektrokardiogramm und Hauttemperatur bei operativ tätigen Gynäkologen. Arbeitsmed Sozialmed Arbeitshyg 7:168–173
5. Woitowitz HJ, Mrusek R, Dittrich H, Leutschaft R, Woitowitz R (1972) Radiotelemetrische Untersuchungen von Herzschlagfrequenz, Elektrokardiogramm und Hauttemperatur während chirurgischer Tätigkeit. Herz Kreisl 4:165–169

Multimodal Monitoring of Evoked Potentials in Subarachnoid Hemorrhage Following a Ruptured Aneurysm

P. Christophis, K. Roosen, A. Hüfner, and J. Dings[1]

Introduction

The most frequent causes of mortality and morbidity after aneurysmal subarachnoid hemorrhage (SAH) are, on the one hand, cerebral ischemia caused by a posthemorrhage vasopathy [3] and, on the other hand, the primary acute increase in intracranial pressure (ICP) due to the rupture [19, 20] and secondary posthemorrhage increase due to swelling or, most frequently, the disresorptive increase in ICP [3, 20].

Examinations on humans indicate that a reduction of the cerebral blood flow (CBF) below 30 ml/100 g per minute causes changes of evoked potentials (EPs), in fact, of the central conduction time (CCT) after n. medianus stimulation [15]. In addition, changes in EPs can also be registered even when the ICP increases [2, 10, 11, 18, 22]. They probably indicate a generalized or regionalized disorder in the CBF.

Measuring the blood flow velocity (BFV) by Doppler sonography after SAH can also be accorded the same significance [6].

Moreover, measuring the BFV in the basal cerebral arteries by Doppler sonography only corresponds to the brain perfusion under certain conditions [2, 9, 21].

In view of these considerations, it would be possible, by recording changes in several EPs, to register changes in the cerebral perfusion disorders or hypoxic conditions. A further intention was to find correlations to changes in BFV in the large cerebral arteries and to neurological outcomes.

In addition, we attempted to make a prognosis concerning survival and the possible occurrence of neurological deficits (ischemic damage) based on the changes in EPs.

Materials and Methods

Forty patients suffering SAH after a ruptured aneurysm were included in our study. Their mean age was 56 years (ranging from 41 to 72); 16 patients were male, 24 female. The aneurysm had been ruptured an average of 1.8 days prior to admission, the range being 0.5–5 days. Using Hunt and Hess grading [7], they tended to be

[1] Neurochirurgische Klinik, Justus-Liebig-Universität Gießen, Klinikstr. 29, W–6300 Gießen, FRG.

Advances in Neurosurgery, Vol. 20
K. Piscol, M. Klinger, M. Brock (Eds.)

classified higher than II (3 patients grade I, 12 patients grade II, 13 patients grade III, 7 patients grade IV, and 5 patients grade V).

Fifteen of the aneurysms established angiographically were detected in the area of the anterior communicating artery, 9 in the middle cerebral artery area, 11 in the internal carotid artery area, and 5 in the region of the posterior circulation including the vertebrobasilar region.

Thirty-five patients were treated operatively with aneurysm clipping, as a rule within 48 h or as soon as their condition had improved to Hunt and Hess grade between II and III. The other patients could not undergo surgery on account of their poor clinical condition.

Methods

In all these patients the acoustically evoked potentials (AEPs), the somatosensory EP after n. medianus (M-SSEP) and n. tibialis (T-SSEP) stimulation, and flash visual EPs (vEP) were examined in accordance with standardized methods [14]. Doppler sonography was used to measure the blood flow in all basal brain arteries [6]. The multimodal monitoring was performed on hospital admission or preoperatively, postoperatively, and on the 1st, 2nd, 6th, 8th, and 10th day after the operation or, in the case of patients who did not undergo surgery, at the same intervals.

Further examinations were carried out at intervals of 3–4 days or sooner if acute neurological deterioration or rebleeding thus dictated.

Comparative Groups

The examination findings of each modality were divided into three groups: those who always had normal findings, those with suspect and transient pathological findings, and the last group who always had clear pathological findings.

These findings were then compared with the Glasgow Coma (GC) scores and the neurological deficit. To facilitate the comparison the GC scale was split into larger groups, i.e., one group with the lowest (3–5 points), another with medium (6–10 points), and another with the best score (11–15 points). The neurological deficit can be classified as a sensomotory deficit/hemosyndrome or as a midbrain syndrome. The latter not only includes the midbrain syndrome in the classic sense of stretch and bend automatism, but also considered the symptoms indicating a nuclear lesion. If there was another simultaneous sensomotor deficit, the midbrain syndrome was given higher priority.

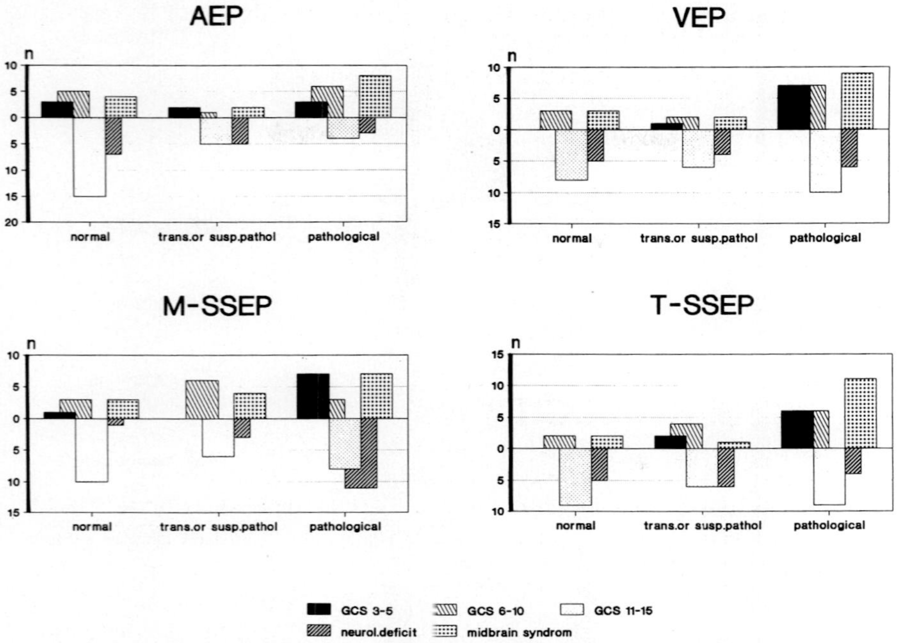

Fig. 1. Correlations of EP changes with clinical findings in patients with SAH following aneurysmal rupture. The best correlation seems to be between the M-SSEP and neurological deficit (including midbrain syndrome)

Results

Only one-third had a clearly pathological AEP. The changes established in AEPs constituted a pathological interpeak latency I–III and I–IV and a reduction in wave amplitude III. A loss of the potential was associated with a bulbary cerebral syndrome or with brain death ($n=4$). No close connection between the AEP changes and the GC score groups or AEP changes and the neurological deficits could be established (Fig. 1). It was, however, often the case that a lower GC score and a more frequent midbrain syndrome was registered when AEP findings were pathological.

Clear changes in the VEP could be established in just over half of the patients (Fig. 1). A comparison between VEP changes and neurological findings did not show a gradual relation. However, when comparing GC scores with VEP changes, lower scores were clearly more frequent, and additionally there was a more frequent incidence of midbrain syndrome in pathological VEP findings. These changes corresponded to an increase in latency and a reduction in wave amplitude P 100 of the VEP.

In three patients these changes were attributable to hemorrhages in the eyeground. VEP loss was found, however, not only in brain death ($n=4$), but also in

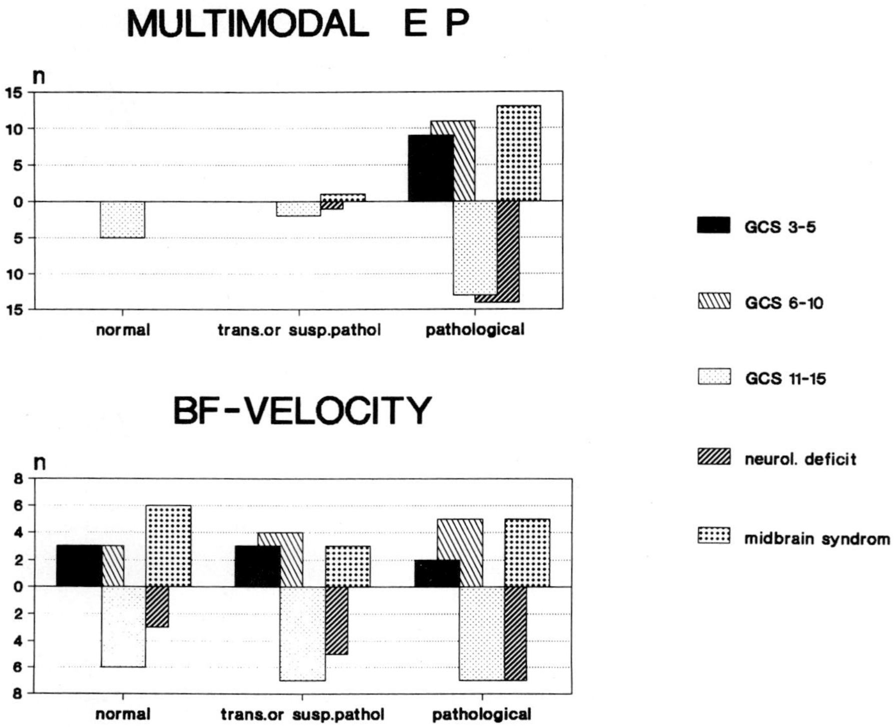

Fig. 2. Correlations of multimodal EP and BFV changes with clinical findings. Multimodal EP changes showed clearly a better clinical correlation in comparison with BFV findings

some cases with midbrain syndrome ($n=3$) and in hemorrhage of the eyeground ($n=2$).

The conditions in T-SSEPs were similar to those of VEP (Fig. 1). The changes recorded were an increase in latency and reduction in amplitude as far as a loss of the cortical potential. The latter could be registered in brain death ($n=4$), midbrain syndrome ($n=2$), or in leg paraparesis.

The best correlation to clinical investigation findings and especially to the neurological deficit was shown by the changes of the M-SSEPs (Fig. 1). Pathological EP findings were always associated with a neurological deficit.

The loss of the bilateral cortical potential of the M-SSEP was connected to a bulbary cerebral syndrome or brain death ($n=4$). After considering all modalities of the EPs (Fig. 2), an improvement in the correlation between clinical findings and EPs was realized so that no more pseudonegative results were found.

When assessing individual developments, it was possible only in four cases to discover or predict a neurological deficit on the basis of the EPs. This means that peristency or deterioration of the pathological EP findings warned of clinically manifest neurological disorders.

Table 1. Quotients of pseudonegative and pseudopositive findings in evoked potentials (EP) and blood flow velocity (BFV)

Quotient	AEP	MSSEP	TSSEP	VEP	BFV
$n_{.np}/n_{.en}$	$\underline{0.49}$	0.28	$\underline{0.64}$	$\underline{0.73}$	$\underline{0.75}$
$n_{.gcps}/n_{.en}$	0.35	0.28	0.18	0.27	$\underline{0.50}$
$n_{.nn}/n_{.ep}$	0.15	0.0	0.21	0.37	0.14
$n_{.gcns}/n_{ep}$	0.30	$\underline{0.44}$	0.37	$\underline{0.42}$	$\underline{0.50}$

Underlined numerals signify high quotients.
gCPS, Glasgow Coma Score 3–10; gCNS, Glasgow Coma Score 11–15; nP, Neurological findings pathological; nN, neurological findings normal; eP, examination pathological; eN, examination normal.

In contrast to the findings of the EPs, the blood flow measured by Doppler sonography showed no clear correlation to the clinical findings, although all basal arteries were taken into account (Fig. 2). A neurological deficit could, however, be registered more frequently in clearly pathological BFVs. No connection could be made between the EP findings and the Doppler sonography findings, as was expected (Fig. 2).

The study thus far makes clear that in the individual modalities of EPs, and also in the Doppler sonographic examinations, pseudopositive and pseudonegative findings can occur.

To compare the individual methods quotients were used. Pseudonegative results were thus expressed by means of a quotient from the number of patients with a GC score from 3 to 10 points ($n_{.gcps}$) or patient group with neurological deficits ($n_{.np}$) and the number of those with clearly normal examination findings ($n_{.en}$) (Table 1). Pseudopositive results were represented by the quotient of the patient group with a GC score above 11 points ($n_{.gcns}$) or with normal neurological findings ($n_{.nn}$) and the total number of patients with findings that were clearly pathological ($n_{.ep}$) (Table 1).

In all EPs, except the M-EP, a high quotient of pseudonegative results was obtained in connection to the neurological deficits, whereas with GC scores, only the blood flow yielded an obviously pseudonegative quotient.

A high pseudopositive quotient can, in contrast, only be found with regard to GC scores (M-SSEP, VEP, and BFV). In other respects, all the methods showed a close correlation between pathological examination findings and actual neurological deficits.

Discussion

Our studies conform to observations of other authors [9, 17, 21] in that only clearly pathological findings in the BFV have a connection to neurological deficits. A correlation can also be easily established between M-SSEP findings and neurological disorders in both our work and that of others [5, 8, 13, 16].

It is by monitoring the VEPs, T-SSEPs, evoked SSEPs, and AEPs and by recording the BFV with Doppler sonography that many pseudopositive and negative results can also be detected in connection to the GS score and neurological disorders. Only by considering all the modalities of the EP monitoring can pseudonegative results be ruled out in our subjects. The number of patients with pathological multimodal EP findings without neurological disorders (pseudopositive findings) is, however, relatively high ($n=6$, ca. 18%).

Whereas the so-called pseudopositive results could be an indicator for the sensitivity of a certain method, i.e., pathological findings could warn of imminently dangerous conditions, the pseudonegative results show that one method is not suitable. Thus, multimodal monitoring of EPs seems to be more valuable than measuring the BFV of all the basal cerebral arteries. The bilateral loss of AEP and cortical M-SSEP as in traumatic brain damage obviously signifies a poor survival prognosis [1, 4, 12]. The bilateral loss of VEP, however, also means in some cases a midbrain syndrome or a retinal hemorrhage connected to the SAH, and the bilateral loss of the cortical T-SSEP additionally means bilateral cortical damage in the supply area of the anterior cerebral artery on both sides.

As far as the prognosis is concerned, we had indications in our own patients that EPs can warn of neurological disorders, or, if pathological findings increase, neurological disorders might ensue. On the other hand, neurological defects or ischemic brain damage could never be established in normal findings after multimodal EPs. The only exception to this is when aphasia or psychosyndrome occur in small, computed tomographically established cortical defects near the motoric speech area or in the regions that normally show no neurological deficits.

Provided that these hypotheses are confirmed by other studies, the multimodal EPs must be accorded a special significance in observing patients with SAH caused by aneurysm rupture. Accordingly, multimodally monitored EPs can warn of imminent ischemia, can complement Hunt and Hess grading, and represent to a large degree the neurological status of patients who are not able to undergo a neurological examination.

Conclusion

Multimodal studies of EPs parallel to BFV measurements in 40 patients with aneurysmal SAH have illustrated that normal findings of single EPs and BFV readings in all basal cerebral arteries cannot completely rule out the possibility of regional ischemia.

Only strikingly pathological findings resulting from these examinations of individual EPs and BFV are relevant and point to vasopathy or generalized or regional ischemia.

Multimodal EPs can expose actual or imminent ischemia and can also exclude the existence of cerebral ischemia. In some cases, they can even be helpful in making a statement on survival prognosis (loss of EPs).

Although in some cases it seems possible to estimate a permanent neurological deficit, more studies on a wider range of patients is required to render the information more precise.

References

1. Adelt A, Bühl G (1989) On the prognosis of severe head injury using multimodal evoked potentials. In: Frowein RA, Brock M, Klinger M (eds) Advances in neurosurgery, vol 17. Springer, Berlin Heidelberg New York Tokyo, pp 107–111
2. Ahmed I (1980) Brainstem auditory evoked potentials in transtentorial herniation. Clinical Electroencephalography 11 (1):34–37
3. Arnold H, Nowak G, Schwachenwald R (1990) Subarachnoidalblutung: Verbesserte Prognose dank Frühoperation, Kalzium-Antagonisten, Vermehrung des zirkulierenden Blutvolumens und Senkung der Blutviskosität. Jahrbuch der Neurochirurgie. Biermann, Zülpich
4. Christophis P, Csécsei G, Klug N (1989) Prognostic significance of somatosensory evoked potentials in traumatic brain stem lesions. In: Frowein RA, Brock M, Klinger M (eds) Advances in neurosurgery, vol 17. Springer, Berlin Heidelberg New York Tokyo, pp 102–106
5. Despland PA, REgli F (1985) Somatosensory evoked response changes in patients with unilateral vascular lesions. In: Morocutti C, Rizzo PA (eds) Evoked potentials, neurophysiological and clinical aspects. Elsevier, Amsterdam, pp 57–66
6. Harders A (1986) Vasospasm and aneurysm surgery. In: Harders A (ed) Neurosurgical applications of transcranial Doppler sonography. Springer, Wien New York, pp 40–64
7. Hunt WE, Hess RM (1968) Surgical risk as related to time of intervention in the repair of intracranial aneurysms. J Neurosurg 28:14–20
8. Jarratt JA, Jakubowski J, Blaszczyk B (1985) The value of somatosensory evoked potentials in the preoperative assessment of patients with subarachnoid hemorrhage. In: Morocutti C, Rizzo PA (eds) Evoked potentials, neurophysiological and clinical aspects. Elsevier, Amsterdam, pp 69–76
9. Laumer R. Steinmeier R, Gönner F, Fahlbusch R, Schramm J, Mück M, Hinkelmann B, Purracker M (1991) Perioperative monitoring of subarachnoid hemorrhage: transcranial Doppler sonography and somatosensory evoked potentials. In: Bock WJ, Lumenta Ch, Brock M, Klinger M (eds) Advances in neurosurgery, vol 19: Springer, Berlin Heidelberg New York Tokyo, pp 17–19
10. Nagao S, Sunami N, Tsutsui T, Honma Y, Monma F, Nishimura T, Nishimoto A (1984) Diagnosis of uncal herniation by auditory brain-stem response. Neurologia Medico-Chirurgica 24:396–400
11. Nagata K, Tazawa T, Mizukami M, Araki G (1984) Application of brainstem auditory evoked potentials to evaluation of cerebral herniation. In: Nodar RH, Barber C (eds) Evoked potentials II. The second International Evoked Potentials Symposium. Butterworths, Boston London Sydney, pp 183–193
12. Papanicolaou AC, Loring DW, Eisenberg HM (1986) Auditory brain stem evoked responses in comatose head-injured patients. Neurosurgery 18 (2):172–175

13. Rosenstein J, Wang AD, Symon L, Suzuki M (1985) Relationship between hemispheric cerebral blood flow central conduction time, and clinical grade in aneurysmal subarachnoid hemorrhage. J Neurosurg 62 (1):25–30
14. Stöhr M, Dichganz J, Diemer HC, Büttner VW (1989) Evozierte Potentiale, 2. überarb erw Aufl. Springer, Berlin Heidelberg New York Tokyo
15. Symon L, Momma F (1987) Relationships between cerebral perfusion and electrical activity in man. In: Wüllenweber R, Klinger M, Brock M (eds) Advances in neurosurgery, vol 15. Springer, Berlin Heidelberg New York, pp 32–34
16. Symon L, Wang AD, Costa e Silva I, Gentili F (1984) Perioperative use of somatosensory evoked responses in aneurysm surgery. J Neurosurg 60:269–275
17. Symon L, Compton J, Redmond S et al. (1986) Bedside monitoring in subarachnoid hemorrhage: evoked responses, hemispheral blood flow, and flow velocity measurements. In: Wilkins RH (ed) Cerebral vasospasm. Raven, New York, pp 73–78
18. Tsutsui T, Avila A, Symon L, Ono M, Wang A, Kalmanchey R (1986) The effects of a supratentorial mass lesion on brain stem auditory evoked potentials and short latency somatosensory evoked potentials. Neurol Res 8 (1):7–13
19. Volby B (1986) Cerebral vasospasm and ICP, cerebral vascular surgery. In: Organizing committee (eds) Proceedings of the EANS course in Neurosurgery, Porto Sept. 6–12. Bial, Porto
20. Voldby B, Enevoldsen EM, Jensen FT (1985) Regional cerebral blood flow, intraventricular pressure, and cerebral metabolism in patients with ruptured intracranial aneurysms. J Neurosurg 62:8–58
21. Wranze-Bielefeld E, Dauch WA, Bauer BL (1990) Discrepancy between the results of TCD and the clinical status of patients after SAH. In: Bushe KA, Brock M, Klinger M (eds) Advances in neurosurgery, vol 18. Springer, Berlin Heidelberg New York Tokyo, pp 276–280
22. York DH, Pulliam MW, Rosenfeld JG, Watts C. Relationship between visual evoked potentials and intracranial presure. J Neurosurg 55:909–916

Necessity of Control Angiography After Aneurysm Surgery

J. Schmitt and A. Spring[1]

Introduction

Recent technical innovations have allowed neurosurgeons to make significant advances in the surgical treatment of cerebral aneurysms, and direct surgical obliteration by clipping is the treatment of choice for most aneurysms. However, cases of failed aneurysm surgery are still published, caused either by slipped or unexpectedly imperfect clip or difficulties which some aneurysms present because of anatomical reasons [4–6, 9, 14].

In spite of these well-known problems, there is no clear statement in the recent literature regarding the necessity of control angiography after aneurysm surgery. Considering the high percentage of incompletely treated aneurysms [6, 9, 15], and confirmed by our experiences we present in the following report, we think that postoperative angiography is still necessary, and it should be routine to check the results and efficiency of surgery.

Material and Methods

Between 1984 and 1990, 84 patients were operated on for 87 cerebral aneurysms following spontaneous subarachnoid hemorrhage (SAH). The mean age was 47.1 years, ranging from 24 to 72. There were 35 males and 49 females. In 48 of the patients hypertension was noticed. The most common location for aneurysms was the anterior communicating artery followed by the middle cerebral artery and the internal carotid artery. In ten patients an additional aneurysm was present; the aneurysm which had ruptured could usually be determined by an irregular angiographic appearance of its fundus and the pattern of SAH on CT scan.

Table 1 shows the preoperative condition according to the classification of Hunt and Hess [10] and the localization of the aneurysms. Our clinical data generally agree with those of the literature [3, 12, 13].

A four-vessel angiography by transfemoral procedure under local anesthesia was attempted initially in all of the patients to verify the location of the aneurysms. In most of the cases the first angiogram showed the aneurysms: in two cases with a

[1] Neurochirurgische Klinik, Leopoldina-Krankenhaus, Gustav-Adolf-Str. 8, W-8720 Schweinfurt, FRG.

Advances in Neurosurgery, Vol. 20
K. Piscol, M. Klinger, M. Brock (Eds.)

negative angiographic exploration, the aneurysms could be confirmed in the control angiogram.

Thirty-five of the patients were operated on within the first 72 h, 19 patients between the 4th and 21st day, and 33 patients later than 3 weeks after the SAH, including 3 additional nonruptured aneurysms treated subsequently by a second elective operation.

The occlusion of the aneurysms was performed with Sugita clips, and the patients were operated on by or with the assistance of the same operator.

Postoperatively in 50 of the 87 cases a control angiography was performed; another control had to be broken off because of temporary neurological deficits. The other patients refused the control. The control angiographies were carried out between 3 weeks and 11 months postoperatively with an average time of 3.2 months.

Results

In 71 of the 87 aneurysms operated, we had the intraoperative impression of a safe clipping. In 16 cases a definite occlusion with a complete exclusion of the sac from the circulation did not seem to be possible, most likely due to a complicated anatomy. In cases of broad-based or fusiform aneurysms or cases where the main branches of the artery embraced the aneurysm, remnants of the base must be accepted to maintain flow in branches supplying critical cortical areas. These aneurysms were partially clipped and coated by pieces of muscle or plastic, stabilized with cyanoacrylate to the clip.

Postoperatively in 50 patients a control angiography was performed. Instead of 42 expected cases, only in 27 was a complete occlusion of the aneurysms shown. Surprisingly, three of the aneurysms considered intraoperatively to be possibly not

Table 1. Localization of the aneurysms according to the preoperative clinical grading of Hunt and Hess

Localization	I	II	III	IV	V	*n*
A. com. ant.	8	11	7	1	–	27
A. cerebri media	4	8	9	3	–	24
A. carotis interna	6	12	3	1	1	23
A. pericallosa	1	1	1	1	–	4
A. cerebri ant.	–	3	1	–	–	4
A. cerebri post.	–	–	2	–	–	2
A. vertebralis	–	2	–	–	–	2
A. basilaris	–	1	–	–	–	1
Total no. of patients	19	38	23	6	1	87

Table 2. Results after aneurysm clipping

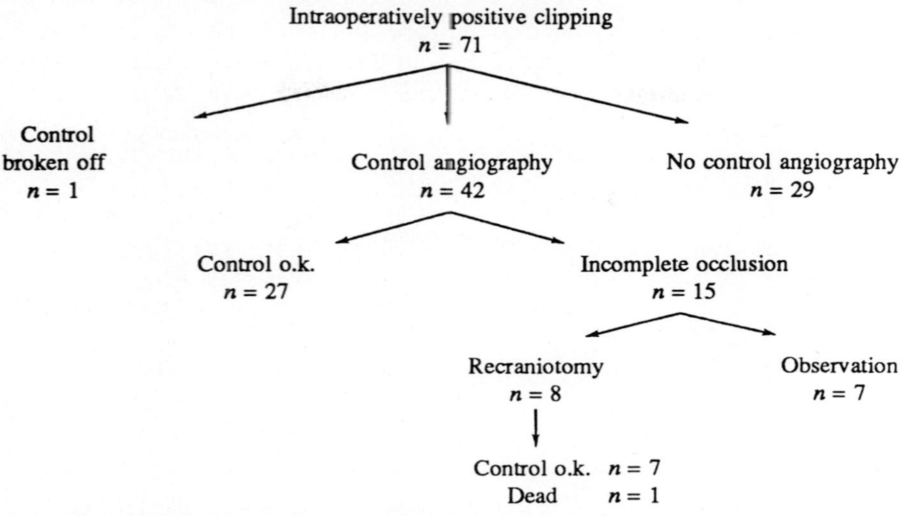

closed were completely occluded in the control angiography. In total, only 30 of the 50 aneurysms controlled (60%) were completely occluded.

In the group of the 20 partially clipped aneurysms, 10 patients were not operated on, but observed. The remnants of the base were either very small (2–3 mm) or a sufficient occlusion did not seem to be possible for anatomical reasons. In the other ten cases a recraniotomy was performed. Intraoperatively in two cases a slipped clip was noticed; in the other eight cases the clips were not well placed, and a significant remnant of the base of the aneurysm was seen. In all these ten cases, it was possible to close the aneurysms totally by clip replacement or additional clip. In nine cases postoperatively, a complete occlusion by control angiography was proved; one patient died of brain swelling. The results are summarized in Tables 2 and 3.

Concerning the 50 control angiographies, the best correlation between the visual intraoperative impression and the objective results of postoperative control angiograms was found for the internal carotid artery aneurysms: 12 of 16 that seemed to be clipped aneurysms were totally occluded. In comparison with the difficulties of occluding the sac, the greatest difficulties were encountered with aneurysms of the anterior communicating artery: only 7 of 15 supposed aneurysms were satisfactorily clipped. Figure 1 shows the results of the 50 control angiographies.

The early postoperative outcome was mainly dependent on the preoperative clinical condition. The result was good in 43 cases, fair in 29 cases, and poor in 3 cases. Seven patients had a rebleeding after aneurysm clipping (8.6%). The mortality was 10.7% ($n = 9$). Five patients died of rebleeding and four of postoperative vasospasm and untreatable brain swelling. One patient died of a recurrent SAH, caused by an

Table 3. Results after aneurysm clipping

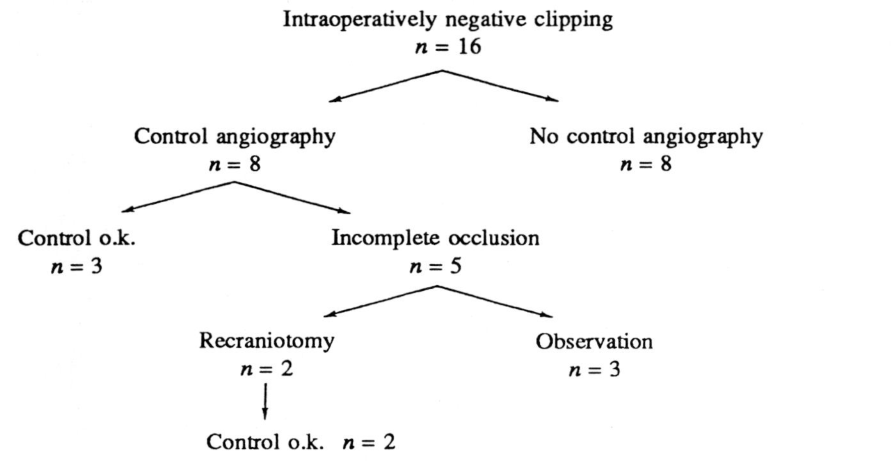

unknown additional aneurysm which was found only at the postmortem examination.

With the improved techniques, cerebral angiography has become a relatively safe procedure. Evaluating 148 angiograms, performed in our 84 patients, the overall incidence of complications was nearly 2% ($n = 3$), and the complications were in all cases light and transient [7, 11, 14].

Discussion

Already nearly 30 years ago the doubts experienced by every brain surgeon about a seemingly well-placed clip on the neck of an aneurysm led Allcock and Drake to urgently demand postoperative angiography [1]. Drake and Vanderlinden reported in 1967 the late consequences of incomplete surgical treatment of cerebral aneurysms [5]. They considered postoperative angiographic control as a part of the surgical treatment and demanded a further operation on incompletely occluded aneurysms.

Confirmed by our results, we also carry out a control angiography some months after aneurysm surgery, even if we were sure that the aneurysms were completely clipped. The control may show, sometimes quite unexpectedly, that the sac has not been completely obliterated. A clip may be merely misplaced, not be closed tightly enough, or slipped. In our series of 50 patients who underwent postoperative angiography, contrast filling of a significant part of the sac or slipped off clips still occurred in 20 cases (40%) despite modern neurosurgery. Recraniotomy was carried out in ten cases with satisfactory obliteration of the aneurysms in all patients. An incompletely obliterated aneurysm with a significant unoccluded remnant of the base should be reoperated as soon as possible, if the anatomical situation promises

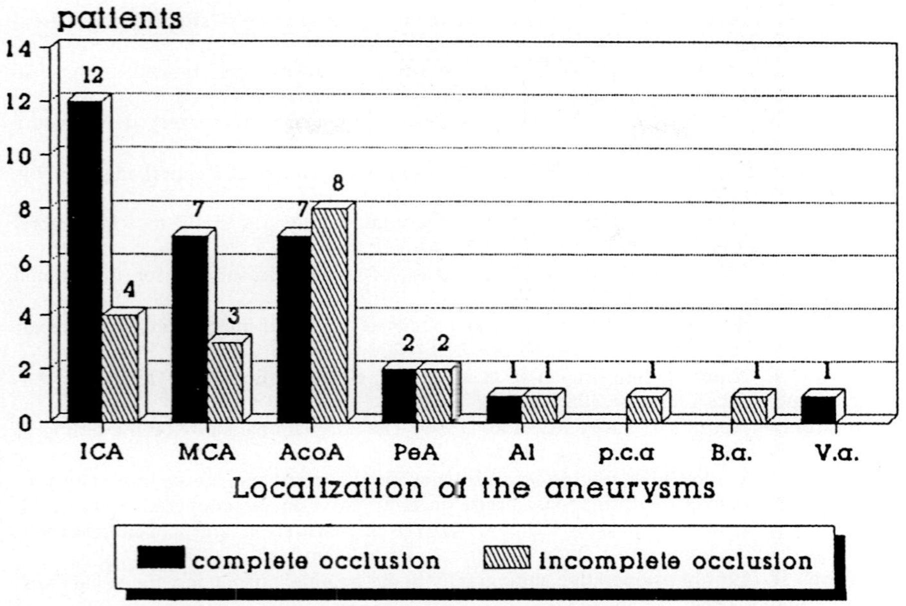

Fig. 1. Results of 50 control angiographic examinations

successful treatment. The risk of reoperation is far less than the possibility of another hemorrhage with awkward consequences [3, 5, 8, 13, 15]. We perform the control angiography not perioperatively as has been published by some authors [2, 8], but some months later. The reasons are, first, that regrowth of the sac may occur from significant remnants of the aneurysm with time, and second, the clips do not slip off early in the postoperative period [3–6, 9]. In selected cases in which visual intraoperative control was unsatisfactory, a control angiogram was performed earlier. In some cases, it was possible to close the aneurysm, which primarily seemed to be insufficiently treatable, completely after control angiography by a reexploration.

Regarding the literature and our results, we think that control angiography should be widely advocated as a routine procedure following surgery for intracranial aneurysms, despite the sophistication of modern operative techniques.

References

1. Allcock JM, Drake CG (1963) Postoperative angiography in cases of unruptured intracranial aneurysm. J Neurosurg 20:752–759
2. Bauer BL (1984) Intraoperative angiography in cerebral aneurysm and AV-malformation. Neurosurg Rev 7:209–217
3. Beverly JR, Sydney JP, Drake CG (1990) Surgical treatment of unruptured aneurysms of the posterior circulation. J Neurosurg 73:165–173

4. Drake CG, Allcock JM (1973) Postoperative angiography and the "slipped" clip. J Neurosurg 39:683–689
5. Drake CG, Vanderlinden RG (1967) The late consequences of incomplete surgical treatment of cerebral aneurysms. J Neurosurg 27:226–238
6. Drake CG, Friedman AH, Peerless SJ (1984) Failed aneurysm surgery. J Neurosurg 61:848–856
7. Earnest F, Forbes G, Sandock BA et al. (1984) Complications of cerebral angiography. AJR 142:247–253
8. Hillman J, Johansson I (1987) Per-operative angiography – a useful tool in cerebral aneurysm surgery? Acta Neurochir 84:39–42
9. Hollin SA, Decker RE (1973) Effectiveness of microneurosurgery for intracranial aneurysms. J Neurosurg 39:690–693
10. Hunt WE, Hess RM (1968) Surgical risk as related to time of intervention in the repair of intracranial aneurysms. J Neurosurg 28:14–20
11. Kachel R, Ritter H, Schiffmann R et al. (1980) Komplikationen bei zerebraler Angiographie. Zbl Chirurgie 105:504–512
12. Kassel NF, Torner JC, Haley EC et al. (1990) The international study on the timing of aneurysm surgery. J Neurosurg 73:18–47
13. Locksley HB (1969) Natural history of subarachnoid hemorrhage, intracranial aneurysm and arteriovenous malformations; based on 6368 cases in the cooperative study. In: Sahs AL, Perret GE, Locksley HB et al. (eds) Intracranial aneurysms and subarachnoid hemorrhage: a cooperative study. Lippincott, Philadelphia, pp 37–108
14. Steven JL (1966) Postoperative angiography in the treatment of intracranial aneurysms. Acta Radiol Diagn 5:536–548
15. Yasargil MG (1984) Efficacy of clipping. In: Yasargil MG (ed) Microneurosurgery, vol I. Thieme, Stuttgart, pp 263–264

Magnetic Resonance Angiography of Cerebral Artery Aneurysms: Present Capabilities and Limitations

B. Ostertun[1], L. Solymosi[1], H. Wassmann[2], and M. Reiser[1]

Purpose

Magnetic resonance angiography (MRA) as a new completely noninvasive vessel imaging modality has undergone continuous improvement over the last few years. Intracranial pathological findings such as arteriovenous malformations and aneurysms are challenging indications for this method due to their complex flow patterns and the smallness of relevant pathological vessels that have to be visualized to give the method acceptable clinical accuracy. Thus, the purpose of this study was the evaluation of MRA's capabilities and limitations in the identification of cerebral artery aneurysms with special respect to conventional X-ray angiography as the gold standard of cerebral vascular imaging.

Material and Method

With knowledge of the findings in cerebral CT, magnetic resonance imaging (MRI), and angiography, 25 patients with 32 cerebral aneurysms were submitted to 31 MRA examinations. Repetitive MRA was performed in five patients as control after operation or balloon occlusion treatment or – with an interval of 6 weeks – after negative result of a first MRA in a case of subarachnoid hemorrhage (SAH). MRA was performed with 1.5T (Philips S15/HP and S15/ACS) as well as 0.5T (Philips T5) systems employing 2D and 3D inflow acquisitions generating projection angiograms after maximum intensity projection (MIP), which can also be viewed as cineloop movies providing a superior spatial impression of anatomy. X-ray angiograms ($n = 28$) were available for comparison in all 25 patients.

Indications for MRA were SAH ($n = 8$), neurological deficits without SAH ($n = 8$), and accidental suspicious findings in CT ($n = 6$), MRI ($n = 2$), and angiography ($n = 1$). Restless patients or those in acute stages of SAH with respiratory insufficiency had to be excluded from this study. Most of them were examined with an interval of 7–10 days after the acute event.

[1] Radiologische Universitätsklinik, Sigmund-Freud.-Str. 25, W–5300 Bonn, FRG.
[2] Neurochirurgische Universitätsklinik, Sigmund-Freud-Str. 25, W–5300 Bonn, FRG.

Advances in Neurosurgery, Vol. 20
K. Piscol, M. Klinger, M. Brock (Eds.)

Table 1. MRA sensitivity and size of aneurysms

Size (mm)	MRA +	MRA –	Sum
< 5	3	6	9
– 10	7	–	7
– 15	2	–	2
– 20	5	–	5
– 25	5	–	5
– 30	2	–	2
> 30	2	–	2
	26	6	32

Table 2. MRA sensitivity and location of aneurysms

Artery	MRA +	MRA –	Sum
Internal carotid	16	–	16
Middle cerebral	5	2	7
Basilar	4	–	4
Anterior communicating	–	2	2
Ophthalmic	–	2	2
Posterior communicating	1	–	1
	26	6	32

Results

Conventional angiography depicted 32 aneurysms of various location and size (Tables 1 and 2). Three patients suffered from two aneurysms; one patient had four aneurysms of the basilar, internal carotid, anterior communicating, and middle cerebral arteries.

The smallest aneurysm detected by MRA was a posterior communicating artery aneurysm 3 mm in size that was not discovered in primary angiography and MRA 10 days after SAH. It was identified with both methods 6 weeks later (Fig. 3).

All aneurysms of more than 5-mm diameter were identified; six smaller ones were missed by MRA. The latter were aneurysms of the ophthalmic, anterior communicating, and middle cerebral arteries.

Signal intensity and signal distribution in the same aneurysm were significantly different in 2D and 3D scans.

In 3D scans the whole imaging volume is simultaneously and repetitively excited, whereas in a 2D scan single slices are subsequently exposed to HF pulses. Thus, blood of a given velocity in 3D is exposed longer to HF pulses with a saturation effect than in 2D scans, which means that slow flowing blood is partly saturated and loses signal in 3D scans.

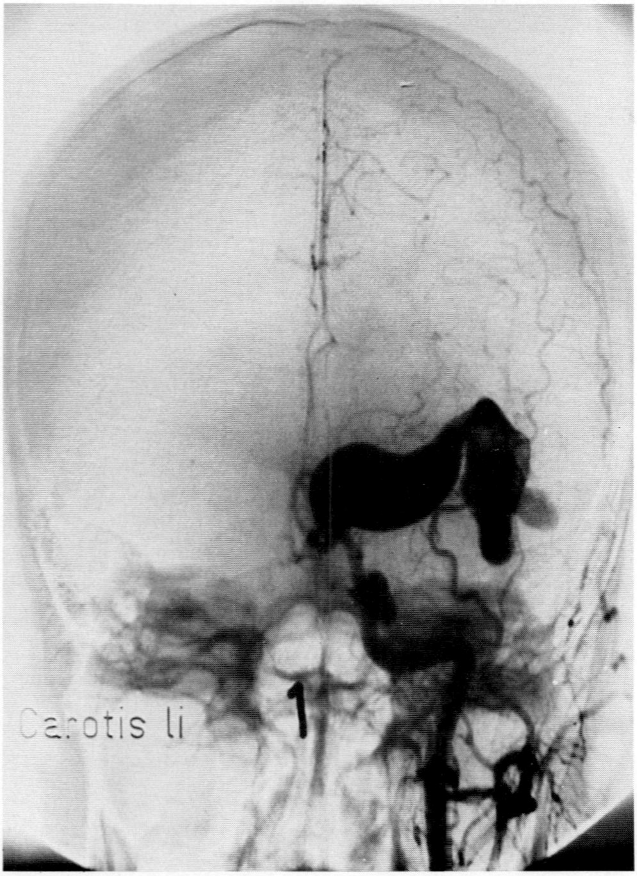

Fig. 1. Giant aneurysm of the left middle cerebral artery: X-ray angiography

2D scans (Figs. 1, 2, and 4) provided superior signal, especially when slow flow in the aneurysm was proved by persisting contrast throughout the venous phase in conventional angiography.

On the other hand, some aneurysms presented higher signal in 3D scans (Fig. 3) with lower echo times (TE). These aneurysms are supposed to have fast and more turbulent flow causing dephasing of spins, which is better visualized with very short TE.

Additional T1-weighted spin-echo images were necessary to detect the whole aneurysm extension in cases with partial thrombosis. In our 25 patients, thrombi were only visualized in these scans; in MRA scans they did not appear with high signal levels that would mimic flow in any case. Thus, high signal areas in MRA scans correlated well with contrasted aneurysm lumina in conventional angiography. In one patient after balloon occlusion of a lobed internal carotid artery

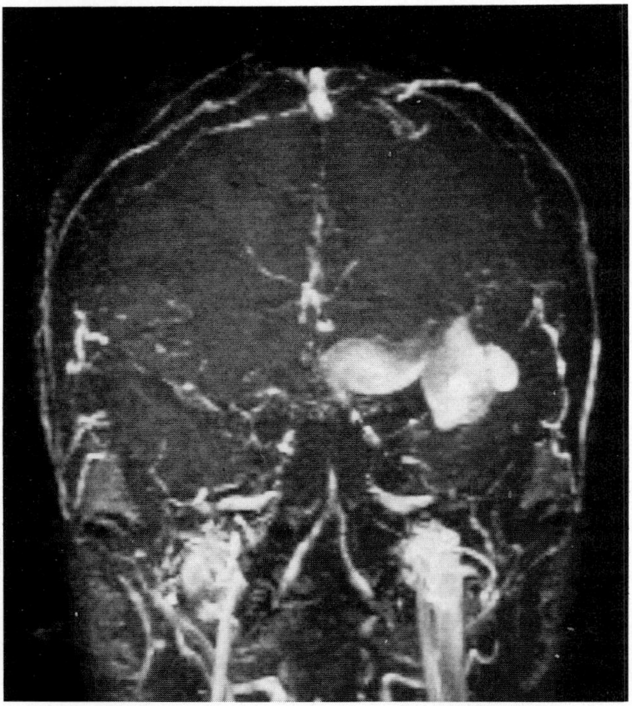

Fig. 2. Giant aneurysm of the left middle cerebral artery: 2D MRA; coronal acquisition; frontal projection

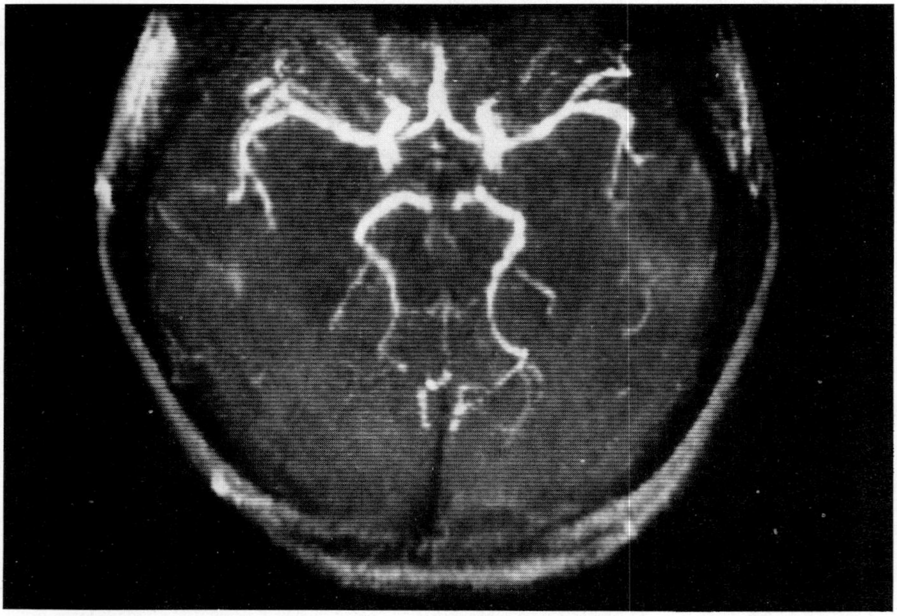

Fig. 3. 3-mm aneurysm of the left posterior communicating artery: 3D MRA; axial acquisition; projection rotated around transverse axis

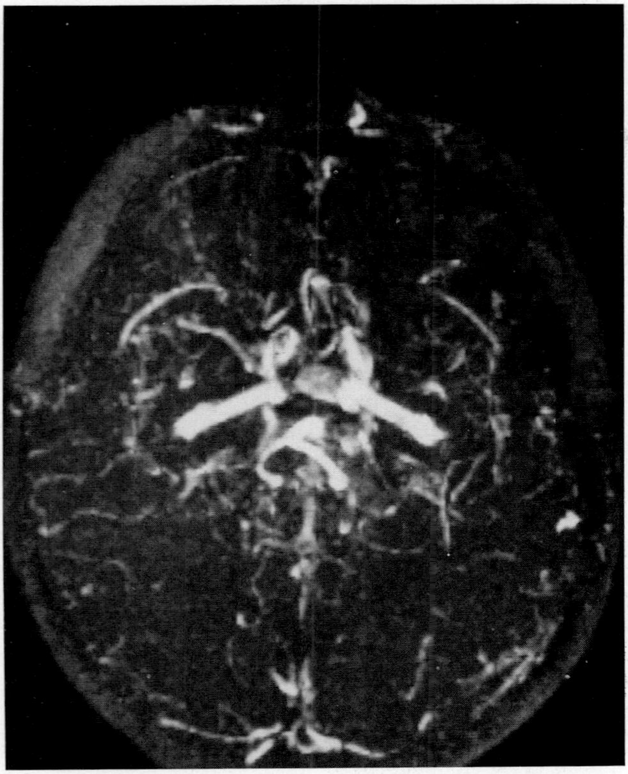

Fig. 4. 12-mm aneurysm of the left internal carotid artery; 2D MRA; axial acquisition; axial projection

aneurysm, a persisting lumen of irregular shape was detected by MRA and proved by conventional angiography.

Conclusion

A combination of 2D and 3D inflow MRA with T1-weighted MRI is highly sensitive in the detection of cerebral aneurysms bigger than 5 mm [2, 3]. 3D acquisitions with short TE and small partitions better depict small aneurysms and those with fast and turbulent flow, whereas 2D acquisitions are superior in detecting large aneurysms with long recirculation of blood. Additional MRI is necessary to evaluate partial thrombosis [1, 5].

Although MRA as a completely noninvasive imaging modality without any risk for the patient is an alternative to invasive angiography in principle, up to now it cannot replace this gold standard in cerebral indications for several reasons.

Presently, there are technical limitations such as an inferior spatial resolution due to an imaging matrix of 256^2 or 512^2, and further reduction of TE and artifacts [4, 6] is necessary to improve accuracy of vessel delineation. Future development of MR hard- and software will solve these disadvantages at least partly. Especially a further increase in sensitivity of MRA in the detection of small aneurysms with diameters below 5 mm is necessary for clinical purposes and can be expected in the near future. Shorter scan times and better access to the head of the patient in smaller magnets such as the T5 system will allow examinations of intensive care patients in acute stages of SAH.

References

1. Biondi A, Scialfa G, Scotti G (1988) Intracranial aneurysms: MR imaging. Neuroradiology 30 (3):214–218
2. Pernicone JR, Siebert JE, Potchen EJ, Pera A, Dumoulin CL, Souza SP (1990) Three-dimensional phase-contrast MR angiography in the head and neck: preliminary report. AJNR 11 (3):457–466
3. Ross JS, Masaryk TJ, Modic MT, Ruggieri PM, Haacke EM, Selman WR (1990) Intracranial aneurysms: evaluation by MR angiography. Am J Roentgenol 155 (1):159–165
4. Ruggieri PM, Laub GA, Masaryk TJ, Modic MT (1989) Intracranial circulation: pulse-sequence considerations in three-dimensional (volume) MR angiography. Radiology 171 (3):785–791
5. Sevick RJ, Tsuruda JS, Schmalbrock P (1990) Three-dimensional time-of-flight MR angiography in the evaluation of cerebral aneurysms. J Comput Assist Tomogr 14 (6):874–881
6. Wagle WA, Dumoulin CL, Souza SP, Cline HE (1989) 3DFT MR angiography of carotid and basilar arteries. AJNR 10 (5):911–919

Differential Disturbances of Memory and Mood Following Striatum and Basal Forebrain Lesions in Patients with Ruptures of the Anterior Communicating Artery

E. Irle[1], B. Wowra[2], J. Kunert[1], M. Peper[1], J. Hampl[2], and S. Kunze[2]

Introduction

For a long time, it has been known that subarachnoid hemorrhage is likely to be followed by Korsakoff's syndrome [13]. However, in many of the patients the syndrome is transient. The remaining patients may show persistent anterograde memory deficits, as well as personality changes. This lasting syndrome is often referred to as ACoA (anterior communicating artery) syndrome because it is observed most often following the rupture and repair of an aneurysm of the ACoA [12].

However, the anatomical basis for the syndrome, especially for the memory deficits, is unsettled. Most authors stress the importance of lesions directly related to the territory of the ACoA (i.e., substantia innominata, diagonal band of Broca, ventral striatum); however, in many cases additional lesions were reported to be situated in the frontal cortex, septu, medial forebrain bundle fornix, anterior hypothalamus, and neostriatum [1, 3, 4 10].

The present study was undertaken to clarify the lesion loci necessary and sufficient to cause amnesia. We chose our subjects on the basis of their lesions from a population of subjects with subarachnoid hemorrhage, all having undergone treatment and follow-up evaluation at the neurosurgical department of the University of Heidelberg. The subjects were investigated neuropsychologically and compared with subjects with brain tumors in similar loci, and with control subjects without brain damage. The resulting samples were representative and indicated that basal forebrain lesions are necessary to cause amnesia, but are sufficient to cause amnesia only in the presence of additional lesions in the neostriatum.

Methods

Subjects

Thirty subjects were drawn from a population of 181 patients with subarachnoid hemorrhage, having undergone treatment (between 1983 and 1987) and follow-up

[1] Psychiatrische Universitätsklinik, Von-Siebold-Str. 5, W–3400 Göttingen, FRG.
[2] Neurochirurgische Universitätsklinik, Im Neuenheimer Feld 400, W–6900 Heidelberg, FRG.

Advances in Neurosurgery, Vol. 20
K. Piscol, M. Klinger, M. Brock (Eds.)

evaluation (in 1988) at the neurosurgical department of the University of Heidelberg. There were five experimental groups, consisting of 5 subjects with striate lesions (group STRIAT), 7 subjects with basal forebrain lesions (group BF), 5 subjects with striate and additional basal forebrain lesions (group STRIAT/BF), 6 subjects with basal forebrain and additional ventral frontal lesions (group BF/FRO), and 7 subjects with lesions of the striatum, basal forebrain, and ventral frontal cortex together (group STRIAT/BF/FRO). From a population of 263 patients with brain tumors having undergone treatment and neuropsychological evaluation at the same department, 20 patients were selected with lesions in the basal forebrain ($n=4$), basal forebrain and ventral frontal cortex ($n=8$), or striatum, basal forebrain, and ventral frontal cortex ($n=8$). All lesion groups were compared with a clinical control group (group CCG; 27 patients with surgery of an aneurysm of the ACoA having no visible lesions) and a normal control group (group NCG) of 30 subjects matched for age and education to all other groups.

Neuropsychological Tests

The testing took place during the follow-up evaluation (aneurysm patients) or 1 week postoperatively (tumor patients). General intellectual abilities were tested with a shortened version of the Wechsler Adult Intelligence Scale. Concentration and psychomotor speed were tested with the Stroop test and the trail making test. Possible receptive language disturbances were examined with the Token test. Special emphasis was laid on the assessment of memory functions. Verbal long-term memory was examined with a paired associate learning paradigm and the selective reminding test. Visual memory functions were assessed with the Benton visual retention test and a perceptual learning paradigm (Gollin's test). Personality and mood measurements included a shortened version of the MMPI and the Profile of Mood States (aneurysm patients), or the *Eigenschaftswörterliste* (tumor patients) (for a detailed description of all tests, see ref. [6]).

Results

Anatomical Findings

Representative lesions of aneurysm and tumor patients are given in Fig. 1. Lesions of the striatum generally covered parts of the head of the caudate nucleus (territory of Heubner's artery). In some cases, small areas of the anterior limb of the internal capsule or the rostral putamen were affected as well. Lesions of the basal forebrain covered parts of the substantia innominata, diagonal band of Broca, and ventral striatum, and in some subjects of groups BF and STRIAT/BF/FRO, also the septal area. Ventrofrontal lesions generally included the rectal and orbital gyri, and in some caes additionally dorsolateral frontal or cingulate areas. For all lesion groups, the lesion laterality (left, right, or bilateral) was represented equally.

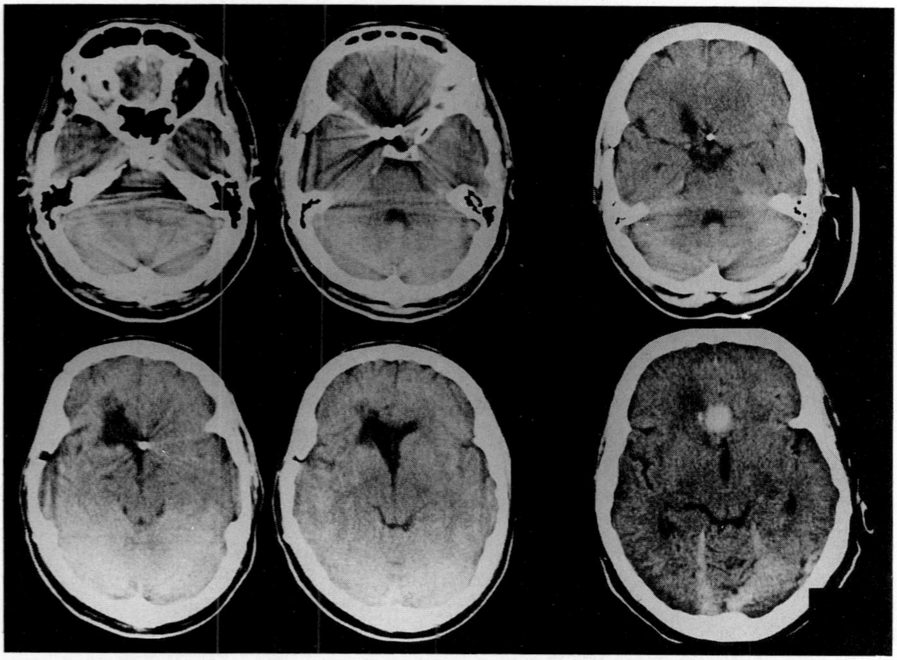

Fig. 1. Illustration of the lesions of one subject of group STRIAT/BF/FRO (aneurysm patient) (*left*) and of the lesions of two subjects of group BF (aneurysm patient, *top*; tumor patient, *bottom*) (*right*). The thickness of the CT scans is 8 mm. The right hemisphere is represented on the viewer's left

Neuropsychological Tests

Concerning the intellectual measures, the most pronounced differences appeared between groups with multiple lesions and those with single lesions. Whereas groups STRIAT and BF (aneurysm or tumor patients) were completely unimpaired in all tests under measurement, groups with multiple lesions were strongly impaired (Mann-Whitney U tests; $P < 0.05$). Concerning the memory designs, the most pronounced deficits appeared in groups STRIAT/BF and STRIAT/BF/FRO (aneurysm or tumor patients) (cf. Fig. 2). The tests for attention and psychomotor speed revealed the strongest deficits in group BF(FRO (aneurysm or tumor patients) ($P < 0.05$) (cf. Fig. 3). The general intelligence was mildly impaired in all multiple lesion groups; language capabilities were entirely normal in all groups studied. Aneurysm and tumor patients differed in that aneurysm patients showed stronger memory deficits and tumor patients stronger attention deficits.

The personality and mood measurements revealed, in contrast to the intellectual measurements, the most pronounced changes in groups STRIAT and STRIAT/BF. Subjects of these groups obtained significantly ($P < 0.05$) elevated scores on the scales "schizophrenia," "hypomania," "psychasthenia," "psychopathic deviate," and

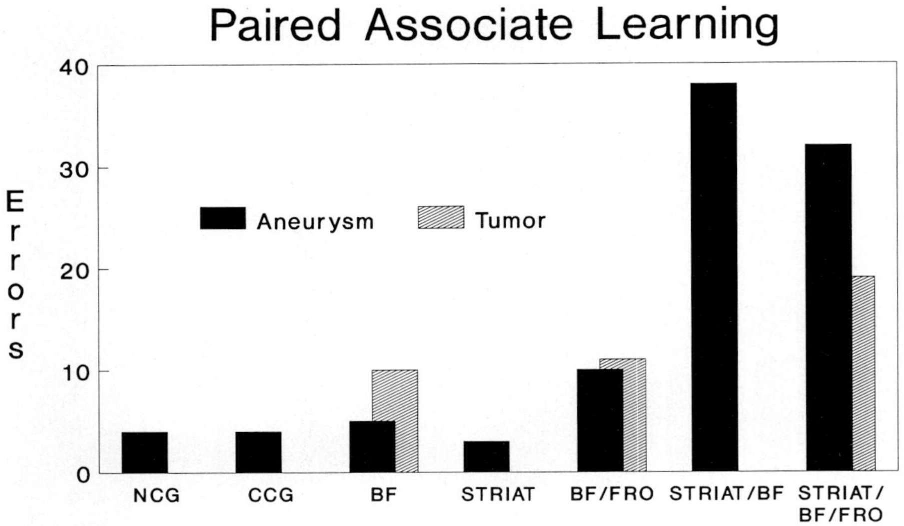

Fig. 2. Results of the paired associate learning. Errors performed during the recall and recognition of ten pairs of words are given. The maximum number of possible errors is 80. *NCG*, normal control group; *CCG*, clinical control group; *BF*, basal forebrain-lesioned group; *STRIAT*, striatum-lesioned group; *BF/FRO*, basal forebrain/ventral frontal-lesioned group; *STRIAT/BF*, striatum/basal forebrain-lesioned group; *STRIAT/BF/FRO*, striatum/basal forebrain/ventral frontal-lesioned group

"anger/hostility" (cf. Fig. 4). The remaining lesion groups, as well as the clinical control group, showed elevated "depression" scores, but normal scores on the other scales mentioned above.

Discussion

Mnemonic Deficits

Our results clearly show that the mnemonic deficits following ACoA ruptures are not solely due to lesions of the basal forebrain region, as suggested earlier [1, 3, 4]. Neither basal forebrain nor striate lesions alone seem to be sufficient to cause substantial mnemonic deficits. In the memory designs, both groups STRIAT and BF were unimpaired compared with the clinical as well as with the normal control group (cf. Fig. 2). However, combined striate and basal forebrain lesions seem to be necessary and sufficient to produce amnesia. Ventromedial frontal lesions seem to add little to the deficit, as suggested earlier [1, 3]. Perhaps the basal forebrain and the striatum form links of different pathways related to mnemonic information processing. Research with nonhuman primates indicates that, besides a corticolimbic pathway using the basal forebrain region as a link between association

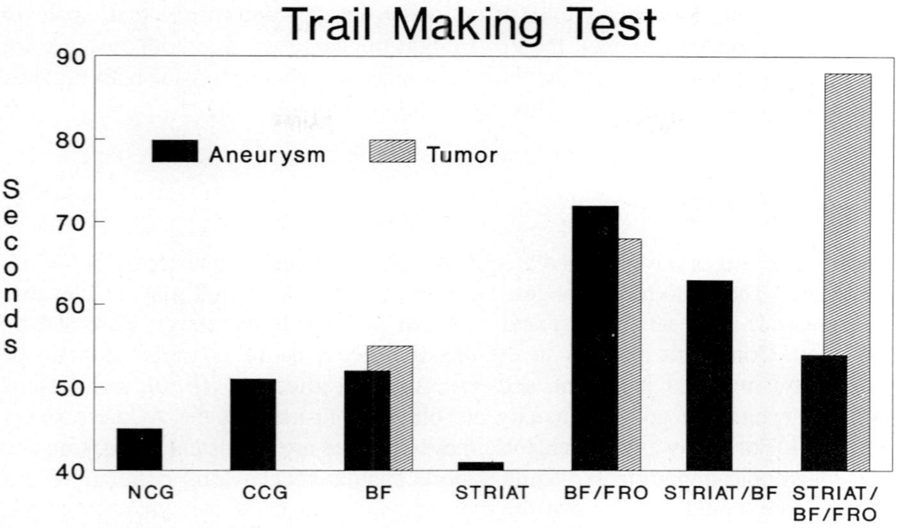

Fig. 3. Results of the trail making test. Seconds needed to complete part A are given. Abbreviations as in Fig. 2

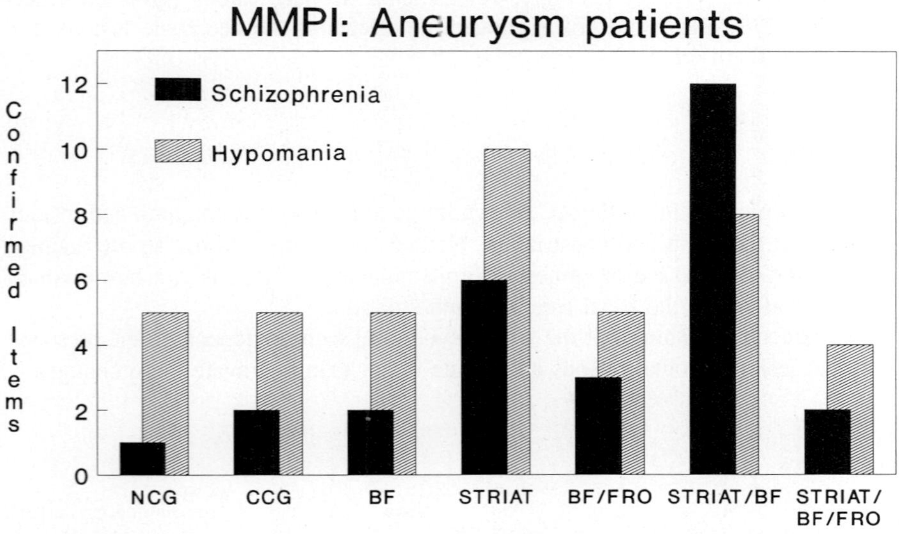

Fig. 4. Results of the MMPI scales "schizophrenia" and "hypomania." Numbers of confirmed items are given. Abbreviations as in Fig. 2

cortex and ventral temporal lobe [8], a corticostriate system may participate in learning and memory as well [5, 9]. It might be suggested that both systems are able to compensate for a dysfunction of the other, but that lesions of both systems together, however small, lead to unrecoverable mnemonic deficits.

Personality and Mood Changes

Emotional changes are observed frequently after the rupture and repair of ACoA aneurysms. The pattern of changes, however, is variable. Mood may be elevated or depressed, interests (e.g., sexual or food) and levels of energy increased or decreased. Consistent changes to the negative occur in the cognitive domain of personality: impaired judgment, self-criticism, and affective control, and loss of social independence and spontaneity are observed in most of the ACoA patients [3, 7, 10]. For many of the patients, these changes are persistent, as is true for their mnemonic impairments. While definite anatomicobehavioral correlations are missing, one would suggest that the motivational changes of the syndrome might be associated to the basal forebrain/hypothalamus/ventral striatum component of the lesion, and the cognitive personality changes to the ventromedial frontal component of the lesion. However, the results of the present study point also to an important effect of neostriate lesions, as suggested earlier for patients with caudate infarcts [2, 11]. Interestingly, ventromedial frontal lesions (group BF/FRO and STRIAT/BF/FRO) did not aggravate the effects of the neostriate lesions, but ameliorated them (cf. Fig. 4).

Summary

The mnemonic deficits of the ACoA syndrome are dependent on combined lesions of the basal forebrain and neostriatum. Neither basal forebrain nor striate damage alone is sufficient to cause amnesia. Similar mnemonic deficits can be provoked by tumors affecting the basal forebrain and striatum.

The personality changes of the ACoA syndrome seem to depend on the presence of striate lesions; frontal lesions ameliorate rather than aggravate these changes.

References

1. Alexancer MP, Freedman M (1984) Amnesia after anterior communicating artery aneurysm rupture. Neurology 34:752–757
2. Caplan LR, Schmahmann JD, Kase CS et al. (1972) Caudate infarcts. Arch Neurol 47:133–143
3. Damasio AR, Graff-Radford NR, Eslinger PJ et al. (1985) Amnesia following basal forebrain lesions. Arch Neurol 42:263–271
4. Gade A (1982) Amnesia after operations on aneurysms of the anterior communicating artery. Surg Neurol 18:46–49

5. Irle E (1990) An analysis of the correlation of lesion size, localization and behavioral effects on 283 published studies of cortical and subcortical lesions in old-world monkeys. Brain Res Rev 15:181–213
6. Lezak M (1983) Neuropsychological assessment, 2nd edn. Oxford University Press, New York
7. Logue V, Durward M, Pratt RTC et al. (1968) The quality of survival after rupture of an anterior cerebral aneurysm. Br J Psychiatr 114:137–160
8. Mesulam MM, Mufson EF (1984) Neural inputs into the nucleus basalis of teh substantia innominata (Ch4) in the rhesus monkey. Brain 107:253–274
9. Mishkin M, Malamut B, Bachevalier J (1984) Memories and habits: two neural systems. In: Lynch G, McGaugh JL, Weinberger NM (eds) The neurobiology of learning and memory. Guilford, New York, pp 65–77
10. Phillips S, Sangalang V, Sterns G (1987) Basal forebrain infarction. Arch Neurol 44:1134–1139
11. Richfield EK, Twyamn R, Berent S (1987) Neurological syndrome following bilateral damage to the head of the caudate nuclei. Ann Neurol 22:768–771
12. Takaku A, Tanaka S, Teruaki M, Suzuki J (1979) Postoperative complications in 1000 cases of intracranial aneurysms. Surg Neurol 12:137–144
13. Talland GA, Sweet WH, Ballantine HT (1967) Amnesic syndrome with anterior communicating artery aneurysms. J Nerv Ment Dis 145:179–192

Treatment of Cerebral Vasospasm with Hypervolemia and Hypertension

A. Unterberg, J. Gethmann, A. von Helden, G.-H. Schneider, and W. Lanksch[1]

Introduction

The term "cerebral vasospasm" is variously defined. Nowadays, the clinically used term stands for the delayed onset of a neurological deficit following subarachnoid hemorrhage, thought to be due to ischemia. There have been many attempts to prevent or treat cerebral vasospasm. The introduction of calcium channel blocking agents, such as nimodipine, has, however, also failed to completely abolish this complication. Cerebral vasospasm remains a challenging clinical problem. It remains the most important cause for mortality and morbidity of respective patients. The best current approach to treat vasospasm is to increase blood volume and to elevate blood pressure [1, 4–6].

The aim of this study was to analyze the occurrence of cerebral vasospasm in patients with a standardized general prophylaxis with calcium antagonists and the efficacy of a so-called hypertensive hypervolemic therapy (HHT).

Material and Methods

From January 1989 to April 1991, 82 patients with a subarachnoid hemorrhage due to a cerebral aneurysm were treated in the Department of Neurosurgery of the Unviersitätsklinikum Rudolf Virchow of the Free University of Berlin. Patients treated in 1989 [34] were analyzed retrospectively, whereas the population treated in 1990/1991 was prospectively studied. All these patients were treated with i.v. administration of nimodipine for 14 days.

Results and Discussion

Occurrence of Vasospasm

Symptoms of a delayed ischemic deficit (vasospasm) were observed in 32% of the retrospectively analyzed group and in 27% of prospectively studied patients (see Table 1). Symptoms of vasospasm were: hemiparesis (82%), drowsiness (69%), or

[1] Abteilung für Neurochirurgie, Universitätsklinikum Rudolf Virchow,
Freie Universität Berlin, Augustenburger Platz 1, W-1000 Berlin 65, FRG.

Advances in Neurosurgery, Vol. 20
K. Piscol, M. Klinger, M. Brock (Eds.)

Table 1. Occurrence of cerebral vasospasm in patients with subarachnoid hemorrhage and effectiveness of hypervolemic-hypertensive treatment (HHT)

	1989	1990/1991
Patients with SAH	34	48
Patients with vasospasm	11 (= 32%)	13 (= 27%)
Patients treated with HHT	–	13
Treatment effective	–	8 (= 62%)
Treatment ineffective	–	5 (= 38%)

dysphasia (17%). These symptoms varied considerably in their expression. There is a trend towards decreased occurrence of vasospasm, especially in the last year. The clinical symptoms of a delayed ischemic deficit were always associated with an increased flow velocity in transcranial Doppler sonography. There were, however, many patients with flow velocity increases and no clinical symptoms.

Hypertensive-Hypervolemic Therapy (HHT)

Since January 1990 all patients with vasospasm were rigorously treated with intravascular volume expansion and induced arterial hypertension, as has been advocated by Kassell et al. [1] and many others thereafter [2–6].

Hypervolemia was induced by infusion of hetastarch and albumin, aiming at a central venous pressure (CVP) of 10–12 cm H_2O. Hypertension was induced by dopamine, Dobutrex, and Arterenol. Arterial pressure was elevated until the clinical symptoms disappeared, up to a systolic blood pressure of 220–240 mmHg maximally. In elderly patients, this aggressive treatment was limited because of cardiac problems in some cases. The efficacy of this therapeutic regimen is given in Table 1. In eight patients, the neurological deficits could be reversed or ameliorated, whereas in five patients this regimen failed. There were two patients who finally died because of vasospasm. These results are in accordance with the findings of Kassell et al. [1] who reported that about two-thirds of patients can effectively be treated by this approach. Thus, hypervolemic-hypertensive treatment of vasospasm is the most effrective therapeutic regimen for symptomatic vasospasm.

Monitoring of Cerebral Blood Flow

Recently, a project of continuous monitoring of cerebrovenous oxygen saturation was started to estimate cerebral blood flow in patients with SAH (grade IV and V according to Hunt and Hess). To date these studies reveal that there are no significant episodes of a global reduction of CBF in patients with vasospasm. Respective

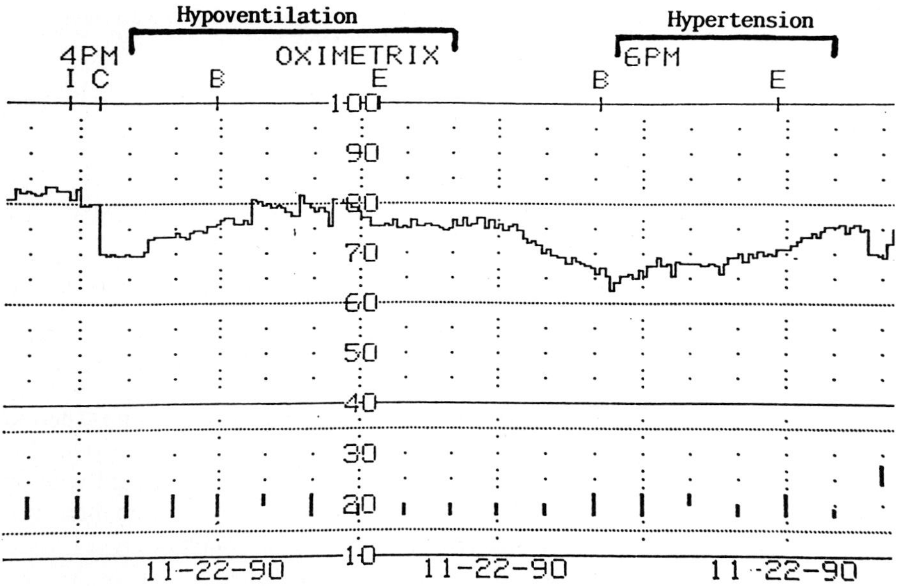

Fig. 1. Cerebral venous oxygen saturation (as measured in the jugular bulb) in a 55-year-old male patient with grade IV subarachnoid hemorrhage during induced hypertension and hypoventilation. The increase of blood pressure from 90 to 110 mmHg was associated with an increase of oxygen saturation from 62% to 69%. This indicates loss of cerebral autoregulation and explains the efficacy of hypertension in patients with severe vasospasm

patients, however, reveal a loss of cerebral autoregulation (Fig. 1). Induction of hypertension is followed by an increase in oxygen saturation, indicating an increased cerebral blood flow [2]. It is hoped that this new monitoring will enable us to better direct therapy and to clarify the significance of the various components of this therapeutic regimen.

Summary and Conclusion

Cerebral vasospasm remains an important complication of subarachnoid hemorrhage due to an aneurysm, even after introduction of a generalized prophylaxis with calcium blocking agents. On the other hand, vasospasm can effectively be treated by induced hypervolemia and hypertension. Clipping of the aneurysm and continuous monitoring of intracranial pressure in drowsy or comatose patients are prerequisites for this treatment.

Taken together, hypertensive-hypervolemic therapy of vasospasm represents an additional argument for early operation of all patients in grade I–IV according to Hunt and Hess.

Acknowledgment. The technical and secretarial assistance of J. Kopetzki and A. Riede is highly appreciated.

References

1. Kassell NF, Peerless SJ, Durward QJ, Beck DW, Drake CG, Adams HP (1982) Treatment of ischemic deficits from vasospasm with intravascular volume expansion and induced arterial hypertension. Neurosurgery 11:337–343
2. Muizelaar JP, Becker DP (1986) Induced hypertension for the treatment of cerebral ischemia after subarachnoid hemorrhage. Direct effect on cerebral blood flow. Surg Neurol 25:317–325
3. Origitano TC, Wascher TM, Reichmann OH, Anderson DE (1990) Sustained increased cerebral blood flow with prophylactic hypertensive hypervolemic hemodilution ("triple-H" therapy) after subarachnoid hemorrhage. Neurosurgery 27:729–739
4. Pritz MB (1984) Treatment of cerebral vasospasm. Usefulness of Swan-Ganz catheter monitoring of volume expansion. Surg Neurol 21:239–244
5. Unterberg A, Marguth F (1988) Aktuelle Konzepte zu Pathogenese und Therapie des zerebralen Vasospasmus. Münch Med Wschr 130:543–544
6. Wilkins RH (1990) Cerebral vasospasm. Critical Reviews in Neurobiology 6:51–77

Value of Transcranial Doppler Sonography in Patients Treated with Nimodipine

R. Laumer, R. Steinmeier, F. Gönner, and T. Vogtmann[1]

Introduction

For more than 8 years, transcranial Doppler sonography (TCDS) has been an important noninvasive tool in detecting vasospasm after subarachnoid hemorrhage (SAH). While initial investigations found a good correlation between the evaluated flow velocities and the neurological status, recent reports were more reserved. Especially the predictive value of TCDS concerning imminent delayed ischemic deficits (DID) was doubted [12, 14, 15]. This fact was mainly due to extremely high flow velocities being tolerated without any neurological deficit.

As all our patients were treated with nimodipine intravenously from the date of admission and many of the statements concerning TCDS are from the era before calcium antagonists were administered routinely, one reason for our investigations was to evaluate the discrepancies between different study protocols.

Patients and Methods

In a prospective study of 100 patients with SAH, flow velocities in basal cerebral arteries were measured by TCDS. All patients were treated with nimodipine from the date of admission. In the beginning, this treatment consisted of an intravenous administration for 7 days, followed by oral therapy for an additional 10–14 days. This regime was replaced by an intravenous administration for about 12 days according to TCDS findings without oral therapy.

The neurological status was documented daily (DID and Hunt and Hess grade). Patients with a CT-proven large hematoma were excluded as were patients developing neurological deficits immediately after surgery. In the remaining 66 cases, the incidence of DIDs was compared with the flow velocities evaluated by TCDS.

To evaluate the role of nimodipine as one explanation for discrepancies in the results, this study was compared with a previous investigation concerning the incidence and severity of DIDs, performed prospectively in the era before nimodipine. Furthermore, the question of normal flow velocities was reexamined in 141 normal subjects.

[1] Neurochirurgische Klinik der Universität Erlangen-Nürnberg, Schwabachanlage 6, W–8520 Erlangen, FRG.

Advances in Neurosurgery, Vol. 20
K. Piscol, M. Klinger, M. Brock (Eds.)

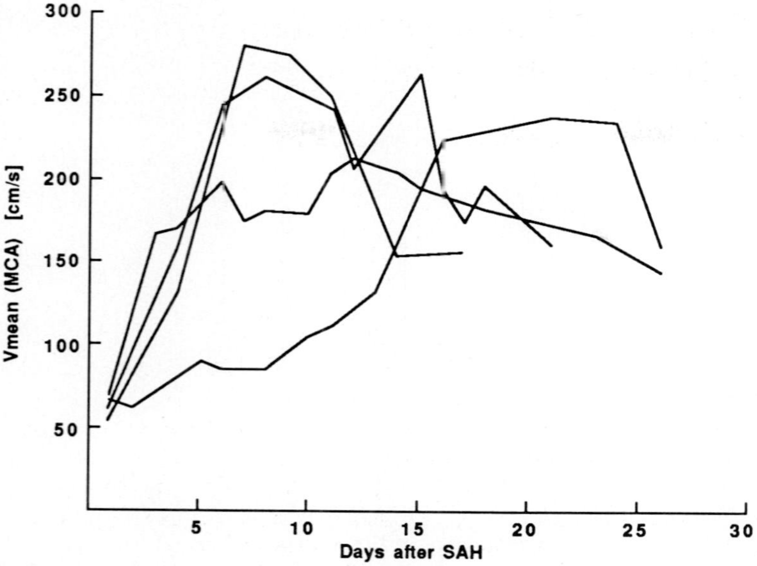

Fig. 1. In a series of 66 patients with subarachnoid hemorrhage, flow velocities (mean) over 200 cm/s were tolerated in 8 cases without any neurological deficit. Four cases are demonstrated as examples

Results

Forty-two patients of this series showed a good correlation between TCDS findings and neurological status, whereas in 24 cases there were discrepancies: (a) 16 patients developed neurological deficits while TCDS showed normal flow velocities and (b) 8 patients developed mean flow velocities in the middle cerebral artery (MCA) over 200 cm/s, in some cases over 250 cm/s, leading to no deficits at all. The time courses of flow velocities of four patients are shown in Fig. 1.

The mean flow velocities evaluated in 141 healthy subjects were higher than described before. Furthermore, a significant age dependency of flow velocities could be demonstrated (Fig. 2). Especially in younger subjects, flow velocities up to 120 cm/s were not unusual. There is a remarkable difference in flow velocities according to the localization on the M1 segment of the MCA. The maximum point was found about 10 mm distal to the bifurcation of the carotid artery. The mean velocity for the MCA was 70.0 ± 21.5 cm/s on the right and 71.4 ± 18.4 cm/s on the left side (Fig. 3).

According to the definition, there were 11 cases (16.7%) in this series developing DIDs. In the series of 123 patients who had no treatment with nimodipine, 25 patients (20.3%) developed DIDs. The difference between the two series is more remarkable in view of permanent deficits where 3.0% and 10.6%, respectively, in the non-nimodipine series were found (Table 1). Two patients developed deficits shortly after changing the route of administration of nimodipine from intravenous to oral therapy.

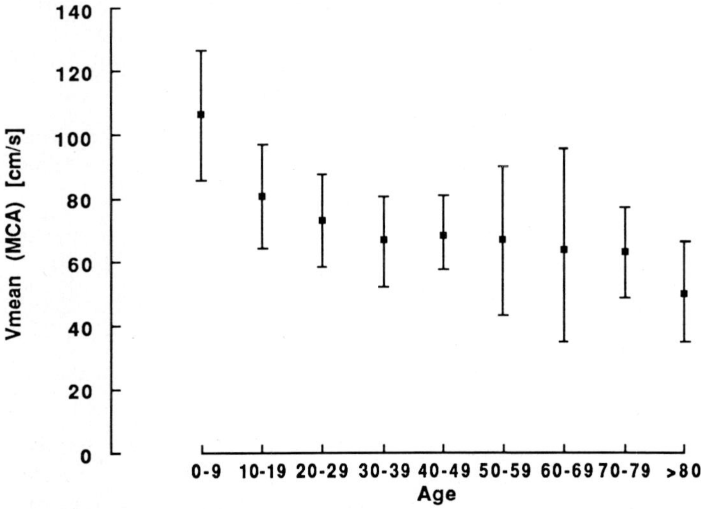

Fig. 2. Flow velocities in middle cerebral artery in 141 healthy subjects related to age

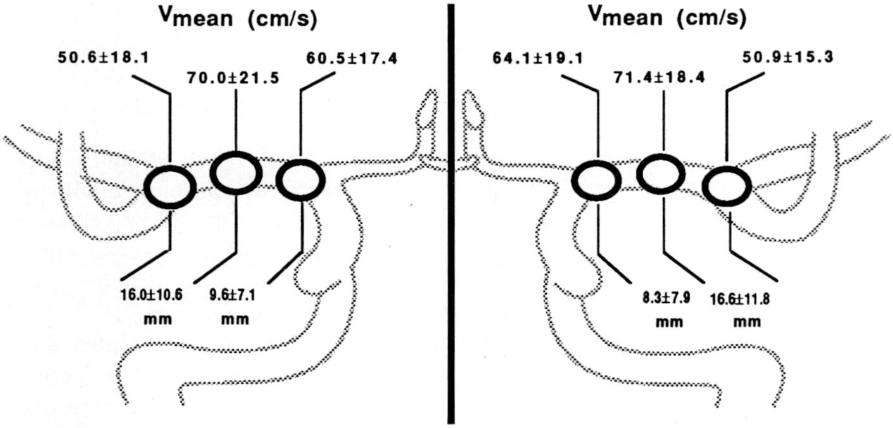

Fig. 3. Flow velocities in right and left middle cerebral artery related to the insonation depth (mm from the bifurcation of carotid artery) in 141 healthy subjects

Table 1. Incidence of delayed ischemic deficits (DID) in two series of patients with subarachnoid hemorrhage: nimodipine vs non-nimodipine treatment

			DID		
Series	*n*	$\sum$	Transient	Permanent	Deaths
Nimodipine	66	11 (16.7%)	9 (13.6%)	2 (3.0%)	0
Non-nimodipine	123	25 (20.3%)	10 (8.1%)	13 (10.6%)	2

Discussion

When we started our own experiments with TCDS in 1986, already within 6 months a preliminary analysis showed that our results differ completely from the results of other groups. Therefore, the definitive results of this prospective study were not surprising, whereas the explanation was not easy.

In about two-thirds of the 455 investigations, there was a good correlation between flow velocities and the corresponding neurological findings, whereas in 24 patients there was a considerable discrepancy in the sense of high velocities associated with a lack of neurological deficits and vice versa. In this series of 66 patients, flow velocities over 200 cm/s in the MCA were tolerated without any neurological deficit in 8 cases; 16 patients developed deficits, while TCDS showed normal values.

The explanation for normal TCDS findings despite neurological deficits seems evident: Only the main branches of the basal cerebral arteries can be investigated, while an isolated vasospasm of more distal parts of the vessels, i.e., A2, M2, or perforating arteries, is not detectable by TCDS. Therefore, the reason for the lack of correlation is the technique itself. The analysis of the opposite constellation, extremely pathological flow velocities with a lack of neurological deficits, is more difficult.

In view of the guidelines evaluated by the pioneers of TCDS [1–3, 6–8, 13], normal values for flow velocities in the MCA of about 50–60 cm/s were reported. The range between 80 and 120 cm/s was found to be critical and over 120 cm/s critical [7]. The risk of neurological deficits was seen either when the daily increase in velocity was more than 20 cm/s [7] or the mean velocity was higher than 200 cm/s [13]. In this series 8 of 66 patients tolerated velocities over 200 cm/s, in some cases up to 300 cm/s.

Investigating the normal values for flow velocities in 141 healthy subjects, the use of a 3D Doppler (Eden Medizinische Elektronik, Überlingen) was of great advantage. It was easily possible to localize and investigate several points on the MCS. The maxinum velocity of around 70 cm/s was found 10 mm distal to the bifurcation of the carotid artery. This value is higher than those reported in the literature and the fact that especially in younger subjects flow velocities up to

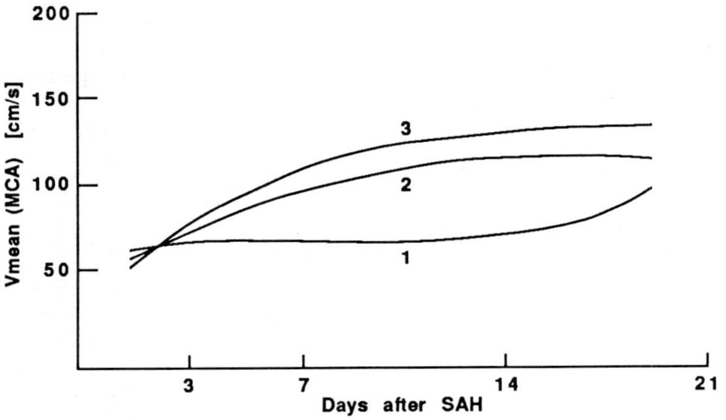

Fig. 4. Time course of flow velocities in middle cerebral artery according to Fisher grading of subarachnoid hemorrhage

120 cm/s were found is at most a hint at the age dependency of flow velocities, but no explanation for the toleration of velocities over 200 cm/s.

A further possible explanation is the compensation via collateral vessels. This fact is more obvious and is sufficient for many cases, but this point does not explain the discrepancy from the guidelines in the early reports of TCDS.

The main difference between this study and investigations before 1986 is the routine administration of nimodipine. Probably this is the main reason for the toleration of high flow velocities.

It is well known that vasospasm cannot be avoided by calcium antagonists, but possibly its incidence and severity. Despite the fact that all patients of this series were treated with nimodipine, a dependency of flow velocities according to the amount of subarachnoid blood in computed tomography [5] was found (Fig. 4). This is proof of the evidence of vasospasm in the sense of elevated flow velocity due to arterial narrowing, also under nimodipine. When compared with the series of 123 patients who had no nimodipine, the incidence of DIDs was less in the treated group. The rate of the reduced incidence of DIDs varies in different studies, but is evident [4, 8–11]. Therefore, the supposed elevated ischemic tolerance of nimodipine is responsible for the toleration of high flow velocities.

This assumption is supported by the observation of DIDs developing shortly after changing the intravenous to oral administration, probably leading to oscillations in the serum level.

References

1. Aaslid R (1986) Transcranial Doppler sonography. Springer, Wien New York
2. Aaslid R, Markwalder T-M, Nornes H (1982) Noninvasive transcranial Doppler ultrasound recording of flow velocity in basal cerebral arteries. J Neurosurg 57:769–774

3. Aaslid R, Huber P, Nornes H (1984) Evaluation of cerebrovascular spasm with transcranial Doppler ultrasound. J Neurosurg 60:37–41
4. Auer LM, Brandt L, Ebeling U et al. (1986) Nimodipine and early aneurysm operation in good condition SAH patients. Acta Neurochirurg 82:7–13
5. Fisher CM, Kistler JP, Davis JM (1980) Relation of cerebral vasospasm to subarachnoid hemorrhage visualized by computerized tomographic scanning. Neurosurg 6:1–9
6. Gilsbach JM, Harders A (1985) Early aneurysm operation and vasospasm. Intracranial Doppler findings. Neurochirurgia 28:100–102
7. Harders A (1986) Neurosurgical applications of transcranial Doppler sonography. Springer, Wien New York
8. Harders AG, Gilsbach JM, Hornyak ME (1988) Incidence of vasospasm in transcranial Doppler sonography and its clinical significance: a prospective study in 100 consecutive patients who were given intravenous Nimodipine and who underwent early aneurysm surgery. In: Wilkins RH (ed) Cerebral vasospasm. Raven Press, New York, pp 73–78
9. Houteville JP (1987) Nimodipine curative treatment of cerebral vasospasm after aneurysmal rupture. Co-operative multicentre study. 8th European Congrtess of Neurosurgery, Barcelona 1987
10. Kazner E, Sprung CH, Adelt D et al. (1985) Clinical experience with nimodipine in the prophylaxis of neurological deficits after subarachnoid hemorrhage. Neurochirurgia 28:110–113
11. Koos WT, Perneczky A, Auer LM et al. (1985) Nimodipine treatment of ischemic neurological deficit due to cerebral vasospasm after subarachnoid hemorrhage. Neurochirurgia 28:114–117
12. Laumer R, Steinmeier R, Vogtmann T, Gönner F, Mück M, Priem R (1989) Stellenwert der transkraniellen Dopplersonographie beim Management der Subarachnoidalblutung. Nervenheilkunde 8:287–303
13. Seiler RW, Grolimund P, Aaslid R et al. (1986) Cerebral vasospasm evaluated by transcranial ultrasound correlated with clinical grade and CT-visualized subarachnoid hemorrhage. J Neurosurg 64:594–600
14. Sekhar LN, WEchsler LR, Yonas H et al. (1988) Value of transcranial Doppler examination in the diagnosis of cerebral vasospasm after subarachnoid hemorrhage. Neurosurg 22:813–821
15. Symon L, Compton J, Redmond S et al. (1988) Bedside monitoring in subarachnoid hemorrhage: Evoked responses, hemispheral blood flow, and flow velocity measurements. In: Wilkins RH (ed) Cerebral vasospasm. Raven Press, New York, pp 73–78

Correlation Between Cerebral Blood Flow Velocity in Basal Cerebral Arteries and Nimodipine Concentration in Serum and Plasma After Acute Subarachnoid Hemorrhage

D. Rosenthal, M. Carvi y Nievas, W. I. Steudel, A. Ricco, and R. Lorenz[1]

Introduction

Calcium channel blockers are being used to an increasing extent in neurosurgery to prevent vasospasm and cerebral ischemia secondary to subarachnoid hemorrhage. However, results reported from open or placebo-controlled studies show a wide variation with regard to the outcome [3, 4, 11, 13–17].

Among other unsolved questions, it is still unclear whether calcium antagonists have some influence on cerebral blood flow velocity (as an indirect way of measuring vasodilatation). Furthermore, the concentration in plasma and cerebrospinal fluid required to achieve therapeutic effect is unknown. The aim of this pilot study was to evaluate the relationship between these variables.

Materials and Methods

During a 3-month period, all patients suffering from an acute subarachnoid hemorrhage due to aneurysm rupture were admitted to our department and included in this study.

Calcium antagonist (nimodipine, Nomotop, Bayer, Leverkusen) administration was started immediately after admission at a rate of 2 mg/kg body weight per hour via central venous catheter and in a continuous perfusion mode.

Samples of cerebrospinal fluid (CSF) were assessed daily and taken via a catheter left in place routinely in the chiasmatic cistern in our clinic after aneurysm clipping.

Serum probes were taken simultaneously by percutaneous tapping of a peripheral vessel. Plasma and CSF probes were immediately centrifugated and deep-frozen at –20°C, avoiding any contact with light. Nimodipine concentration was determined with the gas chromatographic method [18].

Cerebral blood flow velocity (BFV) was determined daily in the middle cerebral artery on both sides, using a transcranial Doppler device (EME, Ueberlingen).

The Hunt and Hess scale [9] was used to assess clinical grading at admission; outcome was determined by means of the Glasgow Outcome Scale [10]. Statistical analysis was performed using the SPSS+PC software.

[1] Neurochirurgische Universitätsklinik, Schleusenweg 2–16, W–6000 Frankfurt/M. 71, FRG.

Advances in Neurosurgery, Vol. 20
K. Piscol, M. Klinger, M. Brock (Eds.)

Table 1. Clinical and surgical data in 24 cases with subarachnoid hemorrhage

Case	Sex	Age	Site	Clinical grade[a]	Outcome[b]
1	F	36	ICA R	III	I
2	F	41	ICA L	II	I
3	F	42	ACA	II	I
4	M	29	ACA	III	I
5	F	33	MCA L	III	II
6	M	30	ICA L	I	I
7	F	45	MCA L	IV[c]	II
8	M	51	ACA	III[c]	II
9	M	45	ACA	IV[c]	V
10	F	43	ICA R	II[d]	II
11	M	45	ACA	III[d]	II
12	F	52	ACA	II	III
13	M	56	ICA L	II	I
14	F	76	ACA	IV	V
15	M	41	ACA	II	I
16	F	47	ACA	I	I
17	F	43	ACA	III	I
18	F	39	MCA R	I	II
19	M	54	ACA	III[c]	III
20	F	30	ACA	III[c]	V
21	F	68	ICA L	III[c]	III
22	F	46	MCA R	III[c]	V
23	M	59	ICA L	I[d]	III
24	F	64	MCA L	II[d]	I

ACA, anterior communicating artery; ICA, internal carotid artery; MCA, middle cerebral artery; R, right; L, left.

[a] Hunt and Hess scale;

[b] Glasgow outcome scale;

[c] Intracerebral hematoma;

[d] Cerebral infraction.

Results

Twenty-six patients were admitted during the study period. Two cases were excluded because of marked vascular instability. The distribution regarding age, sex, aneurysm location, Hunt and Hess grade on admission, and outcome score are summarized in Table 1.

CSF values averaged 0.93 ng/ml and plasma 10 ng/ml. The CSF : plasma ratio was 1 : 15. Two patients had ventricular and cisternal drains simultaneously. The intraventricular nimodipine mean level was 0.257 ng/ml, reaching about one-fourth of the cisternal concentration.

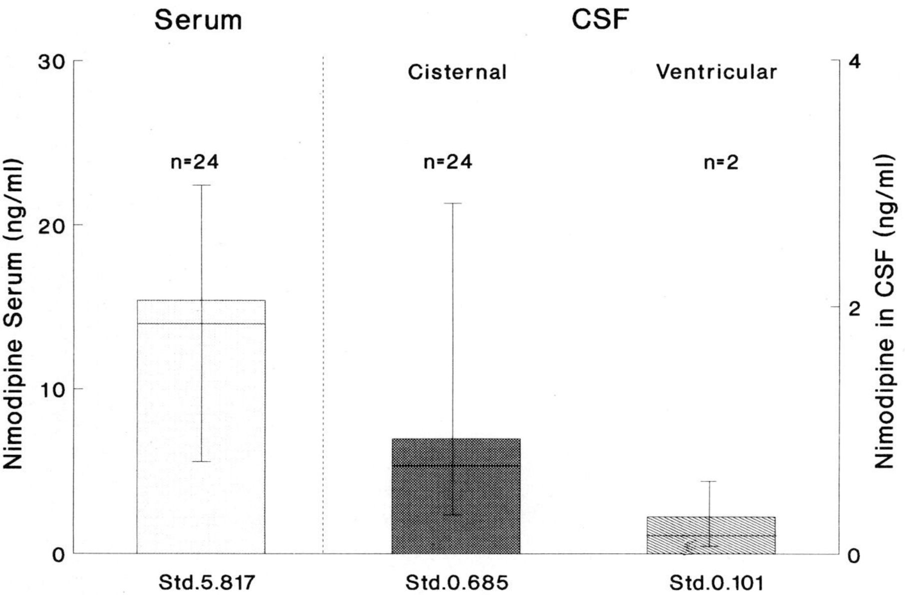

Fig. 1. Mean (*column*), median (—), range (I), and standard deviation (Std.) values of serologic, cisternal, and ventricular nimodipine concentrations

Results with average, standard deviation, median, and range are summarized in Fig. 1. BFV fluctuated between 36 and 220 cm/s on the right and 42 and 190 cm/s on the left middle cerebral artery. Mean values were 97 cm/s for the right and 82 cm/s for the contralateral side. BFV was slightly higher on the side where the surgical approach was made.

There was a marked individual and interindividual fluctuation in serum and CSF concentration values. Changes in nimodipine level did not always run in parallel and sometimes even in opposite directions.

Statistical analysis showed a significant and inverse correlation between blood flow velocity and nimodipine concentration in CSF ($P < 0.01$). This was not found for the serologic values.

Discussion

The relationship between nimodipine concentration in CSF and blood flow velocity has not been reported yet. The fact that CSF and not serum concentration values correlate with BFV suggests that cerebrospinal fluid is the principal route of transport for this drug. Experimental observations have demonstrated that nimodipine blocks about 80%–90% of the available receptors [6]. In our experience with CSF values of about 1 ng/ml or more, blood flow velocity remained under

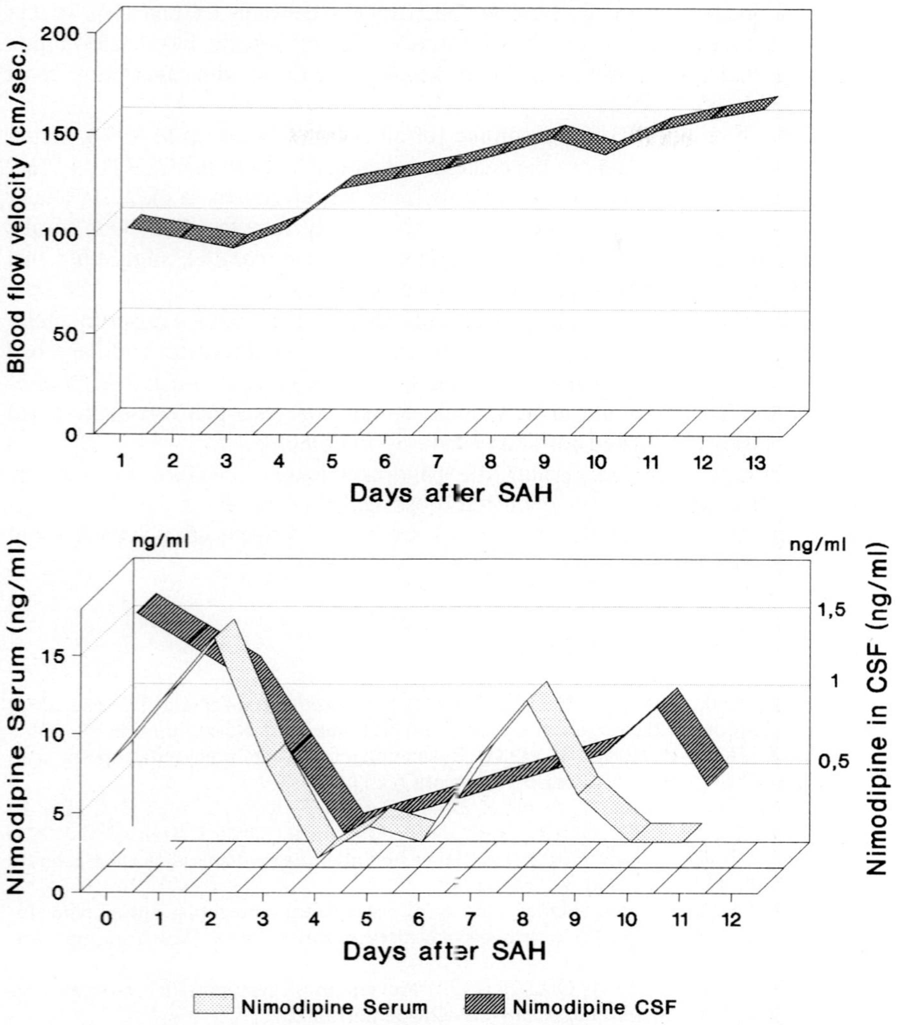

Fig. 2. Example of BFV and nimodipine level in cerebrospinal fluid (case 11, Table 1). Blood flow velocity values stayed under 100 cm/s as long as nimodipine concentration in CSF was above 1 ng/ml. Blood flow velocity was measured at the right middle cerebral artery (*upper part*)

100 cm/s (considered upper normal value in our Doppler laboratory), leading to the conclusion that this may be the ideal therapeutic concentration (Fig. 2).

Induced vasospasm in animal models was reversed by giving calcium channel blockers sublingually [6], but failed when nimodipine was administered orally [7]. Cisternal administration has a preventive effect against vasospasm [5, 8, 12, 13]. Pharmacokinetic studies have demonstrated that nimodipine is degraded in the liver;

due to a major first pass effect, bioavailability ranges between 3% and 10% 10 min after drug administration [18]. The absorption rate or hepatic biotransformation may explain variations in serum and CSF levels. Interaction with other drugs must also be considered.

Due to the high affinity of nimodipine for albumin (it binds up to 90%), serum protein concentration influences the calcium antagonist level in the CSF [19]. Fluctuations of plasma proteins will affect nimodipine concentrations in the CSF. Under normal conditions large molecules do not pass freely into the CSF. Our results show that albumin and nimodipine concentrations run in parallel, suggesting that alterations in the blood-brain barrier may also play a role.

The effect of nimodipine on resistance vessels was demonstrated experimentally [20]. From the physiological point of view, dilatation of the distal capillary bed would only lead to augmentation of blood flow velocity due to a fall in peripheral resistance. The reduction in BFV achieved here suggests that capacitance and resistance vessels are dilated simultaneously by nimodipine.

Further investigations concerning the pharmacokinetics, metabolism, and site of action will clarify concepts about the dose and time at which calcium antagonist therapy should be started to prevent secondary damage after subarachnoid hemorrhage.

References

1. Aaslid R, Markwalder TM, Nornes H (1982) Noninvasive transcranial Doppler ultrasound recording of flow velocity in basal cerebral arteries. J Neurosurg 57:969–774
2. Aaslid R, Huber P, Nornes H (1984) Evaluation of the cerebrovascular spasm with transcranial Doppler ultrasound. J Neurosurg 60:37–41
3. Allen G, Ahn H, Preziosi T, Battye R, Boone S, Chou S, Kelly D, Weir B, Crabbe R, Mellits D, Bertsch L, Boisvert D, Hundley M, Johnson R, Strom J, Transou C (1983) Cerebral arterial vasospasm controlled trial of nimodipine in patients with subarachnoid hemorrhage. N Engl J Med 308:619–624
4. Auer LM (1983) Cerebrovascular activity of the calcium antagonist nimodipine. In: Reivich M, Hurtig HI (eds) Cerebrovascular disease. Raven Press, New York, pp 375–384
5. Auer LM, Ito Z, Suzuki A, Ohta H (1982) Prevention of symptomatic vasospasm by topically applied nimodipine. Acta Neurochir 63:297–302
6. Cohen RJ, Allen GS (1980) Cerebral arterial spasm: the role of calcium in vitro and in vivo analysis of treatment with nifedipine and nimodipine. In: Wilkins RH (ed) Cerebral arterial spasm. Williams & Wilkins, Baltimore, pp 527–532
7. Espinosa F, Weir B, Scnitka T, Overton T, Boisvert D (1984) A randomized placebo-controlled double-blind trial of nimodipine after SAH in monkeys. Part 2: Pathological findings. J Neurosurg 50:1176–1185
8. Giola E, White R, Bakhtian B, Robertson J (1985) Evaluation of the efficacy of intrathecal nimodipine in canine models of chronic cerebral vasospasm. J Neurosurg 62:721–728
9. Hunt W, Hess R (1968) Surgical risk as related to time of intervention in the repair of intracranial aneurysms. J Neurosurg 28:14–19
10. Jennett B, Bond M (1975) Assessment of outcome after severe brain damage. Lancet: 480–484

11. Kazner E, Sprung C, Adelt D, Ammerer HP, Karnick P, Baumann H, Böker DK, Grotenhuis JA, Jaksche H, Istaitih A (1985) Clinical experience with nimodipine in the prophylaxis of neurological deficits after subarachnoid hemorrhage. Neurochirurgia 28 (Suppl 1):110–113
12. Kunz U, Seifert V, Stolke D, Dietz H (1987) Intrathecal administration of nimodipine for treatment of chronic cerebral vasospasm (an experimental study). In: Isamat F, Ferrer E (eds) Proc VIII European Congress of Neurosurg. Barcelona, Spain, p 277 (abstr)
13. Ljunggren B, Brandt L, Säveland H, Nilsson PE, Cronquist S, Andersson KE, Vinge E (1984) Outcome in 60 consecutive patients treated with early aneurysm operation and intravenous nimodipine. J Neurosurg 61:864–873
14. Ohman J, Heiskanen O (1988) Effect of nimodipine on the outcome of patients after aneurysmal subarachnoid hemorrhage and surgery. J Neurosurg 69:683–686
15. Petruk KC, West M, Mohr G, Weir B, Benoit B, Gentili F, Disney L, Khan M, Grace M, Holness R, Karwon M, Ford R, Cameron G, Tucker W, Purves G, Miller J, Hunter M, Richard M, Durity F, Chan R, Clein L, Maroun F, Godon A (1988) Nimodipine treatment in poor grade aneurysm patients. Results of a multicenter double blind placebo-controlled trial. J Neurosurg 68 505–517
16. Philippon J, Grob R, Dagreou F, Guggiari M, Rivierez M, Viars P (1986) Prevention of vasospasm in subarachnoid hemorrhage. A controlled study with nimodipine. Acta Neurochir 82:110–114
17. Pickard J, Murray G, Illingworth R, Shaw M, Teasdale G, Foy P, Humphrey P, Lang D, Nelson R, Richards P, Sinar J, Bailey S, Skene A (1989) Effect of oral nimodipine on cerebral infarction and outcome after subarachnoid haemorrhage: British aneurysm nimodipine trial. Br Med J 298:636–642
18. Raemsch KD, Graefe KH, Sommer J (1985) Pharmacokinetics and metabolism of nimodipine. In: Beth E, Deck K, Hoffmeister F (eds) Nimodipine, pharamcological and clinical properties. Schattauer, Stuttgart New York, pp 147–159
19. Steudel WI, Carvi y Nievas M, Tiyaworabun S, Lorenz R (1990) The prognostic significance of the concentration of nimodipine in the CSF and plasma in subarachnoid hemorrhage. In: Bushe KH, Brock M, Klinger M (eds) Advances in neurosurgery, vol 18. Springer, Berlin Heidelberg New York Tokyo, pp 180–184
20. Takayasu M, Bassett JE, Dacey RG Jr (1988) Effects of calcium antagonists on intracerebral penetrating arterioles in rats. J Neurosurg 69:104–109

Laser Irradiation of Experimental Carotid Aneurysms: Long-term Results and Histological Alterations

F. Ulrich[1], S. Dohle[1], and R. Schober[2]

Summary

Baby aneurysms of the common carotid artery of adult rats were induced by means of the adventitial patch method [4]. The aneurysms which could be demonstrated 8 weeks later were irradiated intermittently with 12.5-W pulses of 0.05–0.1 s duration from the 1.318 Nd:YAG laser in a 0.2-mm focus. In this way, they could be caused to contract without perforation and thrombosis of the common carotid artery.

The objective of the study was to analyze histologically the structural alterations which occur after laser irradiation of the experimentally induced aneurysms. We assume that a structural alteration of the collagen fibers which we have been able to demonstrate is the cause of the contraction of the aneurysm induced by laser irradiation.

Acute and long-term preparations between 1 and 16 months were investigated histologically. In chronic preparations, a pronounced alteration of the irradiated aneurysm wall with proliferation of myointimal cells, fibrosis, and localized calcifications could be detected.

Introduction

Whereas surgical elimination of pedunculated, sacculated cerebral aneurysms has become a largely risk-free operation today owing to the more sophisticated microtechnique with application of an aneurysm clip, broad-based, fusiform and often vesiculated aneurysms cannot be eliminated from the circulation by application of a clip without closing afferent and efferent vessels. Even the encasement or wrapping up of these baby aneurysms may lead to fresh (often lethal) ruptures of aneurysms in the long term.

On the other hand, aneurysm thrombosis induced mechanically, electrically, or by balloon catheters frequently gives rise to uncontrollable thromboses of the vessels branching off from the aneurysms with subsequent development of cerebral infarction. The further development of diverse laser systems (CO_2 laser, 1.32-μm Nd:YAG laser) has made it possible in recent years to employ lasers to an ever

[1] Neurochirurgische Universitätsklinik, Moorenstr. 5, W–4000 Düsseldorf, FRG.
[2] Institut für Neuropathologie, Heinrich-Heine-Universität, Moorenstr. 5, W–4000 Düsseldorf, FRG.

Advances in Neurosurgery, Vol. 20
K. Piscol, M. Klinger, M. Brock (Eds.)

increasing extent at the microvascular level. By modification of the beam geometry using the 1.32-μm Nd:YAG laser (MBB-Medizintechnik, Ottobrunn) in combination with a 200-μm light guide and a micromanipulator coupled to the surgical microscope (OPMILAS YAG Zeiss, Oberkochen), a suitable instrument for microsurgical laser-assisted contraction of aneurysms was produced [5]. This enables the laser beam and the pilot light to be conducted without contact via a micromanipulator directly coupled to the surgical microscope to the vessel or aneurysm to be irradiated.

Materials and Methods

Vesiculated aneurysms of the common carotid artery of adult rats were induced within 3–4 months with the familiar adventitial patch method [4]. Macroscopically, fusiform raised aneurysms of the common carotid artery of the rat which were 1–2 mm wide and 1–2 mm long were found in these cases.

By application of 0.05–0.1 s pulses with the 1.3Nd:YAG laser (MBB-Medizintechnik) of 12.5 W in the 0.2-mm focus, the broad-based aneurysms of the carotid artery of adult rats induced experimentally with the adventitial patch method could be caused to contract completely without perforation of thrombosis of the carotid artery.

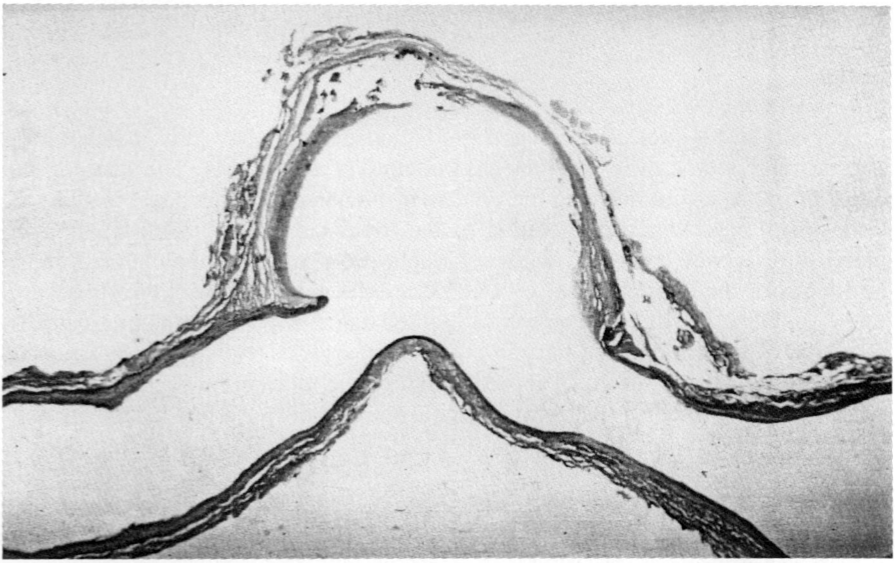

Fig. 1. Vesiculated aneurysm of the common carotid artery of adult rats, which were 1–2 mm wide and 1–2 mm long, were induced with the adventitial patch method [4]

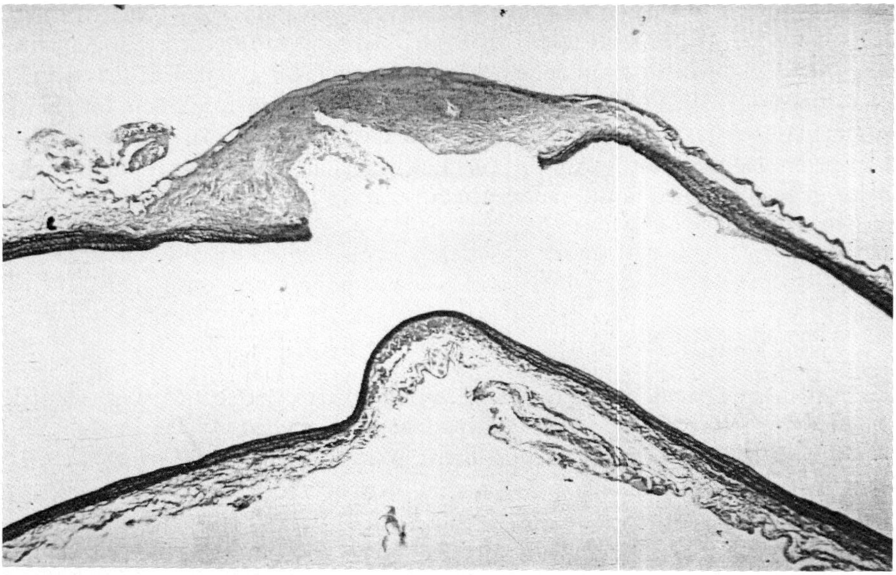

Fig. 2. By application of 0.05–0.1 s pulses with the 1.3 Nd:YAG laser of 12.5 W in the 0.2-mm focus, the broad-based baby aneurysms could be caused to contract without perforation or thrombosis of the carotid artery. The histological evaluation in chronic, 6-month-old preparations demonstrate a pronounced alteration of the irradiated aneurysmal wall with proliferation of myointimal cells and substantial fibrosis

Results

The inspection 4–6 weeks after laser irradiation did not show any indication of fresh sacculations or even spontaneous ruptures of aneurysms. The histological evaluation of subacute and chronic aneurysm preparations after laser irradiation demonstrated a pronounced alteration of the irradiated aneurysmal wall. A substantial fibrosis was combined with a variable proliferation of myointimal cells. The stumps of the incised vessel wall bordering the aneurysm were clearly recognizable, and their elastic lamellae were collapsed due to loss of smooth muscle cells in the area of irradiation. The thickness of the aneurysmal wall was variable, usually increasing toward the base. In occasional cases, more pronounced regressive alterations were present in the form of small rounded or brace-like calcifications.

Discussion

We have demonstrated a laser-induced structural alteration of collagen fibers and consider this to be the reason for the aneurysm contraction attained with laser irradiation [3].

The histological characteristics of the aneurysmal wall play a substantial role in the reaction to laser treatment. In unruptured, small aneurysms, the wall consists of a layer of connective tissue bridging the defect.

If the aneurysms are larger than 2 mm in diameter, the walls become more fibrotic with fewer cell elements and a thin region of the wall at the aneurysm dome. An immediate reduction in the size of the aneurysms in response to laser irradiation can thus be expected in these cases. After rupture of the aneurysm, a membrane in terms of a "false" aneurysm may form around the blood clot. This membrane is increasingly converted into a hyalinized collagen wall with a low content of cells.

The wall in most aneurysms in patients is collagenous and can undergo laser-induced contractive alterations entailing a stabilization of the collagen fibers.

Reports on laser-assisted aneurysm contractions are essentially based on experimental results in artificially induced arterial aneurysms [2]. Surgical experience is confined to observations of individual cases in which a stabilization of the aneurysmal wall by laser irradiation has been demonstrated so that fresh sacculations and aneurysm ruptures were not longer observed [1].

Acknowledgment. The study was generously supported from 1989 to 1991 by the Deutsche Forschungsgemeinschaft (66/2–1). We thank Mrs. Schröter for her excellent technical assistance.

References

1. Fasano VA, Ponzio RM, Benech F, Sicuro M (1983) Effects of laser sources (Argon, Nd: YAG, CO_2) on the elastic resistance of the vessel wall: histological and physical study. Laser Surg Med 2:45–54
2. Maira G, Mohr G, Panisset K, Hardy J (1979) Laser photocoagulation for treatment of experimental aneurysms. J Microsurg 1:137–147
3. Schober R, Ulrich F, Sander T, Dürselen R, Hessel S (1986) Laser induced alteration of collagen substructure allows microsurgical tissue welding. Science 232:1421–1422
4. Ulrich F, Dohle St (1989) The adventitia patch technique. Optoelectronics in Medicine Laser 89:109–111
5. Ulrich F, Nicola N, Bock WJ (1986) A micromanipulator to aid microsurgical removal of intracranial tumors with the Nd:YAG laser. Lasers in Medicine Science 1:131–133

Effects of Intrathecal Thrombolysis on CSF Absorption After Experimental Subarachnoid Hemorrhage

T. Brinker, V. Seifert, and H. Dietz[1]

Introduction

Posthemorrhagic hydrocephalus after subarachnoid hemorrhage (SAH) has been well known since its original description by Foltz [7]. Thereafter, for a long period, acute hydrocephalus after SAH had been regarded to be clinically insignificant, as it was found to be almost mild and transient [14]. Yet, more recently, Bailes and co-workers demonstrated acute hydrocephalus and elevated intracranial pressure in more then 90% of poor-grade patients after SAH. These authors regarded acute hydrocephalus to be responsible for early neurological deterioration in the majority of those patients [1].

Both subarachnoid blood clots within the basal cisterns and a blockade of the arachnoid villi from different blood components have been recognized to cause acute hydrocephalus after SAH [4, 9]. From experimental investigations, Butler found that especially fibrin components may clog the CSF outflow pathways [3]. The resulting impairment of CSF absorption has been regarded to be irreversible so far.

In the present work, it is demonstrated that intrathecal fibrinolysis using recombinant tissue plasminogen activator (rtPA) may restore CSF absorption immediately after experimental SAH almost totally. In addition, intrathecal fibrinolysis was found to prevent subacute hydrocephalus after SAH.

Materials and Methods

The effects of experimental SAH on CSF absorption were investigated in 29 cats which were grouped. The hemorrhage was induced by infusion of fresh autologous, nonheparinized blood into the cisterna magna. During this procedure the animals were intubated, control ventilated, and anesthetized. Intracranial pressure (ICP) was recorded with a ventricular catheter, which was introduced stereotactically. Test solutions were infused into the cisterna magna, which was cannulated percutaneously. The experimental procedures were recently published in more detail [2].

In group 1($n=6$) 2 mg of rtPA were infused into the cisterna magna 30 min after the experimental SAH. The hemorrhage was induced by increasing volumes of

[1] Neurochirurgische Klinik, Medizinische Hochschule Hannover,
Konstanty-Gutschow-Str. 8, W–3000 Hannover 61, FRG.

Advances in Neurosurgery, Vol. 20
K. Piscol, M. Klinger, M. Brock (Eds.)

blood (2–4 ml). CSF dynamics were measured with the methods of Marmarou [10] prior and 30 min after the SAH, and again 30 min later after treatment with rtPA.

In group 2 SAH was induced by infusion of 1 ml of blood per kg body weight in 19 cats. An intracisternal infusion of 3 mg of rtPA was performed 24 h later in 11 of these animals; in 8 animals saline was infused for control. Seven days after SAH CSF dynamics were measured; thereafter, the brains were removed and fixed in 10% formalin for some weeks. Then a coronal brain slice was cut from each brain at the level of the posterior margin of the optic chiasm. Each brain slice was photographed together with square paper and then scanned into a computer for planimetry of both lateral ventricles. For control these procedures were done in addition in four healthy animals.

Results

Effects of Early Intrathecal Fibrinolysis (Group 1)

Immediately after the experimental SAH in all investigated animals a severe impairment of the CSF absorption was observed. Depending on the volume of infused blood, the CSF outflow resistance increased exponentially (for details, see ref. [2]). Intrathecal fibrinolysis normalized in each animal, the CSF outflow resistance almost totally (Fig. 1). Table 1 summarizes the CSF dynamics prior to the SAH, after the SAH, and after fibrinolysis performed 30 min after SAH.

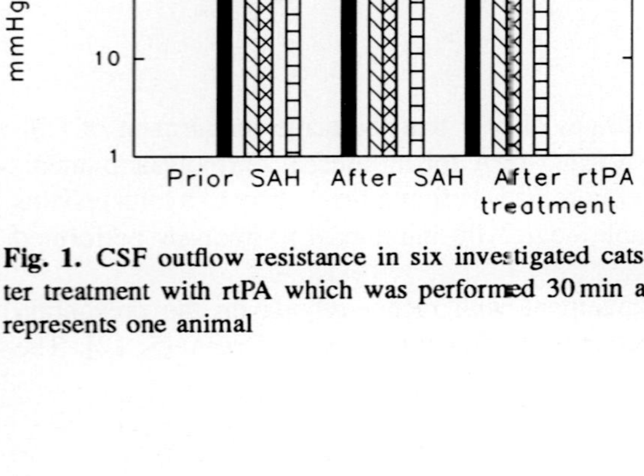

Fig. 1. CSF outflow resistance in six investigated cats prior to SAH, after SAH, and after treatment with rtPA which was performed 30 min after SAH. Each corresponding *bar* represents one animal

Table 1. CSF dynamics of group 1

	ICP	PVI	Ro
Prior to SAH	4.7 ± 0.5	0.94 ± 0.6	74.8 ± 22
After SAH	25.5 ± 13.7	0.45 ± 0.08	2283 ± 2650
After rtPA	11.2 ± 8.3	0.47 ± 0.2	104.2 ± 62

ICP, intracranial pressure (mmHg); PVI, pressure volume index (ml); Ro, CSF outflow resistance (mmHg/ml/min); mean ± SD

Table 2. CSF dynamics of group 2

	ICP	PVI	Ro
Control	7.5 ± 1	0.6 ± 0.03	71 ± 0.5
Nontreated SAH	9.1 ± 1.7	0.44 ± 0.44	265 ± 19.8
rtPA-treated SAH	6.2 ± 1.1	0.38 ± 0.03	151 ± 6.4

ICP, intracranial pressure (mmHg); PVI, pressure volume index (ml); Ro, CSF outflow resistance (mmHg/ml/min); mean ± SD

Effects of Delayed Intrathecal Fibrinolysis (Group 2)

Seven days after experimental SAH the CSF outflow resistance of the nontreated animals was elevated significantly in comparison with the healthy control animals. In the rtPA-treated animals CSF absorption was improved to a considerable degree. Even this improvement was statistically significant ($P < 0.01$, Wilcoxon test); CSF absorption was not normalized totally. CSF dynamics of the investigated animals are summarized in Table 2.

Planimetry of the lateral ventricles of the nontreated animals gave a value of 11.1 ± 3.9 mm^2, which differed statistically from the value of the healthy control group (3.7 ± 2.7 mm^2). In contrast, the ventricular plane of the rtPA-treated animals (3.5 ± 1.1 mm^2) did not differ from the healthy control group (Fig. 2).

Discussion

The present investigation demonstrates clearly that the acute impairment of CSF absorption after SAH is reversible using rtPA for intrathecal fibrinolysis immediately after the hemorrhage. Furthermore, it was found that subacute hydrocephalus may be prevented to a considerable degree by intrathecal fibrinolysis performed 24 h after the hemorrhage.

These findings are in good agreement with recent reports on the prevention of cerebral vasospasm after experimental SAH by the use of rtPA [5, 12]. The

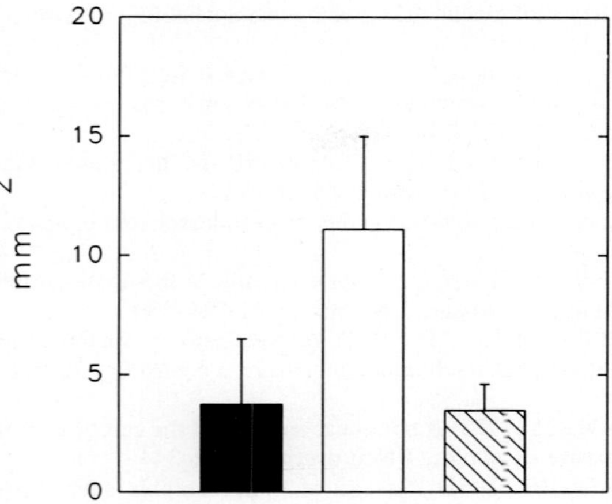

Fig. 2. Bar graph depicting the mean ± SD of ventricular plane of both lateral ventricles in control animals (*blank column*), in nontreated animals 7 days after SAH (*black column*), and in rtPA-treated animals again 7 days after SAH (*hatched column*)

premature lysis of subarachnoid blood clots has been suggested to be the most important pathogenetic mechanism.

From the present investigation, one may conclude that the restoration of CSF absorption should be another decisive factor for the prevention of cerebral vasospasm after SAH. From earlier investigations, it is known that the clearance of proteins and other particles from the CSF space depend on normal CSF absorption [11]. Therefore, we suggest that a normalized CSF flow after SAH enables the more rapid clearance of spasmogenic substances from the CSF space, thereby preventing vasospasm.

These suggestions are confirmed by the well-known increase of vasospasm *and* hydrocephalus after SAH in patients treated with antifibrinolytics [8, 13].

Experimental results demonstrating the prevention of both cerebral vasospasm *and* hydrocephalus after SAH are striking [2, 5, 12]. Whether clinical use of rtPA is possible remains the most important question. The recent report of Findlay and co-workers [6] on the successful treatment of intraventricular hemorrhage in a case of SAH should encourage further clinical work.

References

1. Bailes JE, Spetzler RF, Hadley MN, Baldwin HZ (1990) Management morbidity and mortality of poor-grade aneurysm patients. J Neurosurg 72:559–566
2. Brinker T, Seifert V, Stolke D (1991) The effect of intrathecal fibrinolysis on the cerebrospinal fluid absorption after experimental subarachnoid hemorrhage. J Neurosurg 74:789–793
3. Butler AB, Maffeo CJ, Johnson RN, Bass NH (1980) Impaired absorption of CSF during experimental subarachnoid hemorrhage: effect of blood components on vesicular transport in arachnoid villi. In: Shulman K, Marmarou A, Miller JD, Becker DP, Hochwald GM, Brock M (eds) Fourth International Symposium on ICP. Springer, New York, pp 245–248

4. Ellington E, Margolis G (1969) Block of arachnoid villus by subarachnoid hemorrhage. J Neurosurg 30:651–657
5. Findlay JM, Weir BKA, Steinke D, Tanabe T, Gordon P, Grace M (1988) Effect of intrathecal thrombolytic therapy on subarachnoid clot and chronic vasospasm in a primate model of SAH. J Neurosurg 69:723–735
6. Findlay M, Weir BKA, Stollery DE (1991) Lysis of intraventricular hematoma with tissue plasminogen activator. Case report. J Neurosurg 74:803–807
7. Foltz EL, Ward AA (1956) Communicating hydrocephalus from subarachnoid bleeding. J Neurosurg 13:546
8. Kassell NF, Torner JC, Adams HP (1984) Antifibrinolytic therapy in the acute period following aneurysmal subarachnoid hemorrhage. J Neurosurg 61:224–230
9. Kusske JA, Turner PT, Ojemann GA, Harris AB (1973) Ventriculostomy for the treatment of acute hydrocephalus following subarachnoid hemorrhage. J Neurosurg 38:591–595
10. Marmarou A, Shulman K, Rosende RM (1978) A nonlinear analysis of the cerebrospinal fluid system and intracranial pressure dynamics. J Neurosurg 48:332–344
11. Prickop LD, Schanker LS, Brodie BB (1961) Passage of lipid-insoluble substances from cerebrospinal fluid to blood. J Pharmacol 135:266–270
12. Seifert V, Eisert WG, Stolke D, Goetz C (1989) Efficacy of single intracisternal bolus injection of recombinant tissue plasminogen activator to prevent delayed cerebral vasospasm after experimental subarachnoid hemorrhage. Neurosurgery 25:590–598
13. Van Gijn J, Hijdra A, Wijdicks EFM, Vermeulen M, van Crevel H (1985) Acute hydrocephalus after aneurysmal subarachnoid hemorrhage. J Neurosurg 63:355–362
14. Vassilouthiis J (1984) The syndrome of normal pressure hydrocephalus. J Neurosurg 61:501–509

Malignant Gliomas

The Neurosurgical Treatment of Malignant Gliomas

W. Seeger[1]

Gliomas are, with few exceptions, not amenable to radical surgery. While the tumor may contain a central core composed of pure tumor tissue, its peripheral portion can permeate an entire hemisphere with nests of tumor cells in areas that cannot be safely resected. The problem is greatest with so-called "benign" gliomas, which grow purely by expansion and may not have a core, i.e., an area in which there are no remaining intact cerebral structures. Differentiation of the core and periphery is easiest in the case of glioblastomas, where both surgical exposure and neurologic imaging reveals a clear line of demarcation between the tumor core and the surrounding, diffusely involved tissue.

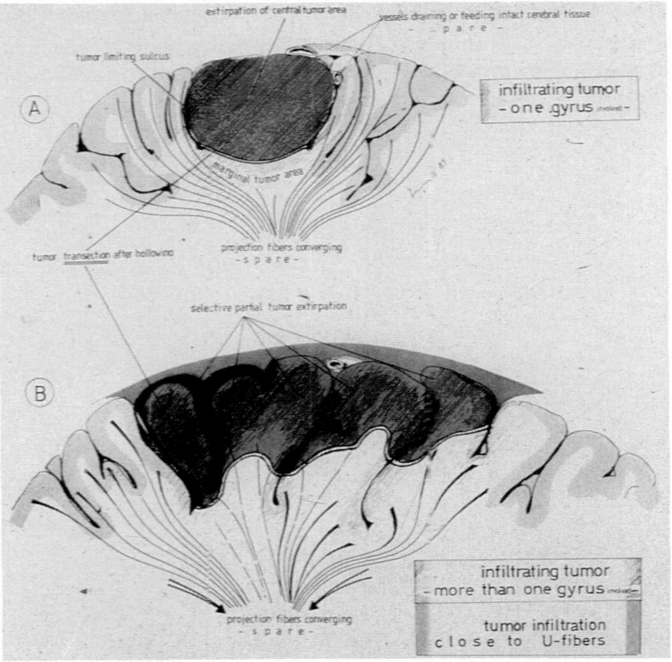

Fig. 1. Tumors that are confined to one gyrus can generally be debulked even in functionally critical areas (*upper part*). A more serious problem is posed by tumors that involve multiple gyri in functionally important regions and have spread to the U fibers (*lower part*)

[1] Klinikum der Universität, Neurochirurgische Universitätsklinik, Hugstetter Str. 55, W–7800 Freiburg, FRG.

Advances in Neurosurgery, Vol. 20
K. Piscol, M. Klinger, M. Brock (Eds.)

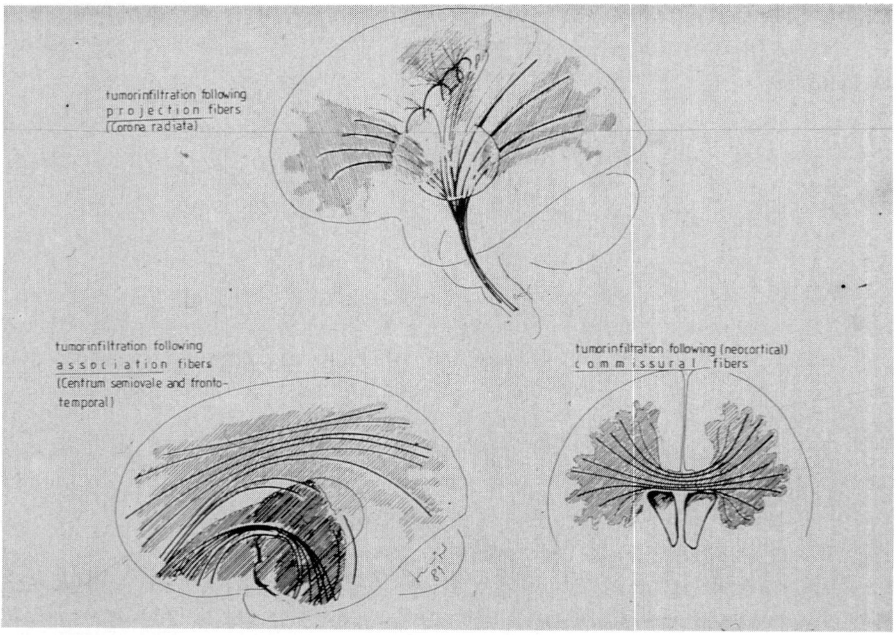

Fig. 2. Many gliomas use the fiber tracts as routes of spread. Depending on its primary site of origin, the tumor may spread along projection tracts, association tracts, or commissural tracts. Gliomas spreading by the latter route are rarely an indication for surgery

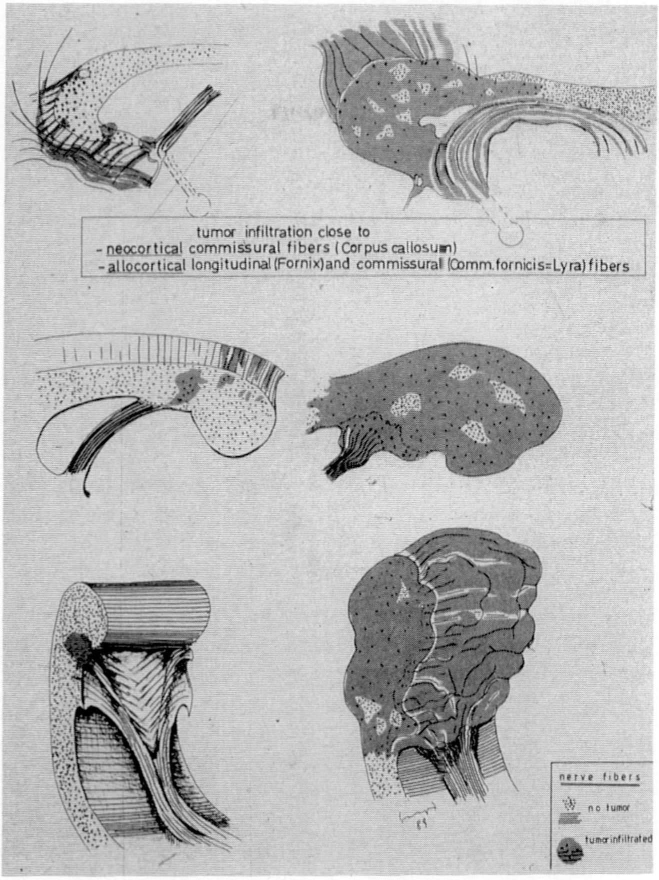

Fig. 3. Midline structures are especially problematic because of the limbic system: the indusium griseum of the corpus callosum with the lateral and medial striate, portions of the cingulum and the fornix columns about the genu of the corpus callosum, the cingular region dorsal to the corpus callosum, and the fornix basal to it in the region of the splenium

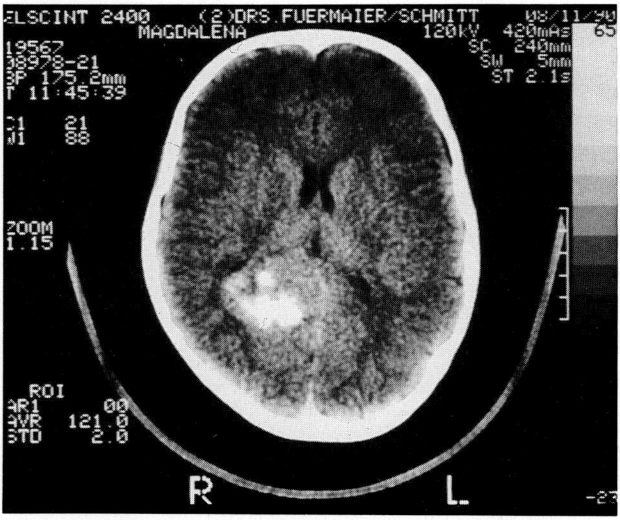

Fig. 4. Unilateral involvement of these structures is also problematic, for we are not dealing with an epileptogenic focus based on a congenital or early childhood lesion, but with tumors that formed later in life. There is, therefore, a greater chance of postoperative mental changes from the unilateral destruction of limbic areas than in operations for epilepsy. A lesion that reaches the base of the atrium and plexus from the occipital side must necessarily traverse the hippocampus and the crus of the fornix. A reductive procedure on this tumor should stop short of the hippocampus

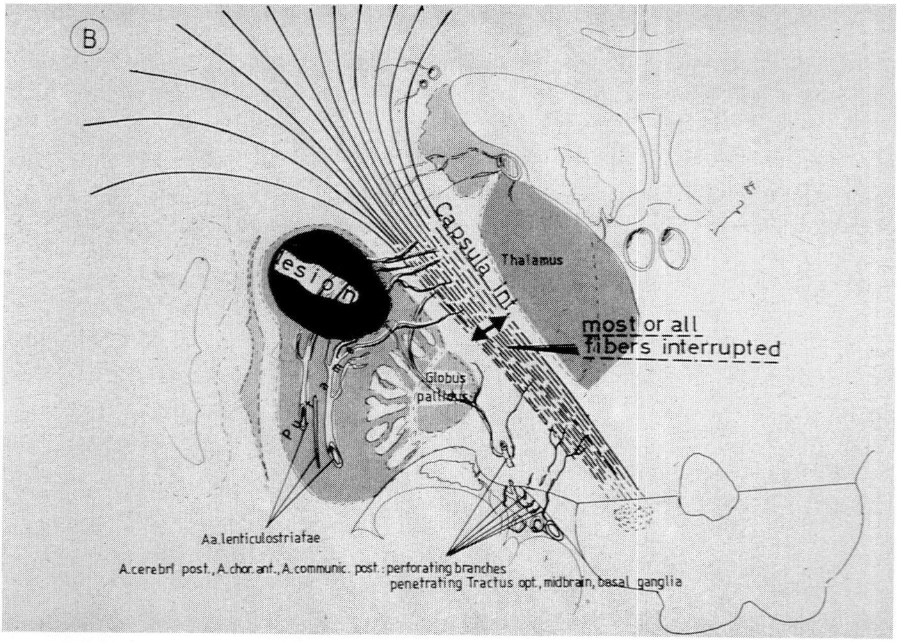

Fig. 5. An operation in the region of the basal ganglia can lead to hemiplegia without damaging the internal capsule if it interrupts the lenticulostriate branches passing from the putamen to the capsule. The same applies to operations for temporo-medial lesions that sacrifice the branches of the anterior choroidal artery

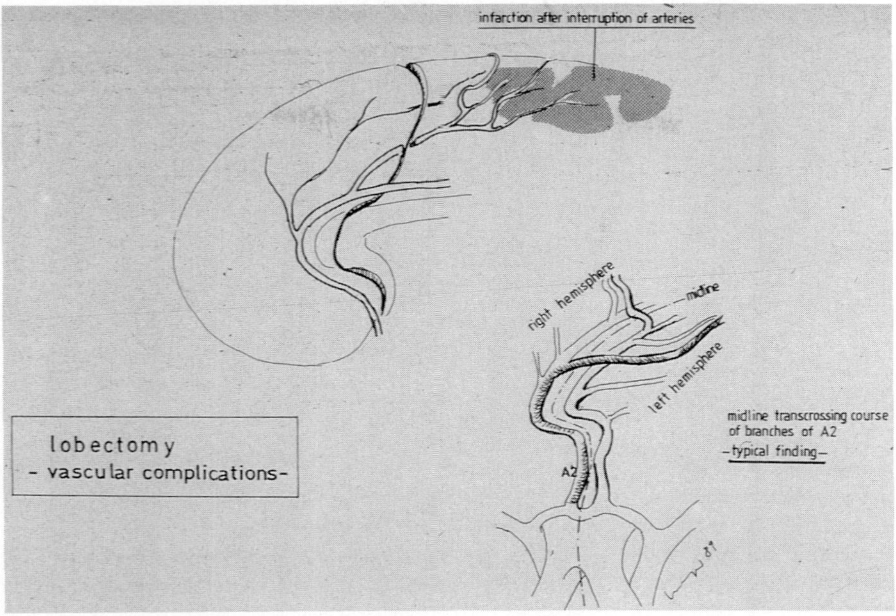

Fig. 6. Other examples of vasogenic insults are lobectomies. Even contralateral malacic foci can develop in the frontal lobe region as it is rare for the anterior cerebral artery to supply just one hemisphere; branches usually pass over the surface of the corpus callosum to the opposite side

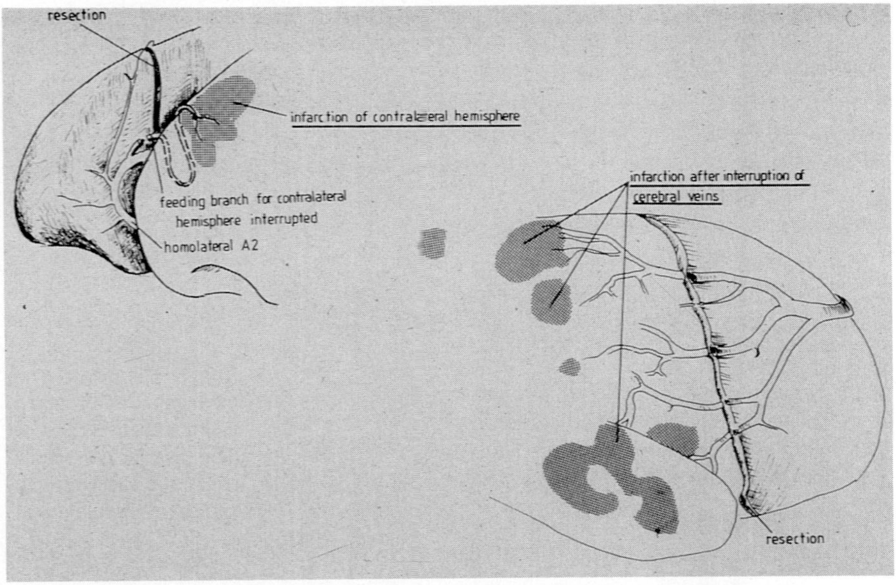

Fig. 7. Venous disruptions caused by lobectomies can also lead to distant foci of cerebral malacia. Given the pattern of spread of gliomas and the vasogenic insult of the operation, there is today essentially no longer a valid reason for performing lobectomy

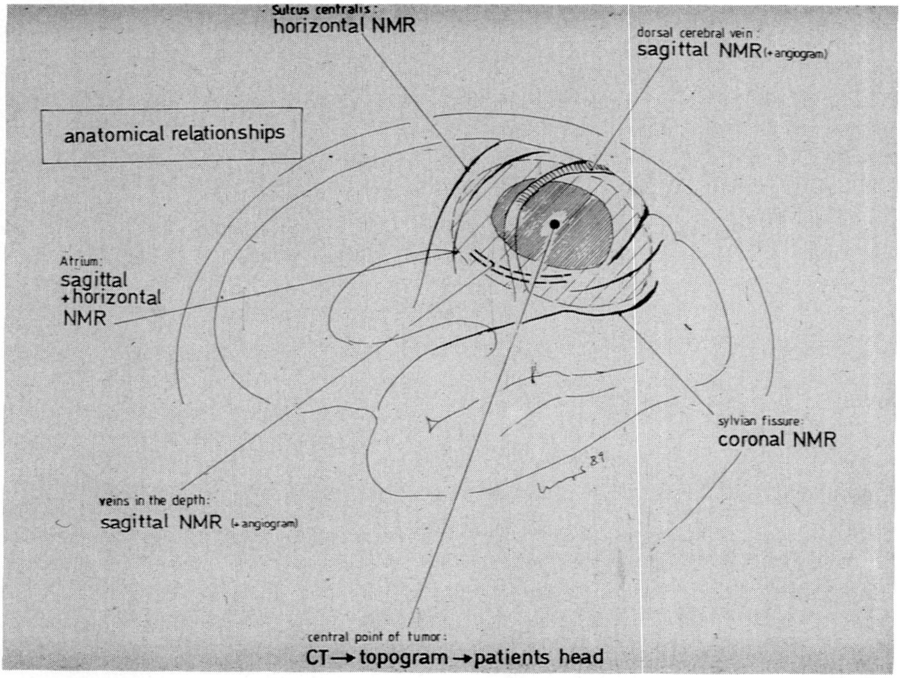

Fig. 8. Example of an oligodendroglioma confined largely to one gyrus behind the central sulcus with no pre- or postoperative deficits

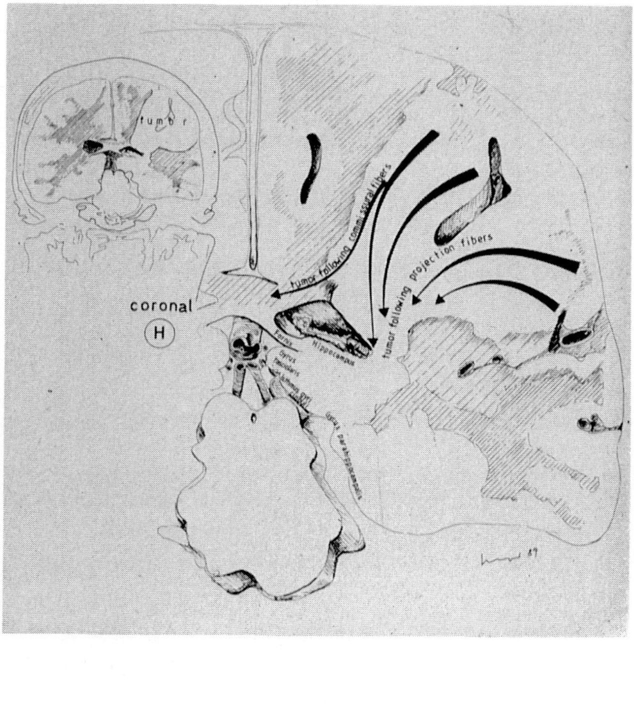

Fig. 9. The magnetic resonance (MR) image and correlative drawing demonstrate tumor extension to the ventricle wall. A recurrence was recently detected at that location following a $2\frac{1}{2}$-year postoperative course

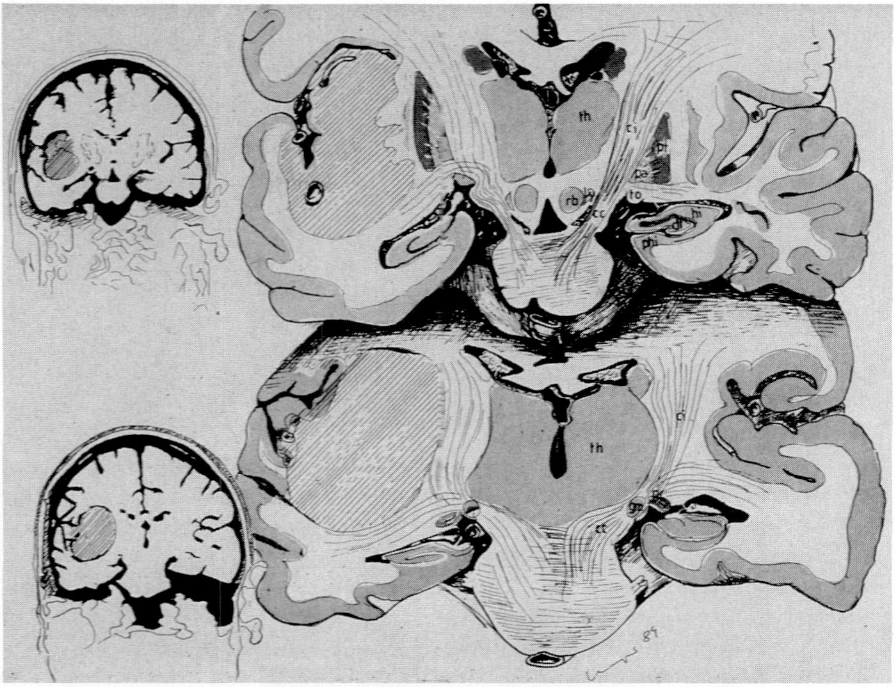

▲ **Fig. 10.** MR appearance of a tumor of the insular cortex spreading to the temporal lobe without involving the hippocampal/parahippocampal region. Reduction in tumor size with no pre- or postoperative deficits

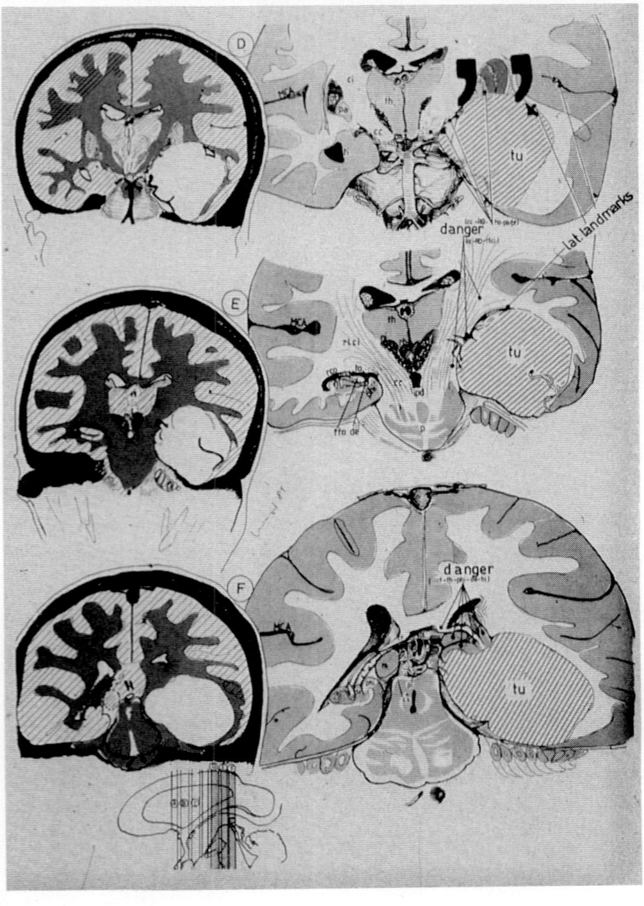

◀ **Fig. 11.** This more temporally located tumor has permeated the hippocampus and the parahippocampal region. Marked personality change did not improve with operative treatment

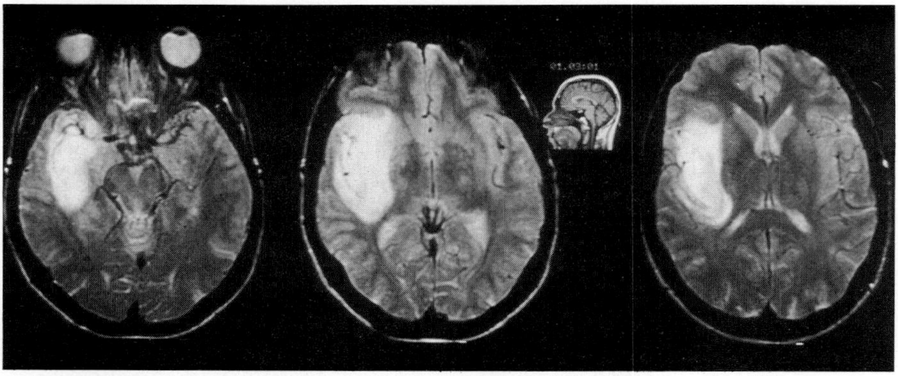

Fig. 12. Subinsular tumor that has invaded the sylvian fissure and encased the middle cerebral artery branches. This tumor was operated on without producing deficits by sparing the basal ganglia and skeletonizing the branches of the middle cerebral artery

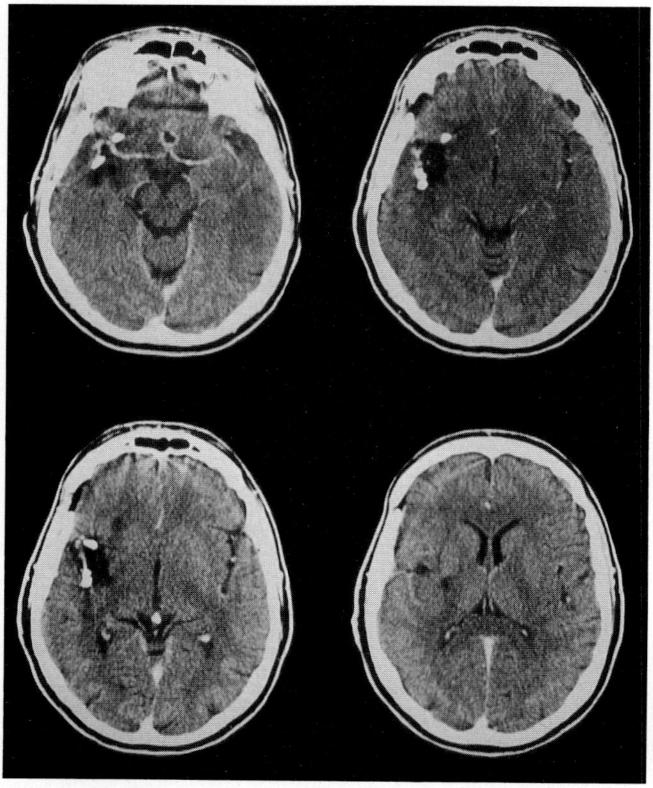

Fig. 13. Postoperative computer tomography (CT) scan with positive enhancement (Ivalon) of the cavity

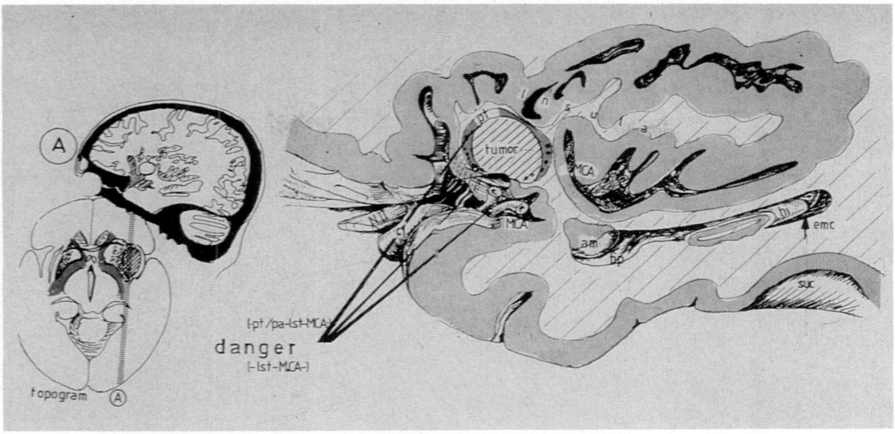

Fig. 14. Glioblastoma of the anterior insular region. Preoperative mixed aphasia regressed after surgery

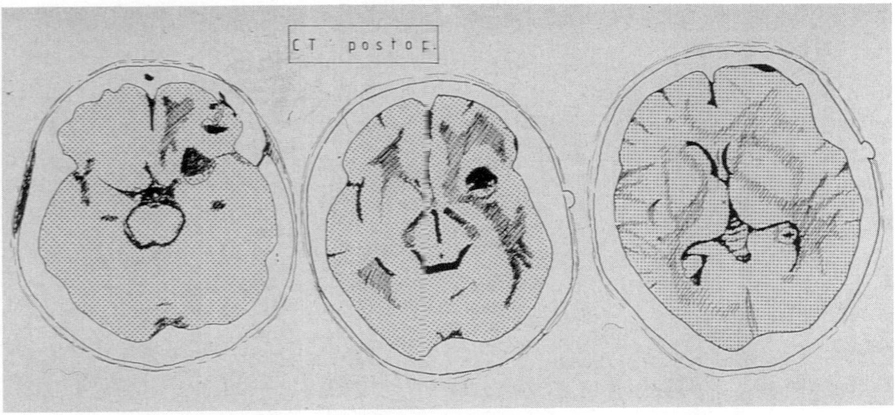

Fig. 15. Postoperative CT scan of the case in Fig. 14

We thank Priv.-Doz. Dr. A. Harders for providing the following compilation of the Freiburg material.

It is apparent that mortality and morbidity have been significantly reduced with respect to earlier operations, but that morbidity is still approximately twice as high as mortality. The survival time in our series has not changed in relation to earlier years.

A comparison of Figs. 17 and 18 shows that surgery was elected with about the same frequency in the functionally critical areas of the left hemisphere as on the right side.

Concern that the tumor core cannot be accurately defined is justified for slow-growing gliomas. With malignant gliomas, the core is much more readily dis-

Microsurgery of Gliomas
Histology (n= 770)

Tumor	%
Glioblastomas	45.0 %
Astrocytomas	28.0 %
Oligodendrogliomas	16.3 %
Mixed Gliomas	8.0 %
Optic Gliomas	1.3 %
Spongioblastomas	1.0 %
Gangliogliomas	0.4 %

Fig. 16

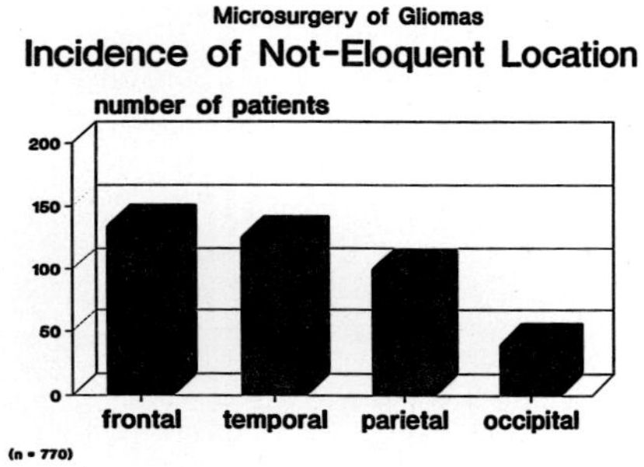

Fig. 17

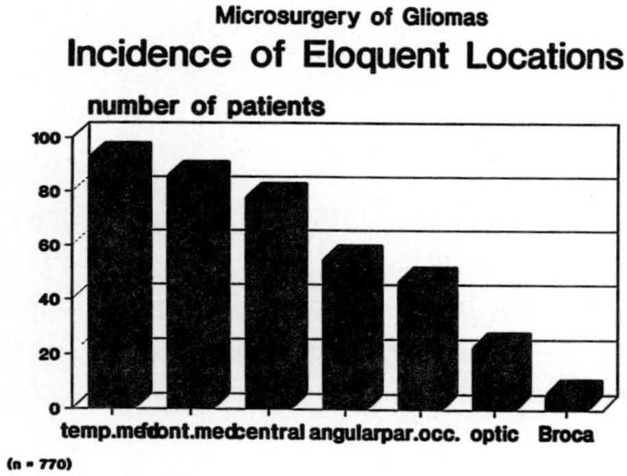

Fig. 18

Microsurgery of Gliomas
1976-1988 (n= 770)

left hemisphere	384	(50 %)
right hemisphere	366	(47 %)
bilateral	20	(3 %)
not eloquent areas	415	(54 %)
eloquent areas	355	(46 %)

Fig. 19. A comparison of the operations on the left and right hemispheres also indicates virtually no preference for the right hemisphere

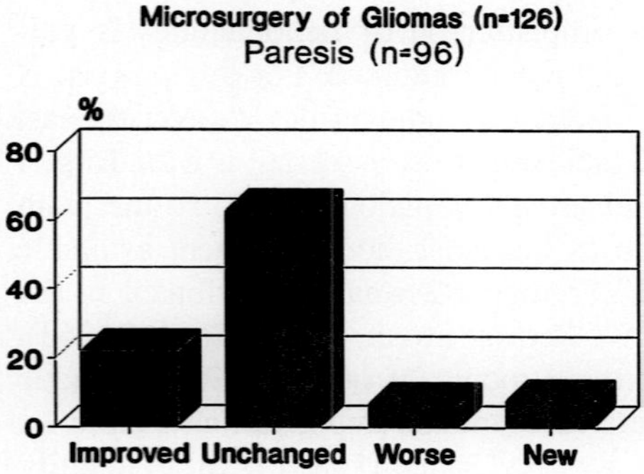

Fig. 20. The best justification for this is provided by an analysis of pre- and postoperative speech disorders, which either remained unchanged or improved but rarely showed exacerbation

Microsurgery of Eloquent Gliomas
Outcome (n=126)

Improved	30 %
Unchanged	65 %
Worse	5 %

Fig. 21. This is also consistent with the overall results of the operations in functionally critical areas

tinguished from peripheral tumor. Thus, the early result is somewhat better for malignant lesions than for benign lesions. The present series includes a slightly higher prevalence of malignant than benign lesions.

If surgery is confined to the principal site of tumor involvement, where one can be reasonably certain that most of the core has been encompassed, there should be no risk of increased postoperative morbidity even in functionally critical areas. The main problem is preservation of the vascular supply. Below the critical cortical regions, limbic structures should be approached with great restraint, even with a unilateral procedure, and should be operated on only if a definite tumor core is present in that region. This also applies to projection tracts, especially those in the capsular region and in the brainstem itself.

Stereotactic Interstitial Brachycurietherapy (Iridium-192 and Iodine-125) in Nonresectable Low-Grade Gliomas

F. Mundinger[1]

Interstitial or intracavitary irradiation using radioisotopes, known as brachytherapy, has become an indispensable part of the intracranial therapy of tumors of the brain and the skull base [3, 4, 10]. Today, the implantation of radionuclides is guided exclusively by the stereotactic image computer technique. For this purpose, I have modified and improved our original Riechert-Mundinger device over the last 20 years to meet the growing number of indications. In association with Birg, I have made the device computer [11] and imaging compatible [1, 12] so that with its large range of software it is referred to as the most modern system available (manufactured by F.L. Fischer MET, 7800 Freiburg, Germany; distributed in the USA by Leibinger and Fischer, Dallas, 8350 Sterling Street, Irving, Texas 75063). The system can be employed in any operating room. Of our 11 439 stereotactic operations (as of 15 April 1991), 2834 were radionuclide implantations (Table 1). In all of these cases, the stereotactic biopsy was performed [5, 8, 15, 16] to identify

Table 1. Bioptically confirmed histology and number of cases in which interstitial irradiation (left) and radionuclei (right) were used at University Hospital and at St. Josef's Hospital, Freiburg, Germany (1952 – 15 April 1991)

Astrocytoma	WHO I–III	1147	^{32}P	32
Oligodendroglioma	WHO II–III	158	^{60}Co	179
Glioblastoma	WHO IV	567	^{90}Y	44
Ependymoma		64	^{182}Ta	21
PNET		87	^{198}Au	129
Meningioma		33	^{125}I	1296
Metastases		191	^{125}I (Brachycurie)	40
Sarcoma		16	^{192}Ir (Gammamed)	401
Pituitary adenomas		265	^{192}Ir	692
Hypophysectomy		57		
Craniopharyngioma		84		
Other lesions		144		
Pallidotomy		21		
Total		2834		2834

[1] St. Josefskrankenhaus, Stereotaktische und funktionelle Neurochirurgie, Hermann-Herder-Str. 1, W–7800 Freiburg, FRG.

Advances in Neurosurgery, Vol. 20
K. Piscol, M. Klinger, M. Brock (Eds.)

Table 2. Life expectancy of patients with low-grade gliomas after brachycurietherapy, dependent on peripheral accumulated tumor dose and volume of tumors (measured in CT [8])

Tumor dose (cGy)	*n*	Mean life expectancy (months)	Survival 2 years (%)	3 years (%)	5 years (%)	10 years (%)
Iridium-192						
12000–18200	7	41.2	42.5	15.5	–	–
12000	104	68.6	67.5	55.0	37.5	25.0
9000–11000	54	72.3	80.0	70.0	45.0	27.5
4000– 9000	6	21.1	57.5	–	–	–
Total	171					
Iodine-125						
12000	83	46.4	62.5	47.5	42.5	–
9000–11000	59	41.8	62.5	55.0	–	–
4000– 9000	42	39.1	65.0	–	–	–
Total	184					

Volume of tumors (cm^3)	*n*	Mean life expectancy (months)	Survival 2 years (%)	3 years (%)	5 years (%)	10 years (%)
0.9– 40	298	66.1	76.9	51.8	43.0	29.4
40 –120	257	38.8	72.2	41.3	27.3	–
≥120	45	26.1	62.5	44.0	–	–

The results of a 10-year follow-up study evaluated in association with Huber-Stentrup, which comprised 600 low-grade astrocytomas and oligodendrogliomas treated between January 1965 and June 1985. For bradycurietherapy with ^{192}Ir the best results were achieved with a peripheral tumor accumulation dose of between 9000 and 11000 cGTy. The dose is also dependent on the volume of the tumor: the smaller the tumor volume, the better the long-term results, as the long-term results of low-grade gliomas show. Therefore, curietherapy should be instituted as soon as possible after the tumor or the tumor recurrence has been detected.

and grade the tumor and to optimize dose planning [8–10]. Out of the large number of radioisotopes available [2–4] 74d-iridium-192 and 60d-iodine-125, which I introduced for intracranial therapy, are the ones now used most commonly [2, 3, 6, 7]. We employ both of these radionuclides for very low dose irradiation (< 2–6 cGy/h). Implantation is usually done with an afterloading catheter, which can be removed to cut off the dose accumulation in the case of severe perifocal reaction. According to evaluations (in association with Huber-Stentrupp) of 650

Table 3. Life expectancy of patients with low-grade gliomas who underwent interstitial irradiation compared with those who had biopsies only (as of June 1985) [10]

	Tumor type	*n*	Percentage of patients surviving at			
			1 year	3 years	5 years	10 years
Iodine-125	Astrocytoma I	67	95	70	55	–
Iridium-192	Astrocytoma I	59	94	86	78	61
Biopsy only	Astrocytoma I	79	73	49	45	21
Iodine-125	Astrocytoma II	106	87	31	28	–
Iridium-192	Astrocytoma II	91	86	45	31	26
Biopsy only	Astrocytoma II	196	86	17	6	–

astrocytomas, the optimal peripheral tumor conformation dose is between 70 and 110 Gy, depending on the location and volume (Table 2).

Underdoses and overdoses worsen the life expectancy. The results of brachycurietherapy using ^{125}I are not as favorable as those obtained with brachycurietherapy using ^{192}Ir, with the exception of tumors in the pineal region and brainstem pons. This is due to the more rapid dose fall-off associated with ^{125}I. Our experience has shown that it is also necessary to reduce the dose around the midline and in the case of recurrent tumors, depending on any previously performed interstitial brachycurietherapy or percutaneous radiotherapy [9, 10].

Since the brain has practically no immunological resistance or regeneration mechanisms, the requirement for a homogeneous dose distribution in the target volume cannot necessarily be satisfied. The radiation necrosis is replaced by a nonfunctioning gliotic scar or cystic liquefaction. For this reason, we do not feel it necessary to distribute the radiation on the low-dose lines as on a grid in an attempt to achieve a homogeneous dose distribution, as is necessary when treating larger tumors with beta emitters such as phosphorous-32 or gold-198 [2, 3, 16]. In most cases ^{192}Ir or ^{125}I implants spaced at a distance of 15–25 mm from one another are sufficient. Depending on the shape of the tumor, they are confined to three, four, or five implantation sites, or sometimes more in bilateral lesions. This also reduces the risk associated with the operation when several emitters have to be distributed.

The various radiobiological responses to low-dose-rate irradiation (curietherapy) and high-dose-rate irradiation (brachycurietherapy) are described in the literature (see [4, 10, 16]).

Radioprotection measures are not required, especially when the soft photon emitter ^{125}I is used. Our long-term results for tumors [6, 7, 10] of the midline, brainstem [16, 17], diencephalon, thalamus [14], pineal restion [15], pituitary [13], and other locations have been presented in a number of evaluations, which I and my coworker compiled in my former institution (Department of Neurosurgery, Freiburg). The therapeutic value for very critical indications is evident, even in patients in whom all other forms of treatment have been unsuccessful. Interstitial brachytherapy without doubt has additionally improved the survival time in patients

Table 4. Brachycurietherapy for various tumors

Malignant tumors		*Recurrence of malignant tumors and/or of irridation necrosis*	
			Tumor conformation dose
– Operation with resection or debulking whenever possible and advisable (quality of life?)		– Reoperation with debulking	
– External irradiation		– Brachycurietherapy	
– Brachycurietherapy (better inverse)		– High-dose-rate iridium-192 or iodine-125 after loading	25–30 Gy
– Chemotherapy		– Low-dose-rate iodine-125	70 Gy
		– Depending on dose time factor, additional local fractioned external irradiation	15–20 Gy
Small corticosubcortical malignant tumors		*Recurrence of small corticosubcortical malignant tumors and/or irradiation necrosis*	
	Tumor conformation dose		Tumor conformation dose
– Open stereotactic biopsy with debulking		– Open stereotactic biopsy with debulking	
– Brachycurietherapy		– Repeated brachycurietherapy with low-dose-rate iodine-125	70 Gy
– High-dose-rate iridium-192 after loading, e.g., Gammamed	30 Gy in min	– Possibly, focal external irradiation	10–20 Gy
– High-dose-rate iodine-125 after loading	30 Gy in 3–7 days	– Continuation of chemotherapy?	
– Low-dose-rate iodine-125 after loading or combined	85–100 Gy in 5–7 min		
– Focal fractionated irradiation starting after 14 days	45–55 Gy		
– Chemotherapy			
Non resectable malignant tumors of the midline (diencephalon, brainstem/pons, central dominant temporal region)		*Recurrence of malignant tumors of the midline (diencephalon, brainstem/pons, central dominant temporal region)*	
	Tumor conformation dose		Tumor conformation dose
– Stereotactic biopsy		– Stereotactic rebiopsy	
– Brachycurietherapy with iodine-125 directly or after loading	40–70 Gy	– Brachycurietherapy with iodine-125 directly or after loading	40–70 Gy
– Possibly, focal fractioned external irradiation	10–20 Gy	– Possibly, focal fractioned external irradiation	10–20 Gy

with high Karnofsky scores. This applies especially for nonresectable midline or hemispheric tumors, particularly low-grade ones. The treatment also has a palliative effect on higher-grade tumors, including recurrent disease. The long-term results of interstitial brachytherapy in low-grade astrocytomas are presented in Table 3.

Table 4 illustrates how, based on our long-term results, image stereotactic brachycurietherapy should be fitted into the therapy regimen and the corresponding tumor conformity doses.

References

1. Birg W, Mundinger F (1973) Computer calculations of target parameters for a stereotactic apparatus. Acta Neurochir (Wien) 29:123–129
2. Mundinger F (1966) Treatment of brian tumors with radioisotopes. In: Krayenbühl H, Maspes M, Sweet W (eds) Progress of neurological surgery, vol I. Karger, Basel, pp 202–257
3. Mundinger F (1970) The treatment of brain tumors with interstitially applied radioactive isotopes. In: Yen Qang, Paoletti P (eds) Radionuclide applications in neurology and neurosurgery. Charles C. Thomas, Springfield Ill, pp 199–265
4. Mundinger F (1982) Implantation of radioisotopes (curietherapy). In: Schaltenbrand G, Walker AE (eds) Textbook of stereotaxy of the human brain. Thieme, Stuttgart, pp 410–435
5. Mundinger F (1982) CT-stereotactic biopsy of brain tumors. In: Voth D, Gutjahr P, Langmaid C (eds) Tumours of the central nervous system in infancy and childhood. Springer, Berlin Heidelberg New York, pp 234–246
6. Mundinger F (1985) Technik und Ergebnisse der interstitiellen Hirntumorbestrahlung. In: Heilmann HP (Hrsg) Handbuch der medizinischen Radiologie, Bd XIX/4: Spezielle Strahlentherapie maligner Tumoren. Springer, Berlin Heidelberg New York, S 179–214
7. Mundinger F (1988) Interstitielle Curietherapie bei Gliomen niedrigen Malignitätsgrades. In: Bamberg M, Sack H (Hrsg) Therapie primärer Hirntumoren. Zuckschwerdt, München Bern Wien San Francisco, S 285–290
8. Mundinger F (1988) Stereotactic biopsy and implantation of radionuclides guided by computed tomography or magnetic resonance imaging for therapy of brain tumors. In: Schmidek HH, Sweet WH (eds) Operative neurosurgical techniques, vol I. Grune & Stratton, New York, pp 491–514
9. Mundinger F (1989) Dosimetry in imaging-stereotactic interstitial Curietherapy (Brachycurie-therapy) with Iridium-192 and Iodine-125. In: Dyck P, Bouzaglou A (eds) Neurosurgery – brachytherapy of brain tumors and related stereotactic treatment, vol 4/Suppl. Hanley & Belfus, Philadelphia, pp 75–94
10. Mundinger F (1991) Imaging-stereotaxic implantation of radionuclides in intracranial tumors (Curietherapy and Brachycurietherapy). In: Sauer R (ed) Medical radiology interventional radiation therapy techniques – Brachytherapy. Springer, Berlin Heidelberg New York Tokyo, pp 67–79
11. Mundinger F, Birg W (1981) CT-aided stereotaxy for functional neurosurgery and deep brain implants. Acta Neurochir 56:245
12. Mundinger F, Birg W (1988) The imaging-compatible Riechert-Mundinger-system. In: Lunsford LD (ed) Modern stereotactic neurosurgery. Martinus Nijhoff, Boston Dordrecht Lancaster, pp 13–25
13. Mundinger F, Riechert T (1969) Hypophysentumoren, Hypophysektomie. Klinik, Therapie, Ergebnisse. Thieme, Stuttgart
14. Mundinger F, Weigel K (1984) Stereotactic Curietherapy of thalamic tumours. J Neurooncol 2:264–278

15. Mundinger F, Weigel K (1988) Die stereotaktische Biopsie und interstitielle Therapie von Raumforderungen der Pinealisregion. In: Bamberg M, Sack H (Hrsg) Therapie primärer Hirntumoren. Zuckschwerdt, München Bern Wien San Francisco, S 361–366
16. Mundinger F, Birg W, Etou A, Mohadjer M (1988) CT/NMR-stereotaktische diagnose und Curie-Therapie von Tumoren des Mittelhirn/Hirnstamm-Brückenbereichs. Vergleichende Studie zur Biopsie allein, perkutanen Bestrahlung und Resektion – 10-jährige Verlaufsbeobachtungen von 148 Patienten (1965–30.6.1985). In: Walter W, Krenkel W (Hrsg) Jahrbuch der Neurochirurgie 1988. Regensberg & Biermann, Münster, S 51–72
17. Mundinger F, Braus DF, Krauss J, Birg W (1991) Long-term outcome of 89 low-grade brain-stem gliomas after interstitial radiation therapy. J Neurosurg 75

Perspectives of Glioma Treatment with Boron Neutron Capture Therapy in Europe

D. Gabel[1]

Introduction

Boron neutron capture therapy (BNCT) is based on the high cross-section of the boron-10 nuclide for thermal neutrons. Upon capture, the boron nucleus disintegrates into highly energetic alpha- and lithium-7 particles. One event liberates enough energy to, in principle, kill a cell. The nuclides that are present in the body (hydrogen, nitrogen, carbon, oxygen) possess such low cross-sections for thermal neutrons that already modest amounts of boron (in the order of several tens of micrograms boron per gram tissue) suffice to deliver a substantially increased dose to that tissue.

Since 1989, the Commission of the European Community (CEC) funds, through their program Europe against Cancer, a Concerted Action European Collaboration on Boron Neutron Capture Therapy.

The European Collaboration has two main goals. Goal 1 is to initiate clinical trials for glioma at the High Flux Reactor, Petten, at the earliest possible time. Goal 2 is to create all necessary conditions to initiate clinical trials for other tumors and treatment at other facilities.

Previously, BNCT had been tried in the United States of America [1] and is presently used in Japan [3, 4] for the treatment of glioma. In both cases, a thermal neutron beam was used. Thermal neutrons possess a half-value layer in tissue of around 1.5 cm and are thus not capable of reaching deeper-seated tumors.

In the approach to clinical trials for glioma in Europe, epithermal neutrons will be used. Whereas epithermal neutrons do not transfer much energy to tissue by themselves, they penetrate far deeper in the tissue, where they are slowed down to thermal neutrons. Thus, problems encountered in the first clinical trials of BNCT in the United States of America with excessive damage to skin might be avoided, while at the same time permitting treatment of glioma through the intact skull.

In this overview the activities of the European Collaboration toward treatment of glioma are summarized, and a proposed treatment scheme is presented. The tasks necessary to achieve before clinical trials can begin are listed in Table 1.

[1] Neurochirurgische Klinik, Zentralkrankenhaus St.-Jürgen-Str., W–2800 Bremen, FRG.

Advances in Neurosurgery, Vol. 20
K. Piscol, M. Klinger, M. Brock (Eds.)

Table 1. Accomplishments necessary before clinical trials with BNCT

Design, construction, and installation of an epithermal neutron beam
Physical and biological characterization of the beam
Installation of a suitable treatment room with corollary facilities
Pharmacokinetic and toxicity studies of boronated tumor seekers
Establishment of a response function for healthy tissue to the treatment intended
Development of an adequate treatment planning modality

Development of a Treatment Facility

The High Flux Reactor of the Joint Research Center of the CEC in Petten, Holland, has been made available for modification for BNCT [8]. The reactor is a 45 MW light water swimming pool reactor. It is used mainly for material testing. The availability of the reactor is very high. A broad-spectrum epithermal beam has been installed at the reactor. The irradiation location is around 5 m from the reactor core, and consequently the beam has little divergence at the treatment location.

The energies of the incident epithermal neutrons are such that they do not deposit large radiation doses in tissue, while permitting thermalization of the neutrons within the target. As shown in Fig. 1, the peak thermal flux for epithermal beams occurs well below the skin.

It was considered important to utilize to as high a degree as possible all the experience that has been gained with other types of radiation therapy. Therefore, the treatment room has been designed such as to permit bilateral irradiations of the head. By then using parallelly opposed fields, tumors in the midline of the brain can still be treated. An observation area and an area for patient preparation will be installed, in accordance with facilities used for conventional radiotherapy.

The facility will allow treatment of patients well in excess of 1000 per year.

Preconditions for Therapy

In Europe, BNCT is planned to be tried clinically by the end of 1991 or beginning of 1992. It is planned to treat glioma patients, with $Na_2B_{12}H_{11}SH$ (BSH) as the boron compound. This compound is presently used by Hatanaka [3, 4] for treatment of glioma with a thermal neutron beam.

Before the treatment can be tried, it must be established that the risk of the treatment is low. To achieve this, the tolerance of healthy tissue to BNCT conditions needs to be determined in animals, and the pharmacokinetics of the boron compound in question needs to be established in both animals and patients.

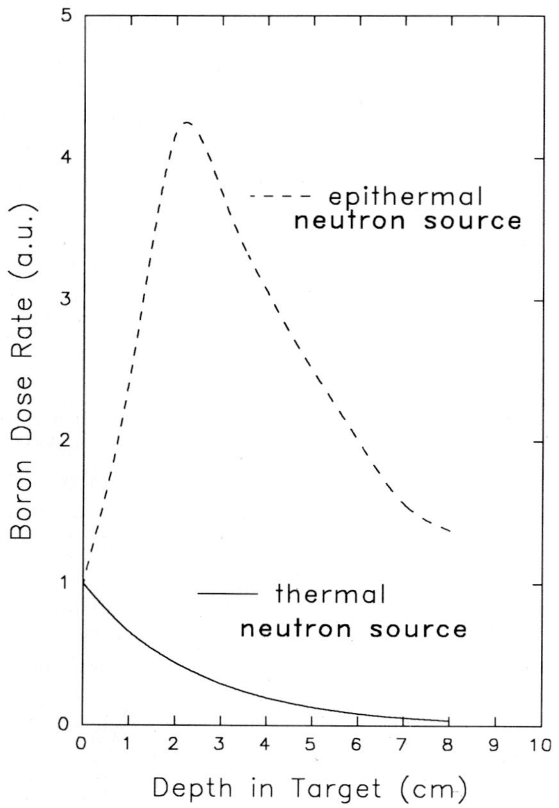

Fig. 1. Comparison of dose rate from neutron capture reactions in a thermal and an epithermal neutron beam. The dose rates (arbitrary units) are recorded along the central axis of a cylindrical phantom filled with tissue-equivalent liquid and normalized to the dose rate at the surface (the skin in case of a patient). Boron is present homogeneously throughout the phantom. Other dose contributions are not shown. They include the dose from incident fast neutrons and from incident and induce γ-photons. The data pertain to the thermal and epithermal beams of the Brookhaven Medical Reseach Reactor. [7]

Healthy Tissue Tolerance

Healthy tissue tolerance will be studied in dogs. The dogs will be given BSH in different amounts, and will then be exposed to different levels of neutron irradiation. From the initial studies on healthy tissue tolerance in dogs carried out in the United States [2], as well as from the dose-depth profiles of such beams in phantoms, the likely tissue at risk is not the skin, but tissue at a few centimeters depth (i.e., brain tissue) (see also Fig. 1). White matter necrosis could occur with such treatment, and this will take several months to develop.

In previous experience of the late 1950s and early 1960s, skin was the most radiosensitive organ. This was caused by both a high boron concentration in the skin and the simultaneous use of a thermal neutron beam. With epithermal beams of moderate mean energy, skin appears to be no longer the dose limiting healthy tissue. Due to the importance of localization of boron [5], the maximally tolerated dose will be dependent on both the compound and the target organ.

Table 2. Glioma treatment with BNCT – Phase I

Selection of patients
Expected Karnovski scale rating > 60 after surgery
Expected survival > 8–12 months
Surgery
BSH administered preoperatively to check uptake
Pre- and postoperative MRI scans
Transport to NKI, Amsterdam, after wound healing
Fractionated BNCT
5–6 fractions in 2 weeks
Infusion of BSH
Transport to Petten by ambulance
Irradiation
Transport to NKI
Return to home
Follow-up
MRI, CT scans
Pituitary gland function
Neurological observation

Pharmacokinetics of BSH

The knowledge of the pharmacokinetics of the boron compound is of paramount importance for treatment planning with the aim of maximizing the neutron dose to be given. Therefore, the European Collaboration has placed great emphasis on a thorough pharmacokinetic study of BSH in brain tumor patients. Data on the boron concentration in different tissues and their time dependence are being collected (see, e.g., [6]). Provided that the study on healthy tissue tolerance does not result in unacceptable damage to the tissue exposed, treatment trials for glioma will be able to start toward the end of 1992.

Proposed Treatment Protocol

The proposed treatment protocol is shown in Table 2. The treatment protocol differs from that currently applied to the treatment of glioma by substituting conventional radiotherapy by BNCT. Thus, patients are first operated upon at the participating neurosurgery department. After wound healing, they are transferred to the National Cancer Institute (NKI) in Amsterdam, which serves as the hospital base for the treatment in Petten. Patients will receive 5–6 fractions of BNCT over the course of 2 weeks. BSH will be infused prior to each fraction. Follow-up after return to home will be with all the means available at the participating home hospital.

Future Perspectives of the European Collaboration

The primary goals of the European Collaboration, as described here, are presently being funded to the middle of 1992. However, the work, and the need for cooperation, will not stop then.

Clinical trials will have begun. The fact that several centers will send patients, and the need for thorough follow-up from the referring institutions, will necessitate a very intense exchange of results and experiences between the centers. For this reason, a follow-up or continuation of the European Collaboration seems desirable and necessary. It may serve as a first example for a European cancer treatment facility and could therefore have an impact on patients in Europe extending beyond the immediate treatment of glioma.

Acknowledgment. I am in indebted to my colleagues of the Collaboration for their enthusiasm. The work of the European Collaboration of Boron Neutron Capture Therapy is supported by the Commission of the European Community. Financial support of national agencies and foundations for the individual projects makes this Collaboration possible. Thanks are due to R. Alberts for skillful and competent organizational and secretarial assistance in the coordination of this project.

References

1. Ashbury AK, Ojemann RG, Nielsen SL, Sweet WH (1972) Neuropathologic study of fourteen cases of malignant brain tumor treated by boron-10 slow neutron capture radiation. J Neuropathol Exp Neurol 31:278–303
2. DeHaan CE, Gavin PR, Kraft SL, Wheeler FJ, Atkinson CA (1991) Acute and late reactions following epithermal-neutron irradiation of the normal canine brain. In: Allen B (ed) Neutron capture therapy of tumors. Plenum Press, New York
3. Hatanaka H (1986) Boron-neutron capture therapy for tumors. Nishimura, Niigata
4. Hatanaka H (1990) Clinical results of boron neutron capture therapy. In: Neuron beam design, development, and performance for neutron capture therapy, vol 54. Plenum Press, New York (Basic Life Sciences, pp 15–22)
5. Gabel D (1990) Approach to boron neutron capture therapy in Europe: Goals of a European Collaboration on Boron Neutron Capture Therapy. In: Proc. European Particle Accelerator Conference EPAC 90. Editions Frontières, Gif-sur-Yvette, pp 283–285
6. Haritz D, Piscol K, Klein H, Gabel D (1991) These proceedings
7. Fairchild RG, Kalef-Ezra J, Saraf SK, Fiarman S, Ramsay E, Wielopolski L, Laster BH, Wheeler F (1990) Installation and testing of an optimized epithermal neutron beam at the Brookhaven Medical Research Reactor (BMRR). In: Neutron beam design, development and performance for neutron capture therapy, vol 54. Plenum Press, New York (Basic Life Sciences, pp 185–200)
8. Moss RL, Stecher-Rasmussen F, Huiskamp R, Dewit L, Mijnheer B (1991) The Petten BNCT project. In: Allen B (ed) Neutron capture therapy of tumors. Plenum Press, New York

Clinical Investigations in Boron Neutron Capture Therapy (BNCT): Pharmacokinetic, Biodistribution, and Toxicity of $Na_2B_{12}H_{11}SH$ (BSH) in Patients with Malignant Glioma

D. Haritz[1], D. Gabel[2], H. Klein[3], and K. Piscol[1]

Introduction

One of the goals of the European Collaboration on Boron Neutron Capture Therapy is to treat malignant gliomas (WHO grade III–IV), using $Na_2B_{12}H_{11}SH$ (BSH) as boron carrier. To treat these tumors with boron neutron capture therapy, it is necessary to accumulate sufficient amounts of boron in the tumor prior to irradiation and at the same time ensure that healthy tissue unavoidably present in the neutron beam contains a minimal amount of boron.

The concentration of boronated compounds in the tissues eventually exposed to the neutron beam is of utmost importance for the prediction of healthy tissue damage and tumor control. In the literature, no detailed information about the biodistribution of BSH in man is found [3]. Therefore, a clinical phase I study has been started. We wish to report here on the pharmacokinetics, tissue distribution, and the possible toxicity of BSH in eight patients with malignant astrocytoma (WHO III–IV) or glioblastoma multiforme.

Protocol

For this study, a coordinated protocol has been established within the European Collaboration. BSH is infused into the patient during the course of 1 h, and blood samples and urine are taken at predetermined intervals. During the operation tissue samples are obtained. These include: skin, muscle, galea, bone, dura mater, cerebrospinal fluid (CSF), normal brain (if available), and tumor tissue. In our study, authorized by the local ethical committee, the patients eligible to enter the study must have a presumed high-grade glioma indicated by CT, MRI, or angiography. The patients are informed about their presumed malignant tumor and the nontherapeutic aim of the study and participate on a voluntary basis. Patients with reduced function of the liver, lung, kidneys, and cardiovascular system are excluded, as are those with major endocrinologic disturbances. The following clinical chemical parameters are among those measured prior to administration and at the 1st, 2nd,

[1] Neurochirurgische Klinik, Zentralkrankenhaus St.-Jürgen-Str., W–2800 Bremen, FRG.
[2] Abteilung für Chemie der Universität Bremen, W–2800 Bremen, FRG.
[3] Institut für Klinische Neuropathologie, Zentralkrankenhaus Ost, W–2800 Bremen, FRG.

Advances in Neurosurgery, Vol. 20
K. Piscol, M. Klinger, M. Brock (Eds.)

7th, and 14th day after the operation to evaluate possible toxic side effects of BSH: complete blood count and clotting, liver enzymes, electrolytes, creatinine, and urea.

BSH is infused through a central venous catheter at a maximal concentration of 15 mg BSH/kg body weight. Blood is taken at predetermined intervals up to 96 h after the start of the infusion. Tissues are removed during the operation either 3, 6, 12, 18, or 24 h after the infusion. Tissues and liquids are frozen rapidly in liquid nitrogen and stored in a freezer at –23°C.

Boron Analysis and Histological Investigations

The concentration of boron in blood and tissues is measured by quantitative neutron capture radiography (QNCR) [1], that in urine and CSF by induced coupled plasma-atomic emission spectroscopy (ICP-AES).

For QNCR, the samples are embedded in 3% carboxymethylcellulose. Cryosections are cut every 1 mm. Standards are prepared from chicken liver, calf brain, or human blood by adding known amounts of boric acid, and 50-μm sections are produced. The sections are mounted onto Kodak Pathé LR 115 Type 1 track detectors and exposed to around 5×10^{12} neutrons $\times$ cm^{-2} at the Neutron Radiography facility in Studsvik, Sweden. The detectors are etched at 60°C in 10% NaOH for around 50 min. The etched detectors are evaluated in an image analyzer, consisting of a microscope, a TV camera, a personal computer with appropriate hard- and software, and a monitor.

By using a bone biopsy needle of 2 mm diameter, small tissue samples are obtained from the exposed surface of the material during cryomicrotomy. After fixation in 10% formalin, embedding, cutting and staining in hematoxylin-eosin, they are examined neuropathologically. The differential diagnoses are reconfirmed, and the type of tissue and density of cells in the sample are described.

Results of the Toxicity Investigation

In none of the eight patients who entered the study to date were measurable acute toxic side effects of BSH found in cardiovascular function, allergenic reaction, bone marrow depletion, liver and kidney functions, and the endocrinologic system. The patients did not complain of any subjective disorders such as nausea or vomiting.

Boron Distribution and Pharmacokinetics

Figure 1 shows the boron concentration in blood of three patients. The boron decrease in blood after the end of the infusion follows biphasic kinetics. For all of the eight patients, the first component had a half-time of around 11 h, whereas the second showed a half-time of around 25 h. Large amounts of boron were found in the urine already shortly after the beginning of the BSH administration. It

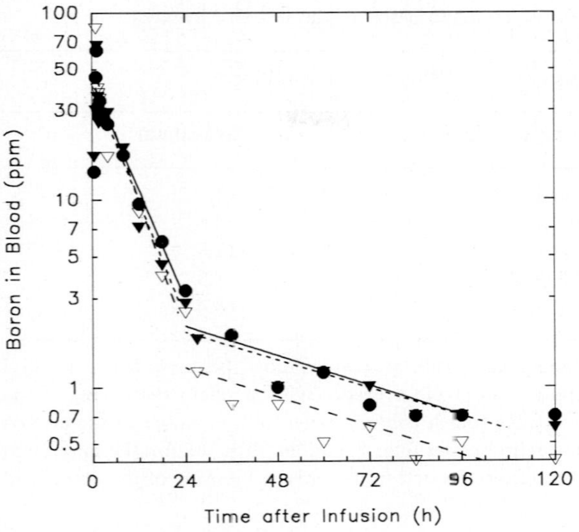

Fig. 1. Pharmacokinetics of BSH in blood of three of the eight patients over the observation period of 120 h after the infusion. The different symbols represent the patients MK (*filled circles*), LK (*open triangles*), and EA (*filled triangles*). The *lines* represent the regression curves for each patient. The boron concentration in blood raises up to values of around seven times more than the administered dose and decreases following biphasic kinetics

is therefore not sure that the first half-time can be equated with the distribution phase and the second with the elimination phase. The evaluation of the QNCRs shows consistently a highly heterogeneous distribution in the neuropathologically reconfirmed tumor tissue [2]. Parts of the tumor tissue accumulate BSH in very high concentrations; this correlates to the histological finding of dense tumor cells with many pathological vessels. In other tissue samples, adjacent areas, less than 1 mm apart, differed by up to one order of magnitude in boron concentration. This corresponds either with spongious formation of tumor cells with only a few vessels or signs of cellular degeneration. In necrotic areas, BSH uptake is very low. In healthy brain, no significant boron uptake is measured. Table 1 shows a summary of the last five patients. The ratio of the boron concentration in tumor to blood increases with a longer interval between BSH administration and sampling of the tumor tissue. Also the maximum values of the tumor to blood ratio are measured at a higher level. Many of the tumor samples, compiled in the fourth column, contained a concentration ratio in tumor to blood greater than 1. For patient FB only 2 of 19 proven tumor samples displayed dense accumulation of tumor cells with a correspondingly high concentration of BSH. The rest of the tissue samples showed a very spongious cell formation and many necrotic areas, which might explain why the measured maximum value of the tumor to blood ratio was very low (see column 5). Figure 2 gives an overview about the ratio of the boron concentration in tumor to blood, and the boron concentration measured in tumor tissue contingent on the

Table 1. Boron concentration ratios of tumor to blood of the last five patients

Patient	Interval (h)	Concentration ratios of tumor to blood		
		Average ± SD	> 1	Maximum
EA	12	0.79 ± 0.56	7/14	1.4
VO	12	1.56 ± 1.80	9/20	4.6
MK	18	8.18 ± 2.80	19/19	11.8
FB	18	0.58 ± 0.21	2/19	1.5
LK	24	3.97 ± 3.48	34/35	18.4

The first column includes the patient code, the second column the time between BSH administration and surgery, the third column the average (with standard deviation) of the concentration ratio of tumor to blood, the fourth column includes the number of the proven tumor biopsies with a concentration ratio greater than 1, and the fifth column the maximum tumor-to-blood boron concentration ratio measured in the proven biopsies of the embedded tissue during cryomicrotomy.

Table 2. Boron concentration ratios in tissues (obtained during surgery at predetermined intervals)

Patient	Interval (h)	Concentration ratios of tissue to blood		
		Muscle	Skin	Bone
VORM	3	–	–	0.1
RUP	3	0.5	0.0	0.0
V	6	–	–	0.1
EA	12	0.1	0.0	0.0
VO	12	0.8	0.5	0.1
MK	18	0.5	0.9	0.1
FB	18	0.4	0.3	0.1
LK	24	2.0	1.3	0.3

For patients VORM and V samples of muscle and skin were not achieved. Uptake of BSH is only very low or reaches up to blood values.

time between BSH infusion and sampling of the tissue. The maximum values are shown for all of the eight patients. For the last five patients, we used the technique to reconfirm the neuropathological status with a biopsy from the exposed surface of the embedded tumor tissue during cryomicrotomy. Therefore, the average values for these patients are specified (see interruptured lines). The initial high uptake of BSH decreases only slowly with time. As the blood is cleared rather rapidly (see Fig. 1), there is a significant increase of the tumor-to-blood ratio with time. This pertains to both the maximum values and the average values.

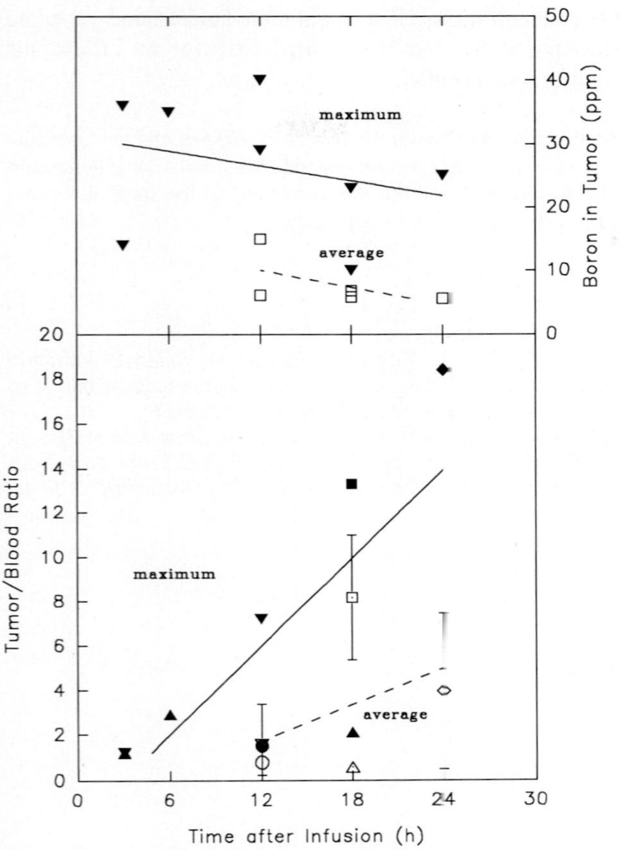

Fig. 2. Boron concentration ratio in tumor to blood dependent on the time after the BSH administration (*lower part*) and the measured boron concentration in tumor tissue (*upper part*). The *lines* represent the regression curve of the maximum values of all of the eight patients; the *broken lines* represent the average values of the last five patients where the obtained biopsies are proven histopathologically. With a longer period between the BSH administration and the tissue sampling, an increase of the tumor-to-blood ratio can be observed, while the decrease of the boron concentration in the tumor tissue is very low over time

For other tissues (see Table 2), boron concentrations are very low (bone, fat, CSF) or it reaches occasionally up to blood concentrations (skin, muscle).

Discussion

In this study, we showed that BSH is taken up in malignant gliomas. In normal brain no significant uptake is measured. By combining QNCR and the histological status, we have the possibility to correlate with a good spatial resolution the type of tissue with an administered boron concentration. Dose escalation studies and repeated administration of BSH are required for building a firm base for an efficacious boron neutron capture therapy in the future.

Acknowledgment. Financial support from the Senator for Health of Bremen and the Commission of the European Communities is gratefully acknowledged. Ms. Orn-Anong Pettersson from the University of Uppsala, Sweden, carried out the irradiation of the track detectors; we say many thanks for her personal contribution to our study.

References

1. Gabel D, Holstein H, Larsson B, Gille L, Ericson G, Sacker D, Somn P, Fairchild RG (1987) Quantitative neutron capture radiography for studying the biodistribution of tumor-seeking boron-containing compounds. Cancer Res 47:5451–5456
2. Haritz D, Gabel D, Piscol K (1991) The distribution of BSH in patients with malginant glioma. In: Allen BJ (ed) Neutron capture therapy for cancer. Plenum Press, New York
3. Hatanaka H (1986) Boron neutron capture therapy for tumors. Nishimura, Niigata/ Japan

Laser-Induced Interstitial Thermotherapy of Malignant Gliomas

M. Bettag, F. Ulrich, R. Schober, M. Sabel, T. Kahn, S. Hessel, and W. J. Bock[1]

Introduction

Interstitial thermotherapy using a low-power Nd : YAG laser is a new therapeutic approach in the treatment of malignant gliomas. The 1.06-μm Nd : YAG laser is an excellent source of local hyperthermia because of its good coagulative properties, its relatively low absorption in brain tissue, and its transmission by an optic fiber. A specially designed laser light guide, the interstitial thermotherapy (ITT) laser fiber, is connected to the Nd : YAG laser and inserted stereotactically in brain tumors. The quartz glass cap at the fiber tip requires no irrigation medium and allows transmission of laser energy up to 10 W, which is sufficient for local hyperthermia.

We studied the effect of interstitial laser irradiation in animal experiments on normal rat brains and on F-98 glial transplantation tumors. Based on these data, laser therapy was performed clinically in a CT, MRI, and PET scan controlled study in patients with malignant gliomas.

Material and Methods

In vivo animal experiments on normal rat brains and F-98 glial transplantation tumors were performed using a 1.06-μm Nd : YAG laser and the ITT light guide. The laser fiber was introduced stereotactically through a right frontal burr hole into the basal ganglia. Laser shots were emitted as continuous waves with an output power of 2–5 W and exposure times of 30 s to 5 min. For histological examination, rat brains were removed immediately, 1 day, 3 days, 1 week, 2 weeks, 4 weeks, and 3 months following laser therapy.

In the first clinical approach, interstitial laser therapy was used in five patients with cerebral gliomas WHO grade III–IV diagnosed by previous stereotactic biopsy. The size of the tumors ranged from 2 to 3.5 cm in diameter. Laser irradiation was performed in one or two foci depending on the size and configuration of the tumor using laser energies of 4–5 W applied over a period of 5–10 min. For evaluation of laser tissue effects we performed pre- and postoperative CT, MRI, and PET scan studies.

[1] Neurochirurgische Universitätsklinik, Moorenstr. 5, W-4000 Düsseldorf, FRG.

Advances in Neurosurgery, Vol. 20
K. Piscol, M. Klinger, M. Brock (Eds.)

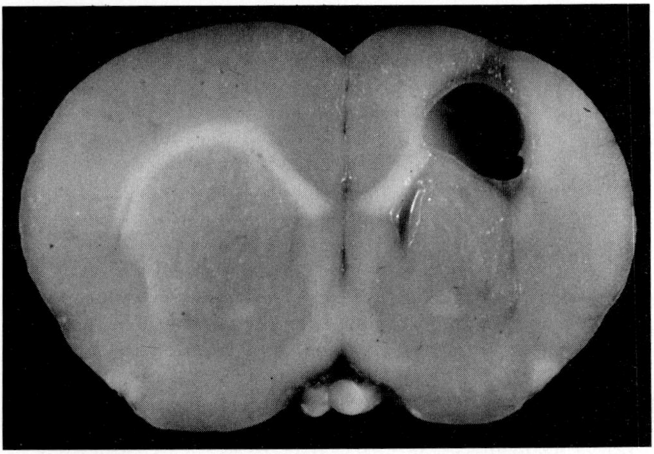

Fig. 1. A frontal cut through a rat brain 4 weeks after stereotactic interstitial laser-induced thermotherapy demonstrates a well-circumscribed cystic lesion at the top of the caput nuclei caudati. Laser parameters used: 3 W, 90 s

Results

Histological examination of normal rat brains showed typical laser-tissue interactions according to the time after laser treatment. Immediate changes consisted in a central zone of necrosis and a sharply demarcated edematous rim toward the unaffected brain. Later on, the necrosis became more evident and the edematous zone subsided. After 1 week we observed marginal granulation tissue, and after 4 weeks histological examination revealed a well-circumscribed cystic lesion (Fig. 1). The histological findings in transplantation tumors were similar. After 3–4 days we found an almost complete destruction of tumor cells and a marked necrosis in the irradiated area. The size of the lesion depend on the laser parameters used and ranged from 4 to 15 mm in diameter.

In our clinical study, MRI and PET scan follow-up investigations were performed 1–3 days, 7–9 days, and 4 weeks after laser thermotherapy. In each MRI examination pre- and post-gadolinium-DTPA 3D-Turboflash sequences were combined with an axial T2-weighted spin-echo sequence. Early postoperative sequences revealed a high intensity region in the center of the tumor in the T1-weighted image and a very low signal in the T2-weighted image. Gd-enhanced images showed a strong decrease of accumulation in the tumor center, while a small, annular uptake could be noticed at the tumor margin (Figs. 2 and 3).

The extent of the lesion increased in size after 7–9 days with no change of Gd enhancement in the tumor center. In the periphery of the tumor, the increased uptake seemed to be more diffuse. After 4 weeks the size of the lesion had slightly decreased. There was still almost no Gd uptake in the tumor center, while the increased accumulation at the tumor margin was clearly less evident.

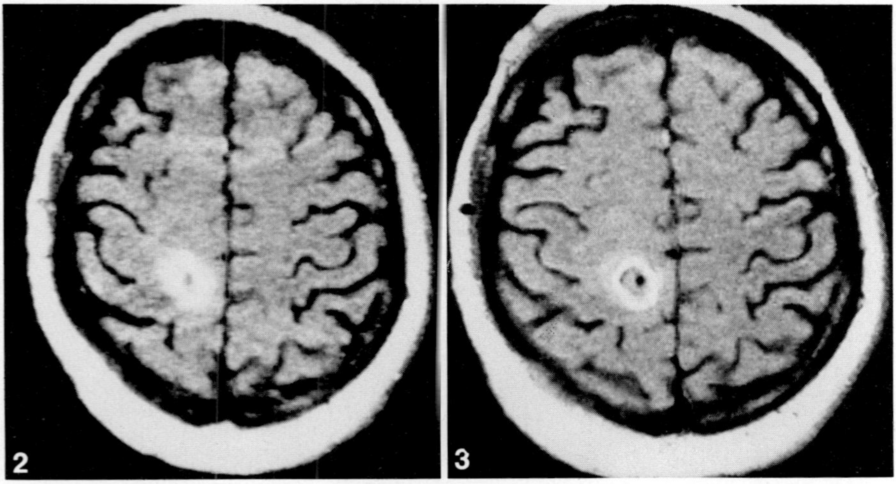

Fig. 2. Gd-DTPA-enhanced MR imaging shows a homogeneous enhancement of an astrocytoma WHO grade II diagnosed by previous stereotactic biopsy

Fig. 3. One day after stereotactic laser-induced interstitial thermotherapy a marked decrease of Gd accumulation in the center of the tumor is noticed. At the tumor margin, a ring-shaped increased enhancement is demonstrated. Laser parameters used: 5 W, 10 min

We suggest that these phenomena represent irreversible necrotic changes in the center of the tumor, whereas the alterations at the tumor margin seem to be reversible probably due to blood-brain barrier disturbance.

PET scan studies measuring the metabolic activity of the malignant gliomas using [^{18}F]2-fluoro-2-deoxy-D-glucose (FDG) revealed very similar results to MRI examinations. Early postoperative scans most clearly showed a profound decrease of glucose uptake in the tumor center due to a necrotic process. Conversely, the volume of distribution of FDG was slightly higher in the border portions of the tumor that probably corresponds to the contrast-enhanced rim seen on the MRI. We think that this area is due to the reactive zone of the surrounding vital tissue that was not destroyed by laser therapy. The fact that the increase of glucose uptake in this region had clearly diminished after 4 weeks underlines our suggestion.

Conclusion

Stereotactic laser-induced interstitial thermal therapy is a new method for inducing local hyperthermia in cerebral tumors [4, 9]. The advantage of lasers is the very precise delivery of energy to tissue and the good instrumental control of total energy deposition [3, 7, 8, 10]. Especially the Nd: YAG laser and its new fiberoptic delivery system, the ITT laser fiber, makes interstitial thermotherapy useful because of its superiority to other application systems in terms of directed circumferential

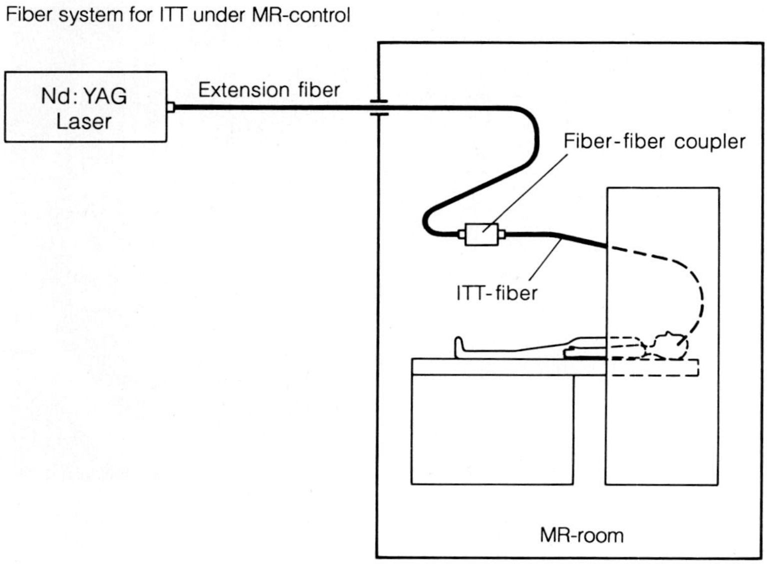

Fig. 4. Schematic drawing of MRI-guided interstitial laser irradiation using a Nd: YAG laser, an extension fiber, and the interstitial thermotherapy (ITT) laser fiber

irradiation, power density at the fiber-tissue transition, biocompatibility, flexibility, geometrical dimension, and compatibility with MRI as a diagnostic and therapeutic control [5]. We found that MRI and PET scan investigations represent powerful tools in evaluating the size and characteristics of structural and biological changes in tissue induced by laser hyperthermia [2]. Also, MRI was useful to demonstrate reversible and irreversible effects after laser thermotherapy. These effects do correspond to the histological findings in rat brain studies. In future, it seems to be possible to use "real time" high-speed MRI sequences during stereotactic interstitial laser-induced thermotherapy (Fig. 4) to obtain improved control of laser energy application [1, 6].

References

1. Ascher PW (1990) Interstitial thermal therapy for brain tumors with ND: YAG laser under real time MRI control. In: Joffe SN, Attsum K (eds) Proceedings of laser surgery: advanced characterization, therapeutics and systems II, SPIE, vol 1200, pp 242–246
2. Bettag M, Ulrich F, Fürst G, Langen K-J, Roosen N, Kiwit JCW, Hessel S, Mödder U, Bock WJ (1991) Gadolinium-DTPA enhanced MRI and positron emission tomography of stereotactic laser-induced interstitial thermal therapy in cerebral gliomas. Neuroradial [Suppl] 33:37–39
3. Cummins L, Nauenberg M (1983) Thermal effects of laser radiation in biological tissue. Biophys J 42:99–102

4. Daikuzono N, Suzuki S, Tajiri H, Tsunekawa H, Ohyama M, Joffe SN (1988) Laserthermia: a new computer-controlled contact Nd: YAG system for interstitial local hyperthermia. Laser Surg Med 8:254–258
5. Hessel S, Frank F (1990) Technical prerequisites for the interstitial thermotherapy using the Nd: YAG laser. In: Optical fibers in medicine V, SPIE, vol 1201, pp 233–238
6. Jolesz FA, Bleier AR, Jakab P, Ruenzel PW, Huttl K, Jako GJ (1988) MR imaging of laser-tissue interactions. Radiol 168:249–253
7. Lajat Y, Patrice T, Nomballais F, Nogues B, Resche F (1987) Effects of 1.06 μm wavelength laser radiation applied stereotactically to brain tissue. Laser Surg Med 3:45–51
8. Mang TS, Dougherty TJ (1986) Use of the Nd: YAG laser for hyperthermia induction as an adjunct to photodynamic therapy. Laser Surg Med 6:237
9. Sakai T, Fujishima I, Tanaka T (1987) Laser hyperthermia for deep seated brain tumor using Nd-YAG laser.J Jpn Soc Laser Med 8:75–76
10. Sugiyama K, Sakai T, Fujishima I, Ryu H, UZemura K, Yokoyama T (1990) Stereotactic interstitial laser-hyperthermia using Nd-YAG laser. Stereotact Funct Neurosurg 54+55:501–505

Interstitial Laser-Assisted Thermal Therapy of Central Brain Tumors: Preliminary Report

P. W. Ascher[1], O. Schröttner[1], F. Ebner[2], and R. Kleinert[3]

Introduction

Tumors of the brain can kill the patient not only by malignancy but also by invading central, surgically inaccessible structures. Biologically benign tumors become in this way malignant. The latter tumors, long considered inoperable, were treated by interstitial brachytherapy.

In 1984 an 8-year-old boy presented at our department with left-sided hemiplegia. A computed tomography (CT) scan showed a tumor of the right posterior thalamus. A biopsy of the tumor was obtained by needle puncture through a newly designed endoscope. Histological examination showed an astrocytoma, grade II. Because the tumor was inoperable according to conventional standards, a 1.06-μm Nd:YAG laser was used to irradiate the portion of the tumor visibly protruding into the posterior horn of the lateral ventricle. A dose of 50 000 J (enough to bring a cup of water to boil) was applied to the surface of the tumor during continuous cooling by irrigation with saline. The surface of the tumor, previously pink, paled visibly during the procedure. Hemiplegia resolved within a week. CT scans 2 months and 4 years after surgery showed no evidence of tumor. A 35-year-old female with a similar tumor was treated the same way a few months later [1].

This therapeutic approach seems appropriate only for paraventricular tumors of the thalamus, which are rare. A potential disadvantage of the procedure is the high-power density at the end of the laser fiber which damages the fiber tip. A further problem is intraoperative temperature control of the radiated tissue.

Two developments occurred in 1986: (a) contact laser tips became available [2] and (b) G. Jako and F. Jolesch [3] demonstrated that the heat effect of laser fibers in the brain could be monitored continuously in nearly real time (3 min delay) by magnetic resonance (MRI) imaging. Clinical studies showed that the heat effect of laser irradiation was visible 2 h later. In the meantime the company MBB-AT has designed a completely new fiber system (Fig. 1) that has proven effective in experiments and clinical practice.

[1] Neurochirurgische Universitätsklinik, Karl-Franzens-Universität, A–8036 Graz, Austria.
[2] Radiologische Universitätsklinik, Karl-Franzens-Universität, A–8036 Graz, Austria.
[3] Pathologische Universitätsklinik, Karl-Franzens-Universität, A–8036 Graz, Austria.

Advances in Neurosurgery, Vol. 20
K. Piscol, M. Klinger, M. Brock (Eds.)

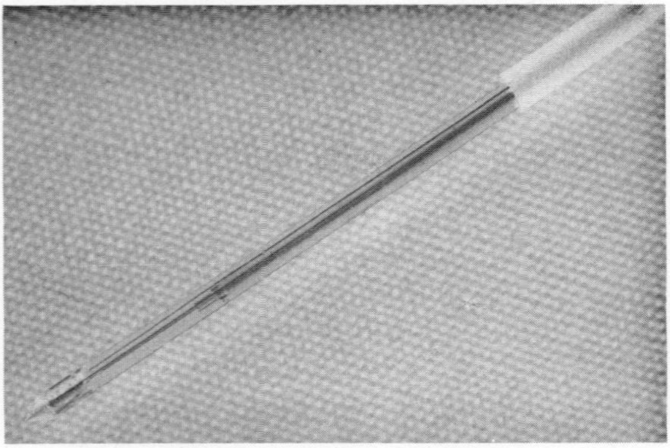

Fig. 1. Laser fiber for interstitial thermotherapy with an air chamber at the end of the fiber

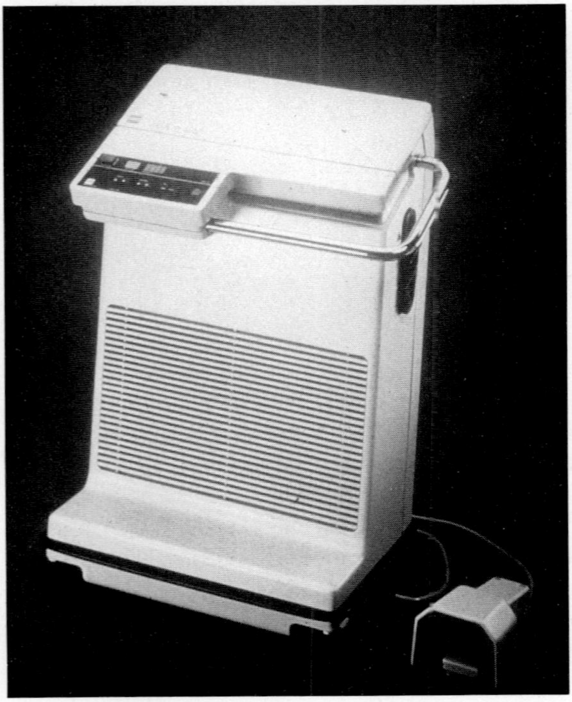

Fig. 2. Nd:YAG 1.06-μm laser, maximum power 50 W (MBB-AT)

In vitro experiments on porcien liver at room temperature showed that 4 W applied over 10 min caused an ellipsoid coagulation necrosis of 12–16 mm. This size is for a single or two fibers not simultaneously heated always repeatable.

Two fibers simultaneously heated do not cause a double volume necrosis but a new geometry and much bigger necrosis. The calibration of the laser source (MBB 50 W laser) was stable during all experiments (Fig. 2).

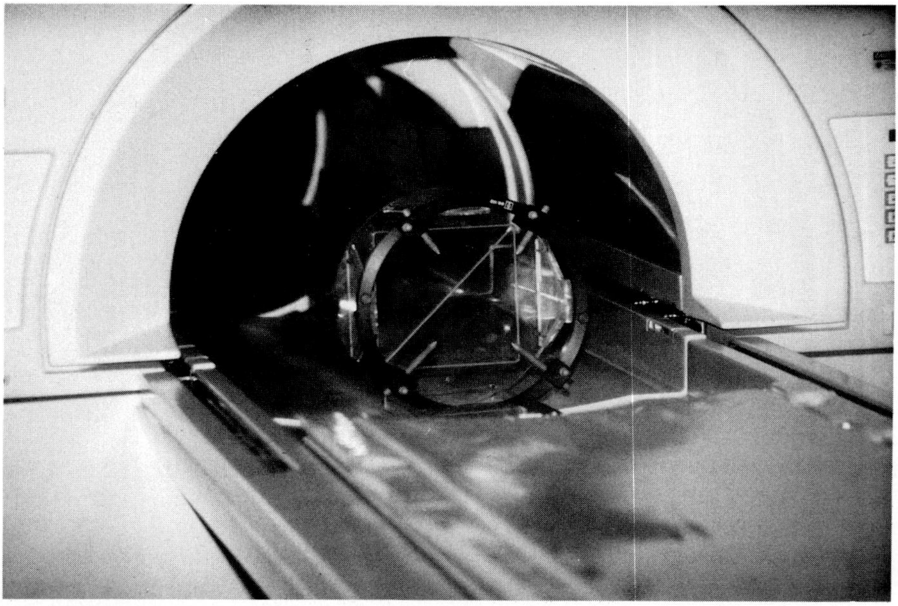

Fig. 3. MRI compatible equipment (Fischer)

Indications

All benign or malignant central brain tumors in patients without neurological symptoms are indications for interstitial laser-assisted thermotherapy (ILTT). ILTT has a number of advantages as compared with interstitial brachytherapy. ILTT is a simple procedure, the heat reaction of the tumor and surrounding tissue can be monitored directly, and ILTT can be performed on all types of tumors. ILTT also has the advantages associated with brachytherapy: only local anesthesia is required, sensomotoric function and speech can be evaluated continuously, the procedure can be repeated, and the stereotactic approach permits minimal damage to the surrounding brain tissue.

Methods

On the morning of surgery a specially designed plastic coordinate ring is placed on the patient's skull. The coordinates of the center of the tumor and those for an appropriate burr hole are plotted by CT. Trepanation is then carried out under local anesthesia. At the same time the coordinates of the target point and the burr hole are plotted on a phantom. An aiming device is adapted and then transferred to the coordinate ring on the patient's head; the probe is then implanted. Afterward the patient is taken to the MRI unit, and the laser fiber is introduced to the calculated length under MRI control.

The laser is then activated (4 W, 10 min). The first changes in the tumor become apparent on the MRI screen after 3 min. Further laser applications are adapted according to the size of the lesion and the observed heat reaction.

The patient is monitored physiologically during the entire procedure. None of the eight patients to date have reported pain or other sensations. The greatest difficulty is the 10-min motionless fixation of the patient.

All of our instruments are now MRI compatible (Fig. 3). Therefore, we do not have to move the patient from the CT unit to the operating room and to the MRI unit. We just prepare our patient in the future in the MRI unit and carry out the whole calculation only in the MRI unit.

Discussion

ILTT permits treatment for otherwise untreatable brain tumors without endangering patient function or life. ILTT is a palliative measure for malignant tumors; for benign lesions it may offer a cure. A number of technical problems (equipment, both instrumentation and MRI), experiments (heat distribution), and clinical studies (histology, long-term follow-up) remain to be done and solved, but ILTT has opened a new vista in the treatment of central brain tumors.

References

1. Ascher PW (1990) Interstitial thermal therapy of brain tumors with the Nd: YAG laser under real time MR control. In: Proceedings of SPIE, vol 1200, Laser surgery advance characterization, therapeutics and systems II, pp 242–245
2. Joffe SN, Tajri H, Oguro Y, Daikuzono N, Suzuki S (1989) Laserthermia, a new method of interstitial local hyperthermia using the contact Nd: YAG laseer. Radiol Clin North America 27:611–620
3. Jako GJ, Jolesz IA (1986) The control of Nd: YAG laser fiber optics hyperthermia with magnetic resonance imaging. In: Parris JA, Scott RS, Joffe SN (eds) Proceedings of SPIE, vol 712, Lasers in medicine, pp 72–77

Transforming Growth Factors-β in Malignant Glioma: Preliminary Studies on Inhibition by Antisense Oligodeoxynucleotides

J. A. Koeppen[1], L. Owen-Schaub[2], E. A. Grimm[2], and R. P. Moser[2]

Abstract

Type β-transforming growth factors (TGF-β) are multifunctional polypeptides that regulate cell growth and differentiation. TGF-β1 and TGF-β2 are closely related and resemble the immunosuppressive effects of malignant gliomas. As TGF-β2 is produced by gliomas, it may contribute to glioma-mediated immunosuppression. To inhibit TGF-β production, a set of 16mer antisense oligodeoxynucleotides (ODNs) was constructed. The glioma cell line U-251 was incubated with 10 μM antisense oligodeoxynucleotides for 24 h. A specific antiproliferative effect was observed for an oligodeoxynucleotide complementary to a region of complete mRNA homology between TGF-β1 and TGF-β2. Inhibition of TGF-β expression could not be verified in a standard Mv-1-Lu bioassay. In this assay TGF-β inhibits proliferation of Mv-1-Lu cells. Direct treatment of Mv-1-Lu with TGF-β1 and TGF-β2 specific antisense as well as unspecific oligodeoxynucleotides resulted in a dose-dependent inhibition of proliferation, indicating direct and unspecific effects of these oligodeoxynucleotides on Mv-1-Lu.

Introduction

TGF-β1 and TGF-β2 both inhibit the generation of specific cytotoxic T cells and lymphocyte activation by interleukin 2 [2, 5, 6].

Depressed T-cell-mediated immunity is well documented in patients with malignant glioma [9], and the cellular immune competence is correlated with the clinical course of disease [11]. As TGFs-β are produced by malignant gliomas and resemble their immunosuppressive effects, secretion of TGF-β may be crucial for gliomas to escape immune surveillance.

Gene expression can be inhibited by antisense RNA or DNA. This inhibition is based on blocking the informational flow from DNA to protein via mRNA by introducing a complementary sequence to a portion of target mRNA. Through base pairing an RNA (or RNA-DNA) duplex is formed. Subsequently, the duplex blocks the processing of mRNA (reviewed in [10]).

[1] Neurochirurgische Abteilung, Universitätskrankenhaus Eppendorf, Martinistr. 52, W–2000 Hamburg 20, FRG.
[2] University of Texas, M.D. Anderson Cancer Center, Houston, Texas 77030, USA.

Advances in Neurosurgery, Vol. 20
K. Piscol, M. Klinger, M. Brock (Eds.)

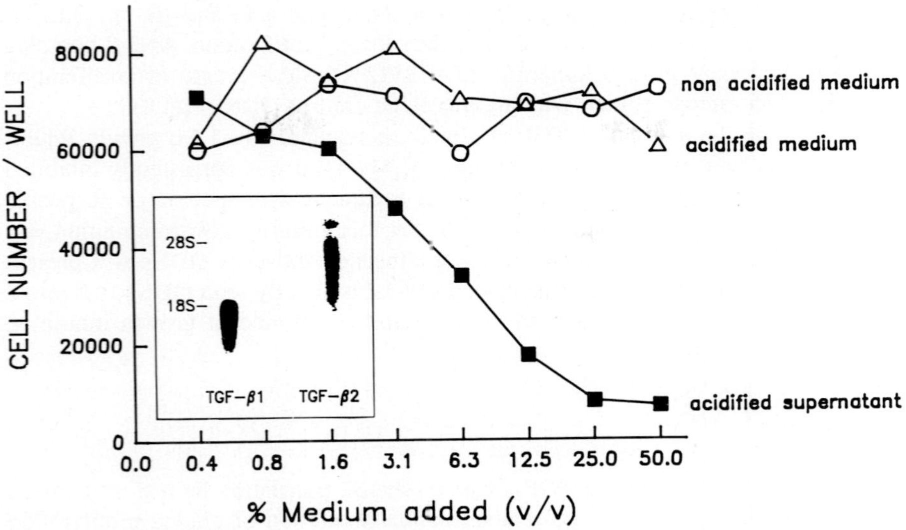

Fig. 1. Detection of TGF-β in an Mv-1-Lu bioassay and Northern blot analysis. Serum-free supernatants from the human glioma cell line U-251 were collected after 3 days of cell culture, centrifuged at 3000 rpm, and transient-acidified by HCl. Mv-1-Lu, a cell line derived from mustela vision lung epithelia (ATCC No: CCL 64), was incubated with glioma-conditioned media in 4% FCS; 48 h later cells were counted in triplicate. All cells were cultured in supplemented Dulbecco's modified Eagle's medium and Ham's F12 (Gibco, Gaithersburg, MD). *Insert,* RNA analysis by Northern hybridization. Total cellular RNA was isolated from U-251 as described in [1]. Electrophoresis, transfer, and hybridization analysis was performed by a procedure from [7]. DNA probes for TGF-β1 and TGF-β2 were labeled using a random primer DNA system (Bethesda Research Laboratories, Gaithersburg, MD)

Results

Transient-acidified supernatants from U-251 inhibit the proliferation of Mv-1-Lu in a dose-dependent manner, indicating the secretion of latent TGF-β (Fig. 1). Expression of TGF-β1 and TGF-β2 was confirmed by Northern blot analysis as shown in Fig. 1 (insert).

To inhibit the translation of TGF-β1 and -β2 mRNA by hybridization arrest, three complementary 16mer ODNs were synthesized. Based on thermodynamic predictions of mRNA secondary structure and antisense binding energies (GENEius sequence analysis software, Bio-Technology Software Specialities based on 3), we prepared ODNs complementary to the initiation codons and the next 13 bases of TGF-β1 and TGF-β2 (TAC GGC GGG AGG CCC G designated anti-β1-ini and TAC GTG ATG ACA CAC G designated anti-β2-ini) as well as complementary to a region of complete cDNA homology between TGF-β1 and TGF-β2 (TG ATG CGG TTC CTC CA hereafter called anti-β-homolog). A 16mer anti-CAT ODN was used as unspecific control. The glioma line U-251 was coincubated with these

ODNs at a concentration of 10 μM for 24 h. Treatment with anti-β1-ini, anti-β2-ini, and their combination resulted in a slightly lower proliferation. Anti-β-homolog led to a significant growth inhibition of U-251. A mild decrease of proliferation was also seen after treatment with an unspecific control ODN (Fig. 2).

To examine the amount of TGF-β protein, a standard Mv-1-Lu growth inhibition bioassay was performed. Proliferation of Mv-1-Lu was consistently inhibited by conditioned glioma media, regardless of treatment with specific or unspecific antisense ODNs (Fig. 3). To determine whether this uniform growth inhibition was due to TGF-β secretion or rather to direct effects of antisense ODNs still present in the conditioned media, we coincubated Mv-1-Lu directly with ODNs. All tested ODNs, including the unspecific anti-CAT, caused a significant growth inhibition (Fig. 4).

Discussion

We have attempted to inhibit TGF-β1 and TGF-β2 translation by use of unmodified 16mer ODNs. We have found a substantial inhibition of glioma proliferation by an ODN complementary to a region of complete homology between TGF-β1 and TGF-β2 mRNA. As TGF-β coregulates cell adhesion [4], TGF-β antisense ODNs may disrupt this regulatory network. Unspecific anti-CAT ODN was almost ineffective. Inhibition of TGF-β protein secretion by glioma could not be verified in a standard Mv-1-Lu bioassay. To validate the Mv-1-Lu bioassay for TGF-β antisense experiments, we examined for direct effects of ODNs on Mv-1-Lu. Significant growth inhibition was observed with all ODNs including the unspecific anti-CAT. This observation may be rationalized by either unspecific DNA/RNA hybridization or toxic contaminations in our ODNs. Given these problems with the Mv-1-Lu bioassay, it is now necessary to determine TGF-β secretion of glioma cells in a antibody-based assay.

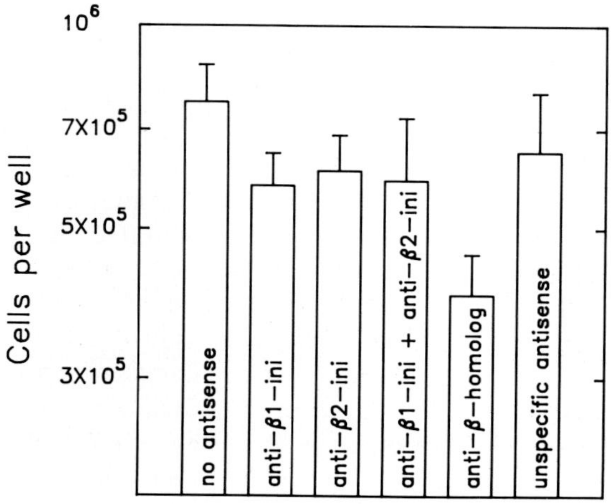

Fig. 2. Proliferation of U-251 glioma cell line treated with antisense oligodeoxynucleotides (ODNs). ODNs were constructed as described in the results and added to subconfluent U-251 glioma cultures without FCS in a concentration of 10 μM; 48 h later cells were counted in triplicate

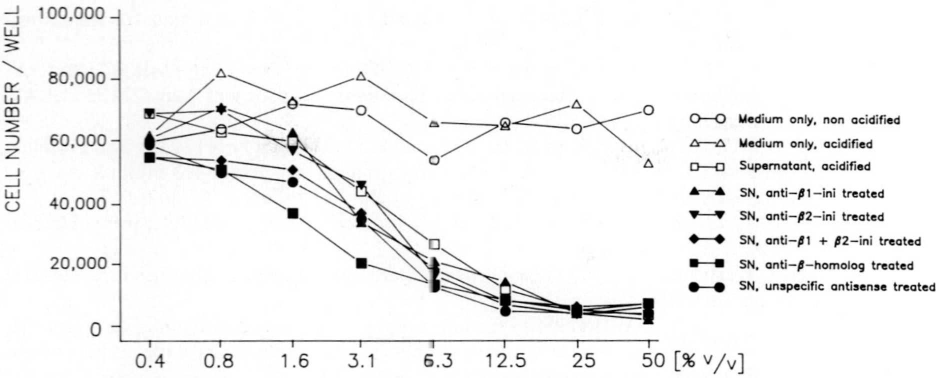

Fig. 3. TGF-β bioassay for conditioned media from antisense treated glioma. Oligodeoxynucleotides were added to U-251 glioma cultures without FCS; 48 h later supernatants were centrifuged, transient-acidified, and tested for TGF-β in a standard Mv-1-Lu bioassay

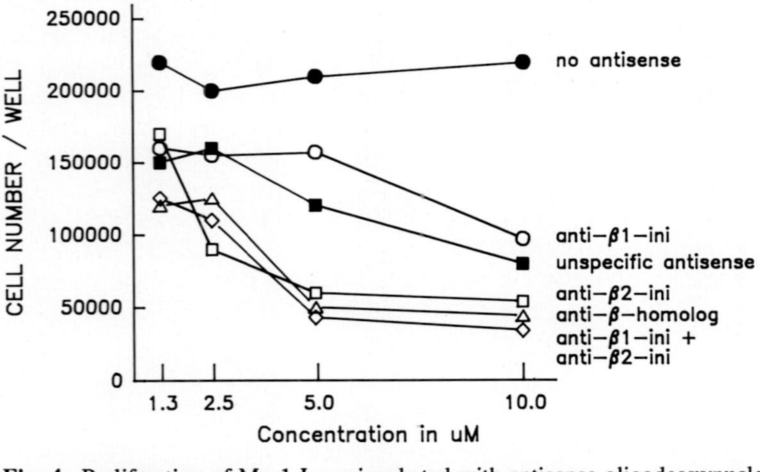

Fig. 4. Proliferation of Mv-1-Lu coincubated with antisense oligodeoxynucleotides. ODNs were added to subconfluent Mv-1-Lu cultures with 4% FCS; 48 h later cells were counted in triplicate

References

1. Ausubel FM, Brent R, Kingstone KR, Moore DD, Seidmann JG, Smith JA, Struhl K (1987) Current protocols in molecular biology. John Wiley & Sons, New York
2. Fontana A, Hengartner H, De Tribolet N, Weber E (1984) Glioblastoma cells release interleukin-1 and factors inhibiting interleukin-2 mediated effects. J Immunol 132:1837–1844
3. Freier SM, Kierzek R, Jaeger JA, Sugimoto N, Caruthers MH, Neilson T, Turner DH (1986) Improved free-energy parameters for predictions of RNA duplex stability. Proc Natl Acad Sci USA 83:9373–9377

4. Ignotz RA, Massague J (1987) Cell adhesion protein receptors as targets for transforming growth factor-beta action. Cell 51:189–197
5. Jin B, Scott JL, Vadas MA, Burns GF (1989) TGF-beta down regulates TLiSA1 expression and inhibits the differentiation of precursor lymphocytes into CTL and LAK cells. Immunology 66:570–576
6. Kuppner MC, Hamou MF, Bodmer S, Fontana A, De Tribolet N N (1988) The glioblastoma derived T cell suppressor factor/transforming growth factor-B2 inhibits the generation of lymphokine activated killer (LAK) cells. Int J Cancer 42:562–567
7. Maniatis T, Fritsch EF, Sambrook J (1982) Molecular cloning. Cold Spring Harbor, New York
8. Ponten J, Westermark B (1978) Properties of human malignant glioma in vitro. Medical Biology 56:184–193
9. Roszman TL, Brooks WH (1980) Immunobiology of primary intracranial tumours. III. Demonstration of a qualitative lymphocyte abnormality in patients with primary brain tumours. Clin Exp Immunol 38:395–402
10. Stein CA, Cohen JS (1988) Oligodeoxynucleotides as inhibitors of gene expression: A review. Cancer Res 48:2659–2668
11. Young HF, Sakalas R, Kaplan AM (1976) Inhibition of cell-mediated immunity in patients with brain tumors. Surg Neurol 5:19–23

Local Adjuvant Adoptive Immunotherapy of Patients with Malignant Gliomas

F. Weber, A. Klein-Struckmeyer, J. Menzel, and U. Pohl[1]

Introduction

During the past years immunotherapy of patients with malignant brain tumors using biological response modifiers (BRM) such as interferons and interleukin-2 has become an area of increasing interest. The current therapeutic concept consists primarily of surgery which is supported by adjuvant modalities such as radiation therapy and/or chemotherapy. Knowing that the brain is an "immunoprivileged" organ, it would be favorable to modulate the natural immunity in such a way as to rebuild the immune surveillance.

Material and Methods

To test the safety, compatibility, and the therapeutic efficiency of the intracerebral injection of natural interleukin-2 (n-IL-2) and lymphokine-activated killer cells (LAKC) as adjuvant therapy after tumor debulking we set up a pilot trial. This study consisted of three groups. One group of five patients was treated by a single administration of n-IL-2 in increasing dosages. The second group of five patients received autologous LAKC. The assignment to each group was randomized. A third nonrandomized group was treated with a combination of LAK cells and the highest tolerated dosage of n-IL-2.

Natural interleukin-2 is identical in its amino acid composition to that of recombinant interleukin-2 with the exception that n-IL-2 is glycosylated.

Four days before surgery, peripheral blood lymphocytes were obtained from a 3- to 4-h leukapheresis. The cells were incubated with n-IL-2 in a completely closed system. Before application the cells were centrifugated to a volume of 10–30 ml.

After tumor resection n-IL-2 (group 1), LAK cells (group 2), or the combination (group 3) of 1×10^6 units n-IL-2 and LAK cells were given. Interleukin-2 was administered in increasing dosages from 1×10^4, 1×10^5, 3×10^5, 6×10^5, and 1×10^6 (group 1).

The amount of LAK cells which could be harvested ranged from 1.5×10^8 to 5×10^9 cells (group 2). The third group received the combination of LAK cells

[1] Neurochirurgische Klinik der Städtischen Krankenanstalten Köln-Merheim, Ostmerheimer Str. 200, W–5000 Köln 91, FRG.

Advances in Neurosurgery, Vol. 20
K. Piscol, M. Klinger, M. Brock (Eds.)

Table 1. Patient profile data

Patient	Sex	Age	Histology[a]	Localization[b]	Therapy	Outcome[c]	Karnofsky
2[d]	M	57	m G3	l/t	3.5×10^8 LAKC	rec	90/80
6	M	50	G3-4	l/t-p	1×10^5 n-IL-2	rem	80/80
7	F	68	G3	l/t	6×10^5 n-IL-2	rem	90/80
8	F	55	G3-4	l/t	3×10^8 LAKC	rem	80/80
9	F	70	GM	l/t-p	1×10^9 LAKC	rem	80/80
10	M	69	GM	r/p	1×10^7 n-IL-2	rem	90/80
11	M	66	m G3	l/f-t	4.5×10^9 LAKC	rem	90/90
12	F	69	GM	l/f	n-IL-2 + LAKC	rem	70/60
13	M	49	G3-4	r/f	n-IL-2 + LAKC	rem	90/70
14	M	44	GM	r/p-o	n-IL-2 + LAKC	ic.rem	50/30
15	F	42	G3-4	l/p	n-IL-2 + LAKC	ic.rem	90/80
1†	M	51	m G3	r/f-p & cc	1×10^4 n-IL-2	ST 20 weeks	
3†	M	70	GM	l/t	4.5×10^8 LAKC	ST 20 weeks	
4†	M	48	GM	l/t-p	1.5×10^8 LAKC	ST 80 weeks	
5†	M	49	GM	r/T-p	3×10^5 n-IL-2	ST 68 weeks	

[a] GM, glioblastoma multiforme; G, glioma; M, mixed.
[b] l, left; r, right; t, temporal; f, frontal; o, occipital; p, parietal.
[c] rec, recurrence; rem, remission.
[d] Complications: patient 2, lung abscess; patient 14, brain edema.
† Dead.

and 1×10^6 units n-IL-2. Postoperatively, a CT scan was obtained as soon as the patient was stable.

Results

Fifteen patients could be evaluated in three groups (Table 1). The mean age was 57 years. Twelve patients had a primary malignant glioma and three a recurrent glioblastoma multiforme. The immunotherapy was well tolerated. There was no complication which could definitively be related to the immunotherapy. There were two complications in all: one lung abscess and one brain edema.

Four patients have died already: one patient who had only received a partial tumor resection and one patient had a heart attack 22 weeks after the first and 3 weeks after the second surgery. The third and fourth patients entered the protocol having a recurrent disease (Table 1).

Eleven patients are alive. The mean Karnofsky score before therapy was 78. At the time of discharge the score was 68.

Discussion

We investigated the safety, compatibility, and as far as possible an efficacy of this adjuvant local immunotherapy.

Our investigation differs from other trials [1–5] insofar as we applied interleukin-2 and LAK cells only one time intraoperatively. Knowing from the reports of Merchant [5] and Barba [1] that multiple applications of the immunotherapy increases the risk of severe side effects such as systemic toxicity, neurological deterioration, and wound infection without giving a greater therapeutic benefit to the patients induced us to a more restricted schedule. The therapeutic efficiency which had been reported up to now is still very unsatisfactory. At this point we can say that the administration of n-IL-2 is safe and consistent if given once after tumor resection. A conclusive evaluation about therapeutic efficacy cannot be made.

In the future, immunotherapy has to integrate other parts of the immune system for a multimodal approach. Another important problem is to overcome the immunosupression which is induced by steroids, prostaglandin E_2, and growth factors.

References

1. Barba D, Saris ST, Holder C, Rosenberg ST, Oldfield EH (1989) Intratumoral LAK cell and interleukin-2 therapy of human gliomas. J Neurosurg 70:175–182
2. Ingram M, Shelden CH, Jacques S (1987) Preliminary clinical trial of immunotherapy for malignant glioma. J Biol Response Mod 6:489–498
3. Jacobs SK, Wilson DJ, Kornblith PL (1986) Interleukin-2 and autologous lymphokine-activated killer cells in the treatment of malignant glioma. J Neurosurg 64:743–749
4. Lillehei KO, Mitchell DHM, Johnson ST, McCleary EL, Kruse CA (1991) Long-term follow-up of patients with recurrent malignant gliomas treated with adjuvant adoptive immunotherapy. Neurosurgery 28:16–23
5. Merchant RE, Merchant LH, Cook HS, McVicar DW, Young HF (1988) Intralesional infusion of lymphokine-activated killer cells and recombinant interleukin-2 (rIL-2) for the treatment of patients with malignant brain tumor. Neurosurgery 23:725–732
6. Yoshida S, Tanaka R, Tahai N, Ono K (1990) Adoptice immunotherapy with LAK cells and interleukin-2 in treatment of recurrent malignant gliomas. Current Therapeutic Research 47:654–664

Intratumoral Administration of Interferon-α in Malignant Gliomas

B. Klun, B. Jereb, J. Petrič, I. Tekavčič, and A. Popadić[1]

Introduction

In spite of extensive research and financial efforts, the prognosis in patients with malignant gliomas remains extremely poor. The life expectancy was increased by about 2 months during the last 3 decades, but it still remains one of the shortest in malignancies of any location. Therefore, it is understandable that any new treatment is embraced with great hope and even enthusiasm. The discovery of interferon seems to be a promising step in the treatment of malignant tumors, and favorable results have been reported from Yugoslavia [2], Sweden [1, 7], and Japan [3–6].

Material and Methods

A series of 24 patients were treated over a period of 6 years. All patients were operated upon. The operations varied from biopsies to lobectomies according to the size of the tumor, its anatomical location, and the condition of the patient. More than half of the patients were operated upon twice and about a third three times. A repeat operation sometimes only meant the implantation of an Ommaya reservoir.

The patients were divided into three groups according to treatment. Group A, numbering eight patients, received postoperative radiation therapy consisting of 30 Gy in 3-Gy fractions during 2 weeks, through two opposing portals to the whole brain, followed by a boost of 3 Gy × 5 locally to the tumor bed. HLI-α was administered locally during the radiation treatment. This group was treated during the period 1985–1986 (Fig. 1).

Group B, numbering nine patients, received the same treatment as above, but in addition chemotherapy consisting of vincristine (2 mg in a 12-h infusion) in combination with cisplatin (60–80 mg in a 12-h infusion) every other week for 6 weeks. This group was treated during 1987 (Fig. 2).

Group C, numbering seven patients, treated during 1989–1990, received less aggressive radiation therapy in terms of doses as well as volume. Only the tumor bed was irradiated with 3600 cGy (200 cGy daily five times per week) with very large margins, including often the entire hemisphere and an additional boost of a "coned down" area of another 1400 cGy in the same daily fractions (Fig. 3).

[1] Neurochirurgische Universitätsklinik, Zaloška 7, YU–6100 Ljubljana, Yugoslavia.

Advances in Neurosurgery, Vol. 20
K. Piscol, M. Klinger, M. Brock (Eds.)

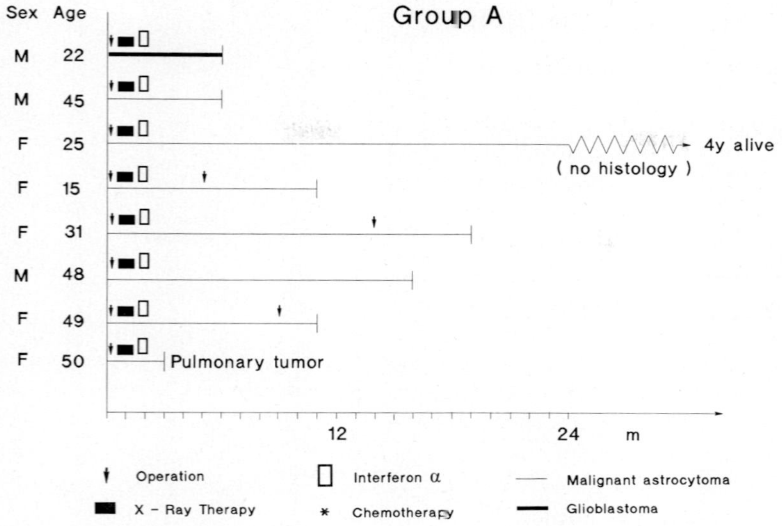

Fig. 1. Group A, treated 1985–1986

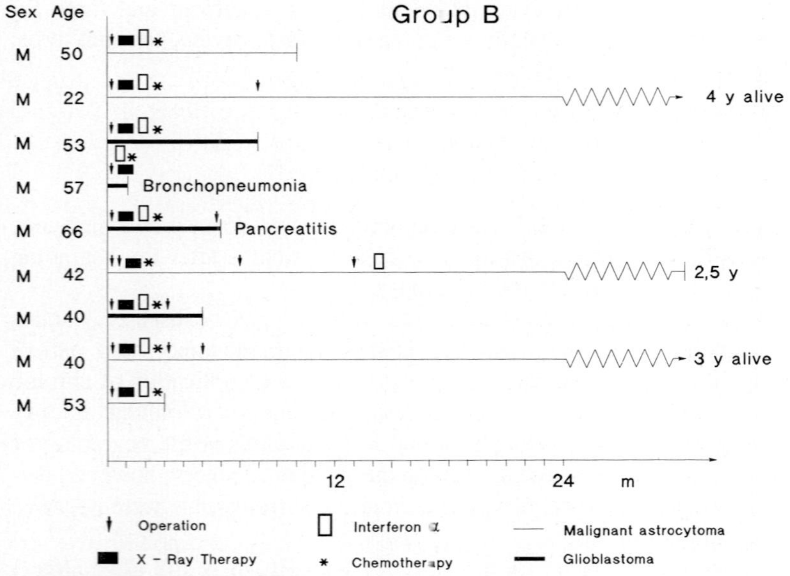

Fig. 2. Group B, treated 1987

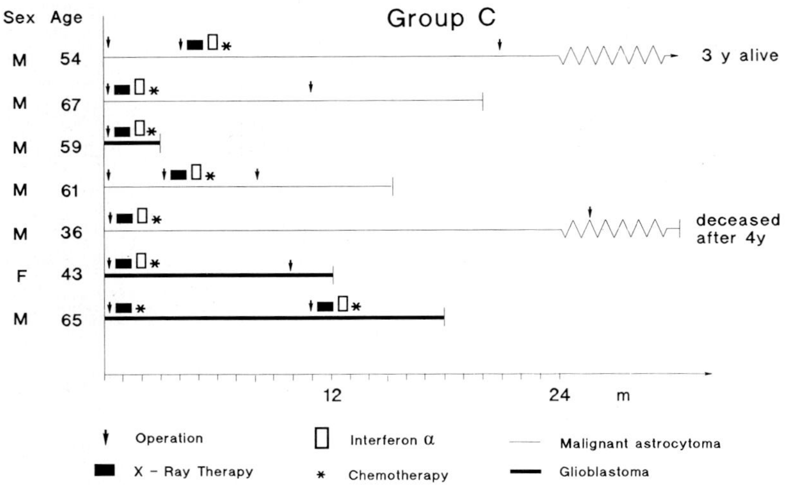

Fig. 3. Group C, treated 1989–1990

Patients with recurrences received additional radiation of 2500 cGy to a volume localized to the tumor bed.

In group A, five patients received HLI-α at the first treatment and three for recurrence; in group B the corresponding figures were, respectively, five and three; in group C, respectively, four and four.

Results

In group A, one patient survived 4 years without signs of disease and has since been lost from follow-up. In one patient who died 11 months after the beginning of the treatment, no tumor was found at autopsy.

In group B, two patients are alive and well, without signs of disease, 3 and 4 years after treatment; one of them was treated for a recurrent tumor. One patient died 2.5 years after treatment because of tuberculosis as a complication of chronic alcoholism. In an additional three patients no tumorous tissue was found at autopsy or at second surgery. The latter was performed in some cases at the beginning of the series for a presumed recurrence as seen on the CT scan. Surgery, however, discovered necrotic tissue, and specimens taken from the surroundings were negative regarding malignant cells.

In group C, one patient treated for a recurrence with HLI-α is still alive after 3 years. Of the six deceased patients, two had no proven tumor at autopsy.

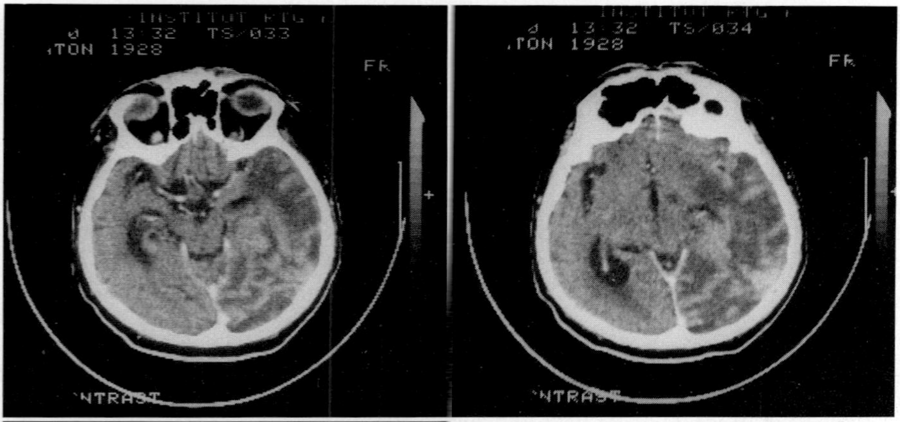

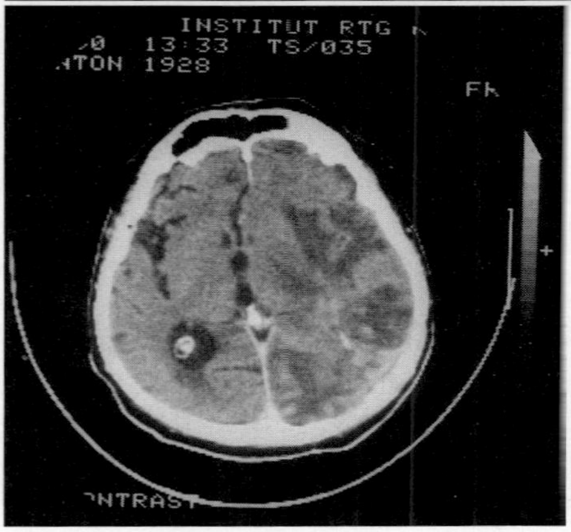

Fig. 4. No signs of recurrent tumor, but scattered necroses and extensive edema 1 year after the treatment

Discussion

Interferon seems today to be an established treatment in some leukemia forms and in the treatment of renal carcinoma, but little is known about its efficacy in brain glioma. Nagai [3] found a 40% response of some kind with local administration of interferon-β in combination with ACNU. Jereb et al. [2] presented 17 patients treated with surgery, HLI-α, and partially with chemotherapy. Five were still alive after 11–30 months and in five who died no tumor or tumor remainders were found. Similar promising results were reported by Salford et al. [7] and Boethius et al. [1]. On the other hand, von Wild [8] did not see a distinct increase in survival in a rather small series of 13 patients treated by intravenous and partially also locally administered interferon-β. He was unable to prove any antitumorous or antiproliferative influence of the given therapy.

It is certainly difficult to evaluate the results in a series where patients were treated with multimodality therapies, all of them quite aggressive. The group of survivors may suggest, however, that at least in some cases it is possible to prolong life.

Most interesting is the group of patients (eight of them) who survived for only a very short time, but in whom no tumor was found at autopsy. The follow-up CT scans were quite similar. There were no clear recurrences; necroses were seen and invariably a severe edema not only around or in the location of the previous tumor, but often involving the entire hemisphere. Figure 1 is a good example of this.

The question arises as to why these patients died. It is possible that the local toxicity of interferon in combination with chemotherapy and radiation resulted in impaired immune response. This was the reason that radiation treatment was modified in group C.

An open question remains regarding the status of the blood-brain barrier. If this is broken down, the concentration of chemotherapy and herewith the toxic effect are much more pronounced than in standard treatment.

Conclusions

Even if an evaluation of a certain drug in a multimodality study is difficult, it seems that HLI-α, administered locally and combined with surgery, radiation, and possibly chemotherapy may prolong life. On the other hand, these therapies are aggressive and run the risk of causing irreversible damage, incompatible with life, even if the tumor is "cured." Early treatment means less treatment, and a standardized therapeutic protocol seems to be imperative to avoid the empirical therapies as in our series. It would be necessary to establish which type of HLI possesses the highest efficacy and the lowest toxicity in the treatment of brain gliomas as well as which route of administration would be most appropriate.

References

1. Boethius J, Blomgren H, Collins VP, Greitz T, Strander H (1983) The effect of systemic human interferon-alpha administration to patients with glioblastoma multiforme. Acta Neurochir 68:239–251
2. Jereb B, Petrič J, Lamovec J, Škrbec M, Šoš E (1989) Intratumor application of human leukocyte interferon-alpha in patients with malignant brain tumors. Am J Clin Oncol 12 (1):1–7
3. Nagai M (1989) Clinical effect on human fibroblast interferon (BM 532) on malignant brain tumors, with special reference to gliomas. Nippon Gan Chiryo Gakkai Shi (English Abstract) 24 (3):638–646
4. Nagai M, Arai T (1983) Treatment of malignant brain tumors with interferon. In: Kiashida I (ed) Interferons. Organizing Committee of the International Symposium on interferon, Kyoto, pp 208–216
5. Nakagawa Y, Hirakawa K, Ueda S (1983) Local administration of interferon for malignant brain tumors. Cancer Tret Rep 67:833–855
6. Oda Y, Konishi T, Suzui H et al. (1989) Efficacy and adverse effects of beta interferon in the treatment of malignant gliomas. Nippon Gan Chiryo Gakkai Shi (English Abstract) 24:2411–2417

7. Salford LG, Stroemblad LG, Nordstroem CH et al. (1981) Intratumoral administration of interferon in malignant gliomas. Acta Neurol 56:130–131
8. Wild K von (1988) Zur Behandlung maligner Hirngliome mit IFN-beta. In: Schmoll HJ, Schöpf E (Hrsg) Lokale und systematische Tumortherapie mit Interferon. Zuckschwerdt, München Bern Wien San Francisco, S 80–86

A Preliminary Study of Superselective Intra-arterial Cisplatin Infusion in the Treatment of Recurrent Malignant Gliomas

L. Cristante, G. Siepmann, M. Westphal, and H.-D. Herrmann[1]

Introduction

Over the past 10 years, there have been a few studies of intra-arterial cisplatin (DDP) administration in patients affected by recurrent malignant intracerebral tumors [2–4, 6]. While the results were encouraging, there were still appreciable instances of systemic (oculo-, otho-, nephro-), and local (CNS) toxicity. The aim of this study was to try to reduce the systemic toxicity and augment the intraneoplastic drug delivery.

Material and Methods

The protocol included

1. Three injections of superselective intra-arterial DDP in 3- to 5-week intervals.
2. The resection of the neoplasia was performed between the first and the second injection.

The patients undergoing this therapeutic regimen were selected according to the following criteria:

1. The patient had, by computed tomographic criteria, a gross totally resectable recurrence of a glioblastoma multiforme or anaplastic astrocytoma.
2. The patient underwent surgery and radiation therapy of the primary lesion.
3. The Karnofsky performance score was at least 50.

Since December 1989 eight patients were selected to undergo this treatment (see Table 1 for an overview of the relevant clinical data). All patients gave written informed consent to the therapy. The work-up before each administration encompassed blood studies, audiography, and current CT scan. Beside a low-dose heparinization, the patient received 10 mg dexamethasone and 100 mg phenobarbital 12 h before each DDP administration, followed by prehydration with 5% glucose/normal saline (1 liter over 4 h). The fluids were supplemented with 12 g mannitol, 12 mval Mg^{2+}, 20 mval KCl, 14 mg metoclopramide, and 40 mg dexamethasone. The superselective catheterization was performed transfemorally with

[1] Neurochirurgische Abteilung, Universitätskrankenhaus Eppendorf, Martinistr. 52, W–2000 Hamburg 20, FRG.

Advances in Neurosurgery, Vol. 20
K. Piscol, M. Klinger, M. Brock (Eds.)

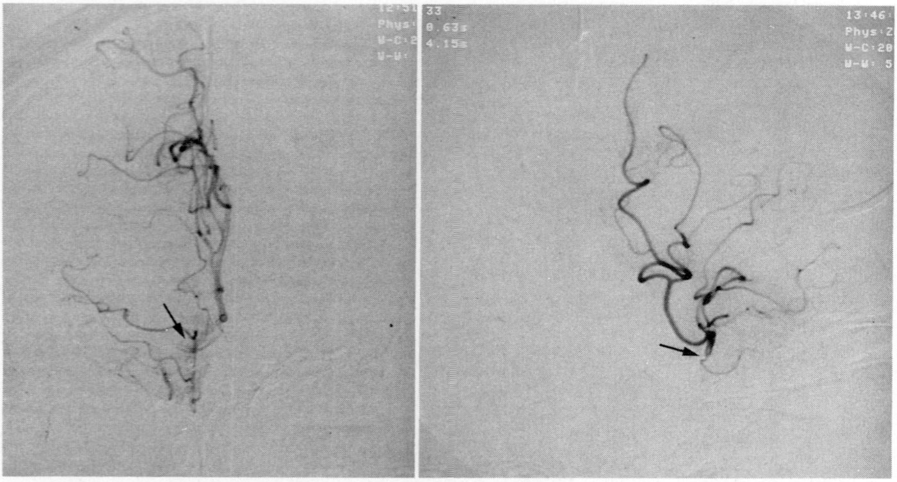

Fig. 1. Angiogram before cisplatin infusion showing the placement of the microcatheter tip in the distal Al (right) and distal M1 segment (case No. 5)

a microcatheter tracker 18. According to the topography of the neoplastic blood supply, one or more vessels were cannulated (Fig. 1). The injection, with the exception of the first two patients, was performed beyond the region of the perforator arteries, i.e., as far as A2, M2, and P2. The DDP (45 mg/m^2 in a normal saline solution 1 mg/3 ml) was administrated with a pump and took some 60 min. During the procedure the hydration of the patient continued at 250 ml/h while he was lightly sedated with 100 mg phenobarbital. After going back to the ward, the infusion therapy was reduced to 80 ml/h for the next 24 h and 1.2–2.5 mg droperidol was administered q 3 h for 12 h.

Table 1. Patient's characteristics

Case	Age/sex	Histology	Localization	Time to failure (weeks)	KPS
1	42/M	GBM	Temporal	35	70
2	56/M	GBM	Parietooccipital	32	70
3	48/F	GBM	Frontal	30	80
4	51/M	GBM	Frontal	64	60
5	57/M	AA	Frontoparietal	34	70
6	43/F	GBM	Frontoparietal	16	70
7	59/F	GBM	Temporal	35	80
8	51/F	GBM	Parietal	30	60

GBM, glioblastoma multiforme; AA, anaplastic astrocytoma; time to failure, evidence of recurrence on CT scan after surgery radiation therapy of the primary lesion; KPS, Karnofsky performance score.

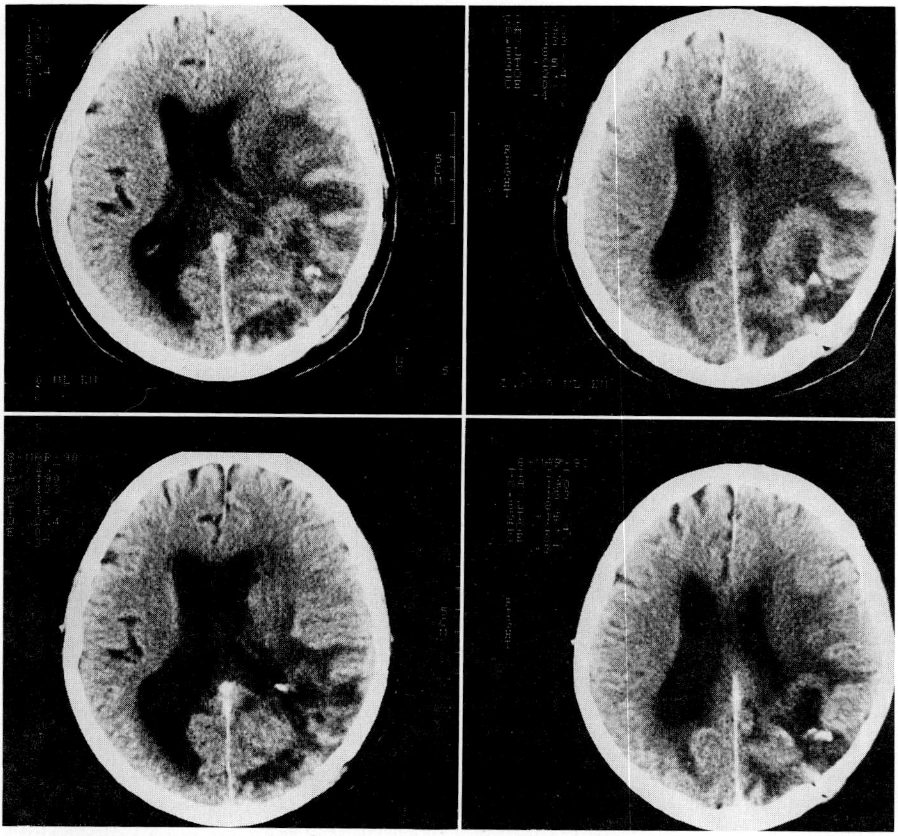

Fig. 2. Contrast-enhanced CT scans before (*upper row*) and 4 weeks after (*lower row*) the first administration of cisplatin. Notice the decreased contrast-enhancing tumor volume and compression of the lateral ventricle (case No. 2)

Results

The control CT scan 4 weeks after the first DDP injection showed that all tumors were responsive. There was either a reduction of the enhancing portion, a decrease of the perifocal edema, cystic regressive changes, or in the majority of the cases a combination of these (Fig. 2). In all patients there was evidence of tumor recurrence either after completing or after interrupting the treatment protocol because of some complication. A summary of the "time to failure," the computed tomographic evidence of a recurrence, and the "survival time" is given in Table 2. Two patients died because of respiratory complications without any evidence of tumor recurrence. The only instance of systemic toxicity, not requiring any therapy, was a transistory anemia and thrombocytopenia in three patients. So far (17 injections), no patient suffered any oculo-, otho-, or nephrotoxic complication. On the contrary,

Table 2. Treatment data/results

Case	Injection site	No. of treatments	KPS	Time to failure (weeks)	Survival time (weeks)
1	M2	3	70	32	36
2	M2 + P1	2	70	–	24
3	M2	3	90	54	66*
4	M1	1	60	34	38
5	A2 + M2	2	60	–	14
6	C. bifurc.	1	50	32	36
7	M2	3	80	26	38*
8	M2	3	60	28	32*

A, M, P, segments of the anterior, middle, posterior cerebral artery; C. bifurc., carotid artery bifurcation; KPS, Karnofsky performance score at the end of the treatment; time to failure, evidence of a new recurrence on CT scan; –, no evidence of recurrence as long as the patient survived; *, the patient is still alive.

after four injections (three patients), we registered clinical evidence of a focal encephalopathy. The deficits complained of by those three patients (the injections were performed in the proximal M1 and P1 segments) were transitory only in two cases and were evident 3–12 h after the injection. Finally, three patients developed epileptic seizures.

Discussion

While the systemic toxicity of DDP did not play any relevant role in this treatment protocol, we still had to register instances of local toxicity. Similar complications have already been reported [1, 4–6]. Because of the preferential involvement of the basal ganglia, their delayed development and the autoptic evidence (one case) of intimal sclerosis in the proximity of the injection site, we believe that either DDP, the solution, or our injection modality harbors a certain vascular toxicity. Therefore, beside performing the injection more peripherally we are now using, in the last patient we treated, DDP-dry substance dissolved in one-third sterile water and two-thirds normal saline (1 mg/2 ml).

Preoperative DDP administration is justified since the tumors at surgery seemed to have a better defined dissection plane. DDP activity in malignant gliomas has been documented once more in this limited series of patients. By and large the palliative value of such a treatment protocol is dependent upon a further reduction of the local (CNS) toxicity of this drug.

References

1. Blalock JB, Wright DC, Dedrick TL et al. (1985) Drug streaming during intraarterial chemotherapy. Sixth International Conference on Brain Tumors Research, Ashville
2. Feun L, Wallace S, Stewart DJ et al. (1984) Intracarotid infusion of cis – diamminoedichloro-platinum in the treatment of recurrent malignant brain tumors. Cancer 54:794–799
3. Mahaley MS, Hipp SW, Dropcho EJ et al. (1989) Intracarotid cisplatin chemotherapy for recurrent gliomas. J Neurosurg 70:371–378
4. Neuwelt EA, Barnett PA, Glasberg et al. (1983) Pharmacology and neurotoxicity of cis-diamminoedichloroplatinum, bleomycin, 5-fluorouracil, and cyclophosphamide administration following osmotic blood-brain barrier modification. Cancer Res 43:5278–5285
5. Stewart DJ, Leavens M, Maor M et al. (1982) Human central nervous system distribution of cis-diamminoedichloroplatinum and use as a radiosensitiver in malignant brain tumors. Cancer Res 42:2474–2479
6. Stewart DJ, Wallace S, Feun L et al. (1982) A phase I study of intracarotid artery infusion of cis-diamminoedichlorplatinum (II) in patients with recurrent malignant intracerebral tumors. Cancer Res 42:2059–2062
7. Stewart DJ, Grahovac Z, Benoit B et al. (1984) Intracarotid chemotherapy with a combination of 1,3-bis(2-chloroethyl)-1-nitrosourea (BCNU), cis-diamminoedichloroplatinum (Cisplatin) and 4-O-demethyl-1-O-(4,6-O-2-thenylidene-β-D-glucopyranosyl) epipodophyllotoxin (VM26) in the treatment of primary and metastatic brain tumors. Neurosurgery 15:828–833

MTT Assay for In Vitro Chemosensitivity Testing of Malignant Intracranial Tumors

J.-C. Tonn[1], G. Nikkhah[2], K. Roosen[1], and W. Schachenmayr[1]

Introduction

Limited benefits of cytostatic therapy for malignant intracranial tumors enforce the need to improve its efficacy until better ways of treatment are found. Several in vitro chemosensitivity tests have been published [1]. The hope of individualizing chemotherapy and screening different drugs prior to their administration has not been fulfilled up to now, mostly due to methodological problems or lack of practicability. The MTT test is based on the conversion of the tetrazolium salt MTT by mitochondrial enzymes only present in metabolically active cells to a blue product, formazan. The assay had been adjusted in previous experiments to improve its application in routine laboratory work [2]. This should allow testing of tumor tissue of every patient operated upon, providing a result within 4 weeks. In this study, we report on a series of MTT tests over a period of 2 years with emphasis on the question of whether the test results are independent from clinical or biological data of the specimen.

Material and Methods

From October 1988 to October 1990, we performed 97 MTT tests on human malignant intracranial tumors. All tests were evaluable. A histopathological classification of each specimen was obtained, usually accompanied by immunohistological examination (GFAP, S 100).

The technique of the assay has been published elsewhere [2]. Briefly, a cell suspension of the surgical specimen was prepared and grown in culture flasks in RPMI 1640 medium with 10% fetal calf serum. When an appropriate number of cells was achieved, the suspension was incubated with a panel of cytostatic drugs at different concentrations. Thereafter, the cells were washed and reincubated in drug-free medium in 96-well plates for another 7 days. Then, 200 μg MTT was added together with fresh medium. After 4 h of incubation, MTT and medium were removed and the formazan crystals were dissolved in 100 μl dimethyl sul-

[1] Neurochirurgische Universitätsklinik, Josef-Schneider-Str. 11, W–8700 Würzburg, FRG.
[2] Institut für Neuropathologie der Justus-Liebig-Universität, Klinikstr. 29, W–6300 Gießen, FRG.

Advances in Neurosurgery, Vol. 20
K. Piscol, M. Klinger, M. Brock (Eds.)

foxide (DMSO). The plates were shaken for 5 min and read thereafter at 550 nm and 630 nm wavelengths in a microplate reader. The extinction of treated cells at clinically achievable tissue concentrations in relation to untreated controls was calculated as relative extinction (RE). In addition, the ratio of the area under the dose-response curve of the treated and the untreated cells was expressed as a sensitivity index (SI). Tumors with an RE under 50% or an SI under 0.5 were classified as sensitive against that drug in vitro.

In this study we report the results concerning ACNU (1–5–25 μg/ml), BCNU (1–5–25 μg/ml), and mitoxantrone (0.07–0.35–1.75 μg/ml).

Statistical analysis was performed with the Wilcoxon test, the log-rank test, the multivariate regression of Cox, and multiple correlation. The statistical software PCS (Topsoft, Hannover, FRG) was used.

Results

The mean age of the patients ($n=97$, 60% male) was 49.8 ± 18.5 years (2–78 years). The most frequent histopathological diagnoses were astrocytoma ($n=31$), glioblastoma ($n=22$), oligoendroglioma ($n=12$), and metastasis ($n=17$). Fifty gliomas had been classified as grade III or more according to the WHO scheme.

The mean weight of the specimen was 2.4 g with a mean viability of 84%. RE and SI correlated very high for each drug (ACNU $r=0.935$; BCNU $r=0.916$; mitoxantrone $r=0.928$). However, in our opinion the SI seems, at least theoretically, to be of more relevance since the dose-response relationship is better represented with the SI than with the RE. The mean SI of both nitrosoureas was far above 0.5, as only few tumors met the criteria of in vitro sensitivity against either drug, in contrast to mitoxantrone (Fig. 1).

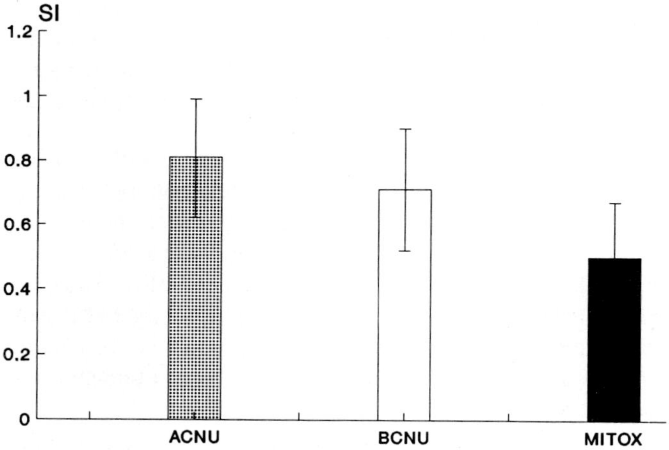

Fig. 1. Mean sensitivity index (SI) of ACNU, BCNU, and mitoxantrone (*MITOX*)

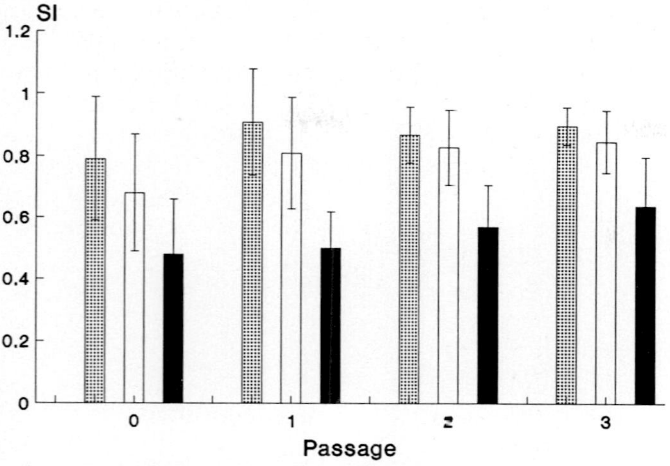

Fig. 2. Mean SI according to the passage of cells. Shading of the *bars* as in Fig. 1

Due to the usually rather large tumor specimen we were able to test 77.3% of the tumors without further passage (passage 0). Regardless of the drug, lower SI values could be obtained in tests of passage 0 cells. No dependency could be detected between the SI and further passages (Fig. 2). The histopathological diagnosis was of no significant influence on the SI, but the drug-dependent differences persisted in all entities (Fig. 3). Within the group of the malignant gliomas, the classification according to the WHO was not linked to the SI. Analysis of the SI in relation to the WHO grading and the drug tested revailed only an influence of the latter. Preoperative treatment (irradiation, former surgery) did not alter either the test results or viability of the cell suspension or the cell density of the specimen.

The Karnofsky performance rate and the extent of surgery were statistically significant prognostic factors in terms of life expectancy in our group of patients. Neither these clinical values nor others (e.g., age, sex) had a significant influence on the test results with regard to the SI (Table 1).

Discussion

The MTT test was evaluated in this study since it fulfills criteria for a test system suitable for routine chemosensitivity testing. It is rather inexpensive, results can be obtained in a reasonable time course, and even small amounts of tumor can be worked up sufficiently. However, the main problem of all systems is whether the test results are valid and reliable [1, 3, 4].

The correlation of the MTT data and the results of a colony-forming assay (CFA) in a subgroup of patients in whom both tests had been performed was rather low. Most of the experience about clinical correlation has been gained with the CFA.

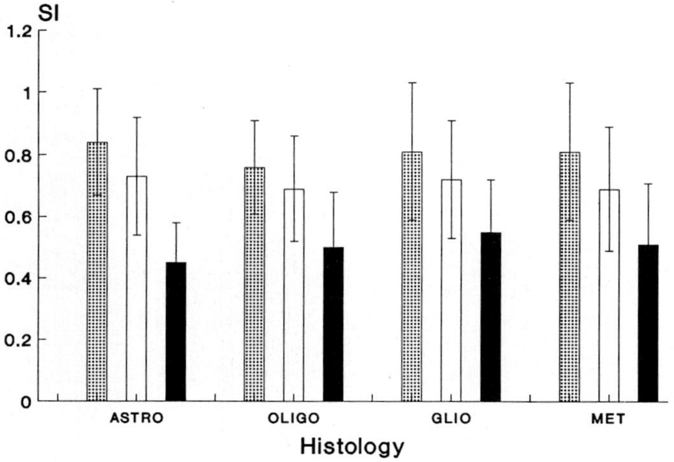

Fig. 3. Mean SI for the four most frequent histopathological entities. Shading of the *bars* as in Fig. 1

Table 1. Multiple correlation (age, sex, Karnofsky score, extent, SI)

ACNU	BCNU	MITOX
0.240	0.262	0.340
0.126	0.102	0.125
0.235	0.253	0.234
0.089	0.112	0.130
0.108	0.148	0.275

Therefore, prospective correlative trials with comparison of these two or more assays should be done. Clinical data of the patients (e.g., age, histology, WHO grading) had no significant influence on the test results – RE and SI seem to be independent variables. Clinical application of any of these tests should only be performed within controlled studies.

Acknowledment. We would like to thank Ms. N. Roetering for her skillful laboratory work.

References

1. Kimmel DW, Shapiro JR, Shapiro WR (1987) In vitro drug sensitivity testing in human gliomas. J Neurosurg 66:161–171
2. Nikkhah G, Darling JL, Thomas DGT (1989) The application of the MTT chemosensitivity assay to short-term cell lines derived from gliomas: characterization and comparison with a ^{35}S-methionine uptake assay. Reg Cancer Treat 2:112–118
3. Rosenblum ML, Dougherty DV, Deen DF, Wilson CB (1981) Potentials and limitations of a clonogenic cell assay for human brain tumors. Cancer Treat Rep (Suppl 2) 65:61–66
4. Thomas DGT, Darling JL, Paul EA, Mott TJ, Godlee JN (1985) Assay of anticancer drugs in tissue culture: relationship of relapse free interval (RFI) and in-vitro chemosensitivity in patients with malignant cerebral glioma. Br J Cancer 51:525–532

Radical Resection of Midline Gliomas in Children

A. Sepehrnia, M. Tatagiba, and M. Samii[1]

Introduction

Tumors of neuroepithelial origin constitute approximately one-half of supratentorial tumors and the vast majority of posterior fossa tumors in children [1, 2]. The clinical presentation and the treatment approach depend considerably on the anatomical location of the tumor. Tumors of the midline are those located in the third and fourth ventricles, in the pineal region, and the cerebellar vermis. Recent technological advances in diagnosis, intraoperative monitoring, microsurgical technique, and treatment modalities had an impact on treatment of the midline tumors [3, 5–7]. However, certain neoplasms located on the midline are still considered unresectable and even "untouchable" due to the complicated neurovascular anatomy of this region [1].

We retrospectively analyzed 57 children with neuroepithelial tumors of the midline operated at the Nordstadt Hospital between 1978 and 1990 to determine the clinical and pathological aspects and to evaluate the possibility of radical resection of these neoplasms. Results of other treatment modalities such as radiotherapy and chemotherapy were not taken into consideration in this study and therefore will not be described.

Patient Population

From 1978 to 1990, 90 patients with tumors of neuroepithelial origin located on the midline were operated on in our department. Fifty-five patients (69%) were 16 years old or younger, with average age of 9 ± 4 years. These latter patients were evaluated concerning the clinical features, the pathological features and location of the tumor, and the surgical treatment applied in each case.

The diagnostic studies included in all cases CT scan and in the most recent cases also MRI. Angiography was performed when the tumor was suspected to involve important vascular structures, most frequently in processes affecting the posterior portion of the third ventricle and the fourth ventricle.

[1] Neurochirurgische Klinik, Krankenhaus Nordstadt, Haltenhoffstr. 41, W–3000 Hannover 1, FRG.

Advances in Neurosurgery, Vol. 20
K. Piscol, M. Klinger, M. Brock (Eds.)

Table 1. Location and pathological findings of 55 midline neuroepithelial tumors in children

Tumor location		*n*	Pathological findings
Third ventricle	Anterior	1	Anaplastic ependymoma
	Superior	2	Low-grade astrocytoma
	Posterior	5	Plexus papilloma, astrocytoma, pineocytoma, pineoblastoma
	Hypothalamus	2	Pilocytic astrocytoma
Fourth ventricle	Roof	6	Oligodendroglioma, ependymoma, plexuspapilloma
	Floor	5	Medulloblastoma, astrocytoma, medulloblastoma
Cerebellum	Vermis	19	Low-grade astrocytoma, oligodendroglioma medulloblastoma
	Other	3	Low- and high-grade astrocytoma
Brainstem		12	Low- and high-grade astrocytoma

Tumor Location and Pathological Findings

Table 1 summarizes the location and pathological findings of the neuroepithelial tumors in the 55 children. The midline tumors were anatomically classified according to their relationship to the third and fourth ventricles and the cerebellar vermis. The region of the third ventricle can be divided in anterior, posterior, and superior portions and the parasellar area (hypothalamus) [3]. In our series only one patient had a tumor in the anterior portion of the third ventricle (one anaplastic ependymoma); two patients had tumors in the superior portion (low-grade astrocytoma), five patients had tumors in the posterior portion (two pinealomas, one astrocytoma, and two choroid plexus papillomas); and two patients had tumors in the parasellar region (both pilocytic astrocytomas).

Twenty tumors were located in the cerebellum [10 astrocytoma (9 low-grade astrocytomas and one anaplastic astrocytoma), one oligodendroglioma, and 11 medulloblastomas]. Eleven tumors were situated in the region of the fourth ventricle [three medulloblastomas, two ependymonas (one anaplastic), two plexus papillomas (one anaplastic), three astrocytomas, and one oligodendroglioma]. Finally, 12 patients had brainstem tumors (ten pilocytic astrocytomas and two anaplastic astrocytomas).

Clinical Presentation

Table 2 summarizes the clinical presentation and the operative characteristics of the 55 children with midline tumors. Patients presenting with tumors located in the hypothalamus usually had visual deficits, which constituted an important factor for decision making favorable to radical tumor resection. In the case of relatively good visual function, partial tumor removal had a decompressive function and improved

Table 2. Clinical and surgical aspects of 55 children with tumors on the midline

Tumor location	Ataxia [%]	Paresis [%]	Hydro-cephalus [%]	Tumor removal		
				Radical	Subtotal	Biopsy
Third ventricle	60	75	70	5	3	2
Fourth ventricle	82	33	73	8	2	1
Cerebellum	86	33	86	18	4	–
Brainstem	58	88	25	5	6	1

preoperative deficit. Radical tumor removal was performed when the patient had considerable visual impairment.

Most of the tumors located in the fourth ventricle and cerebellar vermis caused symptoms and signs of increased intracranial pressure. The patients frequently presented with obstructive hydrocephalus and any grade of ataxia. Papilledema was found in 64% of the cases. Paresis of the limbs was not usually seen. Ventricular drainage or shunting some days or weeks before surgery for tumor removal considerably improved the preoperative clinical deficits.

Patients with brainstem tumors frequently presented with ataxia, paresis of the limbs, and cranial nerve deficits. Hydrocephalus was seen only in 25% of cases. The most common cranial nerves affected were the third, fourth, and sixth nerves (50%). Facial nerve deficit was present in 33% of the patients, and deficits of the vestibulocochlear nerve and the caudal nerves were seen in 25% and 17%, respectively.

Surgical Treatment

Using a microsurgical technique, radical tumor removal was achieved in most of the cases of pilocytic astrocytoma, independently of tumor location – hypothalamus/optic nerve, thalamus, cerebellum, or brainstem (Figs. 1 and 2). Preoperative severe visual impairment was an important factor favorable to radical surgery in cases of hypothalamus gliomas. Exophytic brainstem gliomas into the fourth ventricle could frequently be radically removed without major functional deficits. The initial clinical deterioration observed postoperatively recovered in most of the cases to acceptable results (patient became independent), but required physiotherapy for some weeks or months.

Vermian medulloblastomas were almost always radically removed. In some cases a thin tumor layer infiltrating the floor or the fourth ventricle was left. Postoperatively, an improvement of the ataxia and obstructive hydrocephalus was mostly seen.

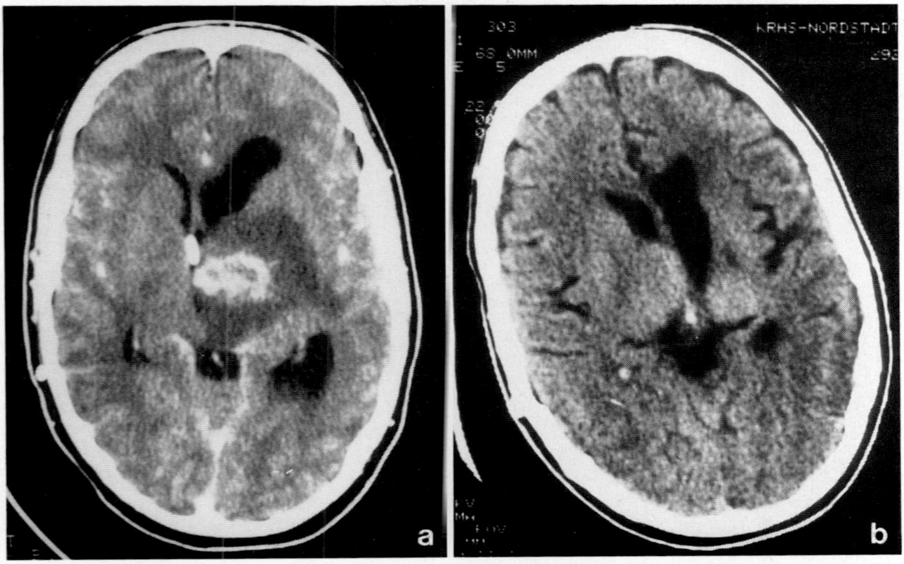

Fig. 1. a Preoperative and **b** postoperative axial CT scan of a thalamus astrocytoma, which was radically resected without additional neurological deficit

Discussion

The management of midline tumors presents special problems to the neurosurgeon and oncologist. Radical tumor resection may improve preoperative deficits due to tumor compression, delay the time to disease progression in older children, and improve the results of adjuvant radio- and chemotherapy [6, 7].

Clinical and radiological studies have better determined prognosis and efficacy of surgical intervention in cases of brainstem gliomas [5]. Patients with cerebellar or fourth ventricle tumors frequently require shunting before operation due to occlusive hydrocephalus. We usually do not operate these patients in a sitting position because of the risk of decompressive subdural hematoma. Hypothalamus gliomas with good visual function may be subtotally removed without major visual deficit. Radical removal is recommended when considerable visual impairment is already present.

With increasing improvement in microsurgical technique and intraoperative monitoring, radical resection of tumors located on the midline has been achieved in a large number of patients with minimal morbidity [4]. However, further clinical studies will probably change in future the concept of operability of some tumors still seen today as unremovable, and new adjuvant modalities show beneficial effect on the residual tumor.

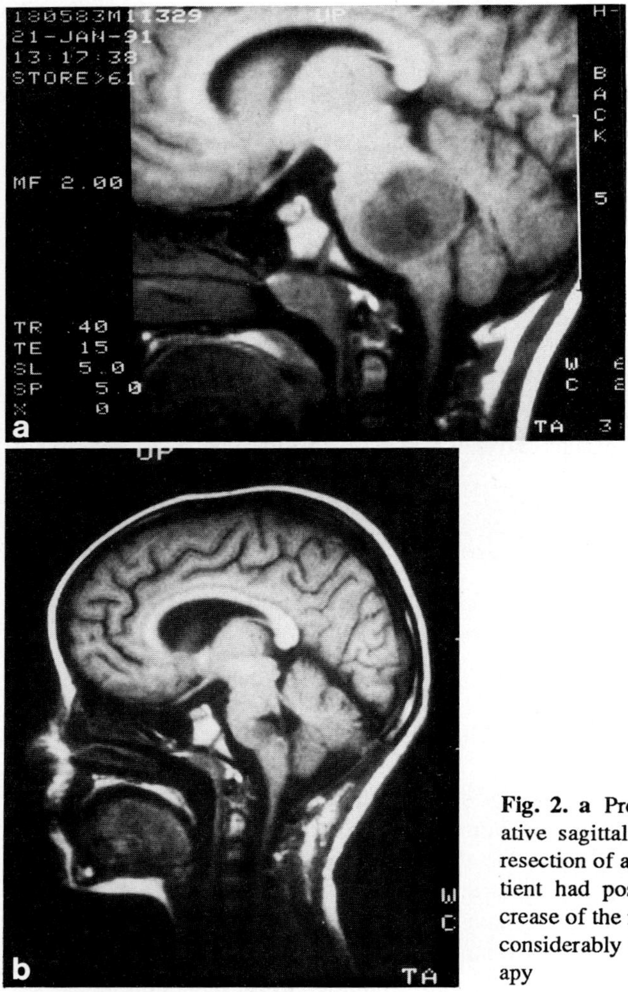

Fig. 2. a Preoperative and **b** postoperative sagittal MRI showing the radical resection of a low-grade glioma. The patient had postoperatively an initial increase of the neurological deficits, which considerably improved with physiotherapy

References

1. Bernstein M, Hoffmann HJ, Halliday WC, Hendrick EB, Humphreys RP (1984) Thalamic tumors in children. J Neurosurg 61:649–656
2. Packer RJ, Shunt L, Sutton LN, Bruce DA (1990) Brain tumors of the posterior cranial fossa in infants and children. In: Youmans JR (ed) Neurological surgery, vol 6, 3rd edn. Saunders, Philadelphia London Toronto
3. Raimondi AJ (1987) Pediatric neurosurgery. Springer, Berlin Heidelberg New York Tokyo, pp 227–264
4. Sepehrnia A, Tatagiba M, Samii M (1989) Mittelliniengliome. Presented at the Arbeitsgemeinschaft Mikroneurochirurgie der Deutschen Gesellschaft für Neurochirurgie, Ingolstadt, November 10, 1989

5. Stroink AR, Hoffman HJ, Hendrick EB, Humphreys RP (1986) Diagnosis and management of pediatric brain-stem gliomas. J Neurosurg 65:745–750
6. Tadanori T, McLone DG (1986) Medulloblastoma in childhood: results of radical resection and low-dose neuraxis radiation therapy. J Neurosurg 64:238–242
7. Wisoff JH, Abbott R, Epstein F (1990) Surgical management of exophytic chiasmatic-hypothalamic tumors in childhood. J Neurosurg 73:661–667

Glioma Surgery Within a General Concept: Ultrasonic Aspiration, Laser Coagulation, Radiotherapy, Relapse Operation, Hyperthermia

J. Schöche[1]

The results obtained in the therapy of brain tumors have an appallingly sobering effect particularly on committed neurosurgeons. This is less a question of temperament or age, but rather a consequence of experience.

Our experience covers 461 brain tumors in 1540 cerebral operations carried out in Chemnitz since 1982. We were able to use angiography from the onset; a CT unit and ultrasonic tumor aspirator were added in 1985. We have had our own intensive care subsection since 1987 and a Nd:YAG laser since 1990.

We have been working according to a general concept for years with neuropathological examinations as an aid in decision making and radiotherapy by means of a linear accelerator that is commendably possibly near at hand.

What are the Results?

1. The complete removal of the tumor remains to be the patients' best help. In this respect, the destruction of the tumor's vascular supply and the preservation of the surviving brain are the most difficult problems, but this is the only chance – in addition to removal – to stop further growth. The reserves provided by the operation are important with regard to the situation during radiotherapy and the beginning of the final compression.

2. Partial removal of brain tumors is of uncertain value and only acceptable when – proceeding from the grading – reliable success from radiotherapy can be expected. Host-tumor balance disturbances and the activation of proliferation zones in the periphery of the tumor have to be considered in a different way, especially when applying the ultrasonic tumor aspirator.

3. Palliative operations do not normally prolong a life worth living, but rather suffering. As a rule, we disapprove of these operations on malignant gliomas as they have not brought about better outcomes.

4. As far as the operation itself is concerned, the ultrasonic tumor aspirator is most helpful to use on malignant gliomas as the tumor can also be removed from regions where removal around the tumor is impossible. The potential preservation of the preformed vessels, e.g., the anterior and the media, is favorable, whereas that of the central arteries is uncertain.

[1] Neurochirurgische Klinik, Kreiskrankenhaus, O–2001 Chemnitz, FRG.

Advances in Neurosurgery, Vol. 20
K. Piscol, M. Klinger, M. Brock (Eds.)

The system decompression is always prepared and in any case highly important for maintaining control and clarity in pursuing the operative schedule. It has stood the test in more than 300 cases and depends on a high monitoring standard with the most important medical quantity being PO_2.

5. Application of the laser is regularly carried out up to the end to reduce the risk of continued growth or the nidation potency on blastomas (and also metastatic tumors). Wattage rarely exceeds 25 W, pulses are never longer than 1 s, and total energy input is rarely higher than 1500 J when applying the Nd: YAG laser.

6. All patients with tumors grade II–IV are recommended to undergo postoperative radiotherapy; the patients' relatives are included in this decision. As for grade II astrocytoma, the patients' age and physical condition, the relation between the tumor and the dominant cortical areas, and the patients' and their relatives' mental attitude are important factors to be taken into account.

Radiotherapy is carried out by a high-voltage linear accelerator up to a total dosage of 60 Gy. The beginning of radiotherapy is scheduled for the 10th day after the operation; this applies particularly to tumors with relations to the subarachnoid or spinal space.

7. Unfortunately, the relapse operation is the most important therapeutic element. As a rule, a planning CT is carried out after the operation of a blastoma, on discharge for radiotherapy, and a CT at the end of the radiotherapy. For the last consultation the patient is required to present himself at the outpatient department of the neurosurgical clinic if this is possible. Another visit to the doctor is arranged for 3 or 6 months in advance of which a CT has to be made (this is still a scheduling problem in our institution and involves waiting in nonacute cases). If there is no recurrence after 9 months, the covering of the bone defect, which is normally existing, will be discussed with the patient. Otherwise, the removal of the conglomerate of radiation scar or tumor recurrence will be scheduled if the patient's state permits.

This general concept is outlined to the patient in advance of the first operation, as we have to explain our recommendation to leave out the bone plate for improving the tolerance of potential radiotherapy.

The majority of the patients are surprisingly reasonable, and group dynamics work just as well here as in neurosurgery. The patients know each other, find fellow sufferers, take comfort from good examples, or find they are better off than others. The neurosurgical consultation hours are frequented and do not avoid the term "brain tumor," thus hypothetically contributing to reducing the patients' anxiety.

8. This concept is also carried out in this or a modified manner elsewhere, and the better the prognosis is on which the histological findings are based, the better the results brought about by this concept will be.

There are some tumor patients in whom an operation seems to offer little promise owing to their age, constitution, other diseases, extension, or histological findings which can be reliably prognosticated. Here, CT-based biopsy is carried out if reduction of the tumor has a good chance. Some of these patients were later radiated and subsequently operated. It was remarkable that after a longer period a grade IV glioblastoma could be changed into a grade II oligodendroglioma.

Apart from these quite rarely appearing possibilities of preoperative tumor conditioning, we have been working on a project since 1986 which implies intratumoral hyperthermia – as it is presently being carried out intraoperatively – to be established in advance and instead of other methods. At the same time, we would like to consolidate and develop our contacts to like-minded colleagues in Düsseldorf or Graz.

The results of therapeutic possibilities achieved in the field of brain tumors will remain sobering. What at all remains to be done by the physician than to prolong life with the quality of the medical work being decisive for the general quality.

Local Administration of Chemo- and Radiopharmaceuticals

H. W. Pannek[1], F. Oppel[1], and R. Schnabel[2]

Introduction

During the past years, disillusionment has characterized the therapy of malignant glioma. Survival rates determined by Walker [7] in the BTSG of 1978 have almost been supported by Krauseneck et al. [4, 5] in the German-Austrian Glioma Study of 1987. Obviously, neither a change of the systemic combination of chemopharmaceuticals nor the latest procedures in imaging diagnostics (MRI technique) or operative high tech (CUSA, Laser) could improve the success of the patients' treatment. As the classic treatment of glioma (operative resection, radiation, and if possible chemopharmaceuticals) does not offer essential progress, there is now a search for new concepts [2, 6].

The therapy described in this article consists of a local administration of chemo- and radiopharmaceuticals. It is intended to complete and improve the conventional treatment in special cases of cystic malignant gliomas. It is not important, however, whether there is a primary, pseudo- (necrosis) or secondary (operative resection) development of cysts.

This treatment is presented on the basis of a retrospective study of 20 patients with astrocytomas grades III–IV (WHO) and a gliosarcoma (1984–1990).

Method

The maximum patient age was fixed at 65 (in good physical condition without secondary illness). In addition, the following demands should be fulfilled: a Karnofsky index of 90%, a positive, subjective self-determination of the patient; all gliomas must be astrocytomas grades III (with necrosis) – IV or gliosarcomas with supratentorial localization.

The treatment was carried out in three phases:

1. Operation with maximum resection, in primary cystic gliomas implantation of an Ommaya reservoir in the resection cave or cystic cave. Postoperative radiation and (if not rejected by the patient) systemic chemotherapy.

[1] Neurochirurgische Klinik, Krankenanstalten Gilead, von Bodelschwinghsche Anstalten, Burgsteig 4, W-4800 Bielefeld 13, FRG
[2] Institut für Neuropathologie, Krankenanstalten Gilead, von Bodelschwinghsche Anstalten, Burgsteig 4, W-4800 Bielefeld 13, FRG

Advances in Neurosurgery, Vol. 20
K. Piscol, M. Klinger, M. Brock (Eds.)

2. In the case of visible tumor progression in CT or MRI examinations and a Karnofsky index of > 70%, local chemopharmaceuticals BCNU, methotrexate, or Alexan were given in a cycle of 3 weeks on 3 subsequent days. If there was no effect or hypersecretion (> 20 ml/day), a liquid nuclide 32-P colloid gel was given. Before each treatment the tumor and cystic liquid were aspired and examined cytologically. If there was no regression of tumor cells (in vivo observation), a change of chemotherapeutics was necessary.
3. In the case of manifest proof of a progression of the patient's clinical state and a Karnofsky index of > 70%, another operation was carried out as ultima ratio, and the combination of therapeutics mentioned above was continued.

Throughout phases 2 and 3 a flexible application of the above-mentioned treatments and reoperation were determined, each dependent on the individual clinical state of the patient.

Results

Because of an underdeveloped cystic cave in 8 of 20 patients, an effective aspiration and instillation was not possible so that they underwent only two to three cycles. Thus, they could not be considered in the results. The age of the remaining 12 patients ranged from 24 to 64 years (mean = 45 years); the female : male ratio was 1 : 5.

In the first operation the histological findings were astrocytomas grade III WHO in five patients, astrocytomas grade IV WHO in six patients, and in one patient gliosarcoma. In six cases the localization was the right or left side, with the lobus frontalis, partietalis, and temporalis being affected. The mean diameter of the extirpated tumor was 3.5 cm (range: 2–5 cm). The mean period between the first operation and the reoperation was 10 months; the transformation of an astrocytoma grade III to grade IV was observed in one case. A comparison between the Karnofsky indices of the first operation and the reoperation showed a mean decrease of 20%. Two patients could not be reoperated; one of them died of fulminant pneumonia in the course of systemic BCNU treatment. The second patient has not shown any progress. Eight patients received systemic BCNU therapy, in four cases in combination with VM-26.

In all patients, Alexan was given via an Ommaya reservoir, in two cases 32-P colloid gel, because of heavy secretion, and BCNU, as well as methotrexate, was given in one case.

In the course of giving Alexan any test of aspiration was positive in six cases (cytological proof of regressive tumor cells); in two patients the evidence was mostly positive, in four cases only occasionally. Two patients who received BCNU both showed positive results only occasionally; thus, a change to Alexan was made. Two patients were given 32-P colloid gel, which led to positive results in every test. The mean survival rate was 77 weeks.

Discussion

Because of the small group of 12 patients, a comparison with other studies is only partially possible. There are, however, similarities: the time between the first and the reoperation, the survival rate in general, and the significantly longer survival rates of younger patients [1, 3]. The aim of this study was to provide a basis for discussion of the innovative aspect of this treatment.

References

1. Ammirati M et al. (1987) Reoperation in the treatment of recurrent intracranial malignant gliomas. Neurosurgery 21 (5):607–613
2. Beierwaltes WH (1985) Horizons in radionuclide therapy: update. J Nucl Med 26:421–427
3. Harsh, Griffith R IV et al. (1987) Reoperation for recurrent glioblastoma and anaplastic astrocytoma. Neurosurgery 21 (5):615–621
4. Krauseneck K, Mertens HG (1987) Results of chemotherapy of malignant brain tumors in adults. In: Jellinger K (ed) Therapy of malignant brain tumors. Springer, Wien New York, pp 349–395
5. Müller H et al. (1985) Long-term survival and recurrence-free interval in combined surgical, radio- and chemotherapy of malignant brain gliomas. Clin Neurol Neurosurg 87–93:167–171
6. Pannek HW, Brock M, Franke A (1987) Die direkte intratumorale Applikation von radioaktiven Substanzen (32 P-Gel) und Zytostatika (BCNU) bei der multimodalen Behandlung von Hirntumoren. Tumor Diagnostik und Therapie 8:225–229
7. Walker MD et al. (1980) Randomized comparisons of radiotherapy and nitrosureas for the treatment of malignant glioma after surgery. New England J Med 303:1323–1329

Combined Radiotherapy of High-Grade Gliomas with Stereotactic Implanted Iodine-125 Seeds and Fractionated Low-Dose Rate Beam Irradiation: Preliminary Results

J. Voges, H. Treuer, W. J. Schlegel, O. Pastyr, and V. Sturm[1]

Introduction

External fractionated irradiation if administered after neurosurgical tumor resection can significantly improve the survival of patients with a cerebral malignant glioma [6, 11]. However, the high risk of brain necrosis precludes the administration of more than 6000–7000 cGy. To achieve local tumor control, interstitial irradiation for the treatment of brain neoplasms was established during the past 30 years [8, 13]. The steep dose gradient around the implanted isotopes and the development of an integrated CT-guided, computerized stereotactic operation and irradiation – planning system allows highly precise local radiotherapy also in functionally important or deep-sited areas of the brain with doses potentially sufficient for tumor destruction [1, 10, 12].

Patients and Methods

From 1982 to 1990, 160 patients with a cerebral glioma were treated with stereotactically implanted iodine-125 seeds and interstitial irradiation. For retrospective analysis, 39 patients with a high-grade lesion were selected according to the following criteria: (a) tumors had been sufficiently demarcable in contrast-enhanced CT scans, the maximal diameter not exceeding 5 cm, (b) the histopathological diagnosis had to be established before seed implantation, and (c) patients with permanent iodine-125 seed implantation should have follow-up times of more than 18 months.

After fixation of a modified, CT-compatible Riechert-Mundinger stereotactic frame [12] and administration of contrast medium (Solutrast 300, Byk Gulden, Darmstadt, FRG), a CT investigation was performed. CT data were transferred by magnetic tape into a computer (VAX 11/700 or VAX-Station 3500, Digital Equip, Corp., USA), and the tumor borders were demarcated manually at the computer screen. Determination of target points as well as the treatment planning for interstitial irradiation were carried out with a special software described elsewhere [1, 10].

During the first 3 weeks after stereotactic surgery, all patients with permanent implanted iodine-125 seeds (3M Deutschland GmbH, Neuss, FRG) and four patients

[1] Abteilung für Stereotaxie und funktionelle Neurochirurgie,
Neurochirurgische Universitätsklinik Köln, Joseph-Stelzmann-Str. 9, W–5000 Köln 41, FRG.

Advances in Neurosurgery, Vol. 20
K. Piscol, M. Klinger, M. Brock (Eds.)

with an implantation time of 90 days (dose rate 1.1 Gy/day) additionally received a fractionated external beam irradiation (boost dose 23.7 + 8 Gy) to increase the dose rate to values equivalent to those achieved with conventional radiotherapy (Table 1).

The iodine-125 sources were implanted under general anesthesia. Immediately before implantation and during the first days after the stereotactic operation, dexamethasone was administered orally. With one exception none of the patients received systemic or local chemotherapy. CT scans without and with contrast medium as well as neurological examinations were performed 6, 12, and 36 weeks after implantation and later on in yearly intervals.

Results

Thirty-nine patients with a high-grade glioma and treated with stereotactically implanted iodine-125 seeds for interstitial irradiation were analyzed retrospectively. In group A, 29 patients received interstitial (permanent implanted seeds) and external

Table 1. Characteristics of 39 patients

Parameter	Group A	Group B
Age (years)		
Range	1–65	25–76
Mean	30	48
Sex (*n*)		
Female	9	6
Male	20	4
Sites (*n*)		
Cortex	10	6
Diencephalon	11	4
Brainstem	6	–
Cortex and brainstem	2	–
Histological findings (*n*)	(Kernohan)	(WHO)
Astrocytoma III	18	–
Oligoastrocytoma III	1	–
Astrocytoma IV	3	1
Glioblastoma	7	9
Implanted volume (ml)		
Mean	29.2	34.3
Iodine-125 activities (mCi)		
Mean	9.2	18.7
Tumor dose (Gy)		
Mean	55	60
Dose rate (cGy/day)		
Mean	0.69	1.2

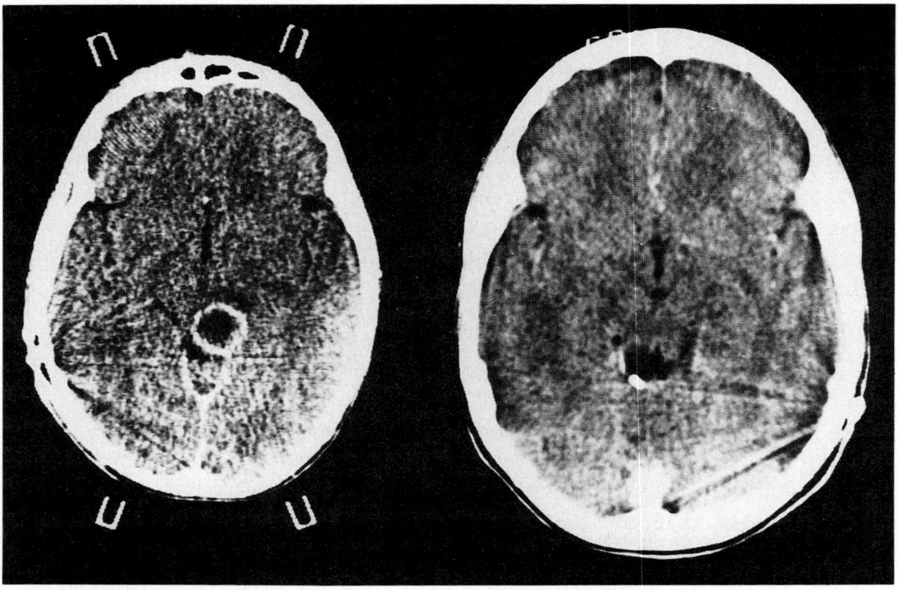

Fig. 1. CT examination of a patient with a glioblastoma (Kernohan classification). *Left*, preoperatively; *right*, 4 years after combined interstitial (iodine-125, permanent implantation, 60 Gy) and external beam irradiation (boost dose 15 Gy)

fractionated beam irradiation. In group B (10 patients), the seeds were implanted temporarily (42 or 90 days) (Table 1). Before iodine-125 seed implantation, the tumors were diagnosed histopathologically by previously resected material (10 patients) or stereotactic biopsies (29 patients). In group B, five patients were preirradiated with a mean dose of 56 Gy. The Karnofsky performance status of all evaluated patients ranged from 75% to 100%.

Postoperatively, the tumor volumes were measured in a CT scan and the patients classified as responders (significant volume reduction) and nonresponders (tumor growth). In group A, 3 months after seed implantation the response rate was 79% for patients with a glioma grade III and 20% for patients with a grade IV lesion or glioblastoma; 42 or 90 days postoperatively a response rate of 80% could be registered for highly malignant gliomas in group B (Figs. 1 and 2).

Survival was defined as the time from seed implantation until the end of the retrospective analysis (November 1990) or the patient's death. In group A, the estimated mean survival probability (Kaplan-Meier [5]) is 64.9 months (mean follow-up: 53.5 months) for patients with a glioma grade III and 12.7 months for patients with a grade IV tumor or glioblastoma, respectively (Fig. 3). In group B, the estimated mean survival probability is 62 weeks (mean follow-up: 46 weeks). There was no operative or perioperative morbidity or mortality. The death of one patient with an astrocytoma grade III in the thalamus/midbrain region 89 months after combined

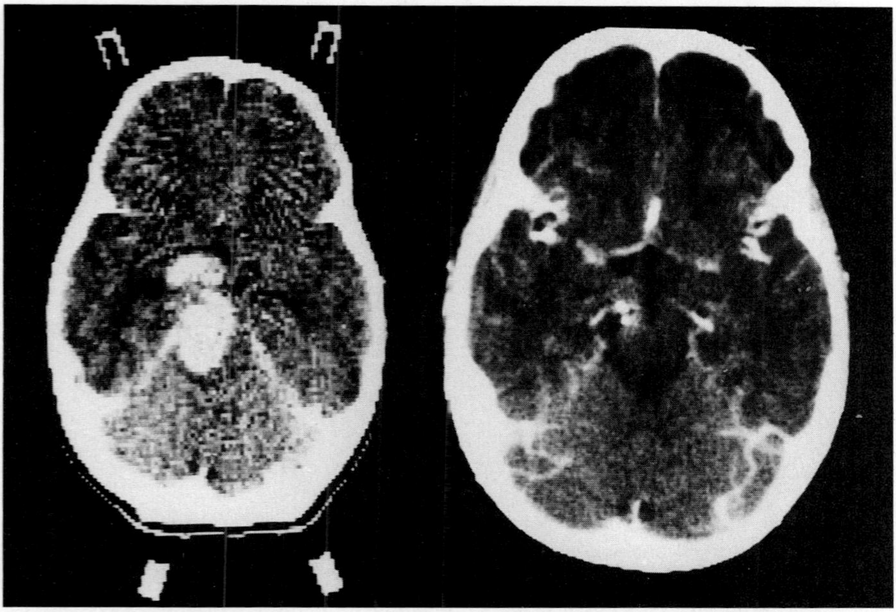

Fig. 2. CT examination of a patient with an astrocytoma grade III (Kernohan classification). *Left*, preoperatively; *right*, 6 years after combined interstitial (iodine-125, permanent implantation, 50 Gy) and external beam irradiation (boost dose 20 Gy)

interstitial and external irradiation probably was caused by radiation necrosis (an autopsy was not allowed). No other treatment-related side effects occurred.

Discussion

With a follow-up of 53.5 months, the estimated mean survival probability of patients with a grade III glioma analyzed in this study is 64.9%. In comparison with conventional treatment schedules, the combined interstitial and external irradiation seems to improve the prognosis of patients with these tumors. In the literature the 3-year survival rates for grade III lesions after surgery and external fractionated irradiation range from 18% to 27% [7, 9, 14]. As evaluated in our study, the estimated mean survival probability of patients with a glioma grade IV or glioblastoma is 12.7 months after combined interstitial and external beam irradiation or 15.5 months after temporary seed implantation and comparable to conventional therapy schedules [7, 9, 11, 14].

With temporary iodine-125 implantation (42 or 90 days) and dose rates ranging from 0.7 to 2.1 Gy/day in our study 80% of the patients with a glioma grade IV or glioblastoma responded to therapy without severe decrease of their performance status. Gutin et al. [2] combined ultrashort brachytherapy (tumor dose:

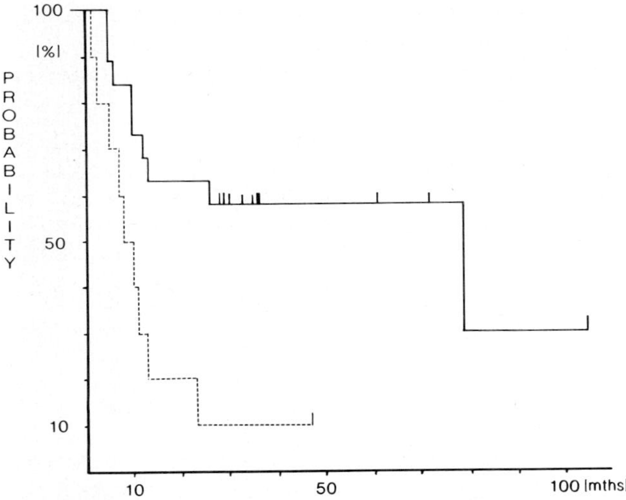

Fig. 3. Kaplan-Meier representation of the probability of survival after combined interstitial (iodine-125, permanent implantation) and external fractionated beam irradiation (group A). *Solid line*, patients with an astrocytoma grade III (Kernohan classification, 19 cases); *broken line*, patients with an astrocytoma grade IV or glioblastoma (Kernohan classification, 10 cases). *Ticks* represent censored patients

5740–12000 cGy, dose rate: 25–100 cGy/h) with external irradiation (tumor dose: 4400–7050 cGy). The response rate was 29.2%. In 41% of their patients, persistent mass lesions or space-occupying radiation necrosis required reoperation [2]. With one exception (death due to localized radiation necrosis) in our series interstitial irradiation had been well tolerated by all patients.

The following facts make the interpretation of the favorable results difficult: (a) the study is retrospective without a control group, (b) the number of patients is rather small, and (c) most of the patients had been young and had had a relatively high Karnofsky score. Despite the possible bias due to the mentioned drawbacks of this analysis, our data show the effectivity and benignity of low-dose rate interstitial irradiation in circumscribable malignant gliomas also if combined with moderate fractionated beam irradiation. An indispensable prerequisite is the use of modern stereotactic treatment planning and implantation techniques, which enable the application of any radiation dose to any intracranial target volume with highest precision and optimnal sparing of the surrounding tissue [1, 10, 12].

Results of multiple in vitro and in vivo studies showed that the critical factor for the inhibition of mitosis is the amount of radiation absorbed per cell cycle rather than the fixed dose rate per minute. The minimal dose seems to range from 720 to 990 cGy per cell cycle [3]. Considering the estimated cell cycle time of a glioblastoma (3 days) [4] and a mean dose rate of 69 cGy/day delivered by permanently implanted iodine-125, each tumor cell received at least 207 cGy per cell cycle. With these dose rates, the growth of highly malignant neoplasms theoretically could not be stopped by permanently implanted iodine-125 seeds alone. External fractionated irradiation additionally applied with doses not affecting normal brain tissue and temporary seed implantation raises the dose rate per cell cycle at the beginning of the treatment.

A radical shortening of the implantation times as used by Gutin et al. [2] necessitates a tumor location which allows reoperation of necrotic masses without damage of surrounding brain tissue. In cases with gliomas located in the midline or eloquent cortical areas, this treatment schedule bears a high risk for decrease of the patient's performance status, and lower dose rates should be delivered. However, optimal surface dose, dose rates, and protraction of the interstitial irradiation are not yet known.

References

1. Bauer-Kirpes B, Sturm V, Schlegel W, Lorenz WJ (1988) Computerized optimization of 125-I implants in brain tumors. Int J Radiation Oncol Biol Phys 14:1013–1023
2. Gutin PH, Leibel SA, Wara WM, Choucair A, Levin VA, Philips TL, Silver P, Da Silva V, Edwards MSB, Davis RL, Weaver KA, Lamb S (1987) Recurrent malignant gliomas: survival following interstitial brachytherapy with high active Iodine-125 sources. J Neurosurg 67:864–873
3. Hall EJ (1978) Radiobiology for the radiologist, 2nd edn. Harper & Row, Maryland/USA
4. Hoshino T, Barker M, Wilson CB, Boldrey EB, Fewer D (1972) Cell kinetics of human gliomas. J Neurosurg 37:15–26
5. Kaplan EL, Meier P (1958) Nonparametric estimation from incomplete observations. J Am Statist Assoc 53:457–481
6. Kornblith PL, Walker MD, Cassady JR (1987) Neurologic oncology. Lippincott, Philadelphia
7. Marsa GW, Goffinet DR, Rubinstein LJ, Bagshaw MA (1975) Megavoltage irradiation in the treatment of gliomas of the brain and spinal cord. Cancer 36:1681–1689
8. Mundinger F (1985) Technik und Ergebnisse der interstitiellen Hirntumorbestrahlung. In: Diethelm L, Heuck F, Olsson O, Vieten H, Zuppinger A (Hrsg) Handbuch der medizinischen Radiologie, Bd XIX, Spezielle Strahlentherapie maligner Tumoren, Teil 4. Springer, Berlin Heidelberg New York Tokyo, S 179–214
9. Scanlon PW, Taylor WF (1979) Radiotherapy of intracranial astrocytomas: analysis of 417 cases treated from 1960 through 1969. Neurosurgery 5:301–308
10. Schlegel WJ, Scharfenberg H, Sturm V, Penzholz H, Lorenz WJ (1981) Direct visualization of intracranial tumours in stereotactic and angiographic films by computer calculation of longitudinal CT-sections: a new method for stereotactic localization of tumour outlines. Acta Neurochirurgica 58:27–35
11. Sheline GE (1977) Radiation therapy of brain tumors. Cancer 39:873–881
12. Sturm V, Pastyr O, Schlegel W, Scharfenberg H, Zabel HJ, Netzeband G, Schabbert S, Berberich W (1981) Stereotactic computer tomography with a modified Riechert Mundinger device as the basis for integrated stereotactic neuroradiological investigations. Acta Neurochirurgica 68:11–17
13. Szikla G, Peragbut JC (1975) Irradiation interstitielle des gliomes. Neurochirurgie (Suppl 2) 21:187–228
14. Wara WM (1985) Radiation therapy for brain tumors. Cancer 55:2291–2295

Malignant Glioma of the Brain: Not in Every Case a Poor Prognosis?

S. Victor and G. Lausberg[1]

Introduction

Since Bennett and Godlee (1884) reported about the first operation of a glioma of the brain, the operative technical standard developed with multifarious innovations [4, 7, 8, 14, 20]. Numerous postoperative adjuvant ways of therapy such as radiation, chemotherapy, and recently immunotherapeutic strategies followed in addition to operation [1, 3, 4, 7, 11, 12, 15, 17, 21, 30]. Nevertheless, in the case of malignant glioma of the brain, a hopeless prognosis is valid up to now [13, 16, 22]. Our own clinical analysis of 100 operated patients with supratentorial malignant gliomas (WHO grades III–IV and IV) resulted from the intention to find out important prognostic characteristics in the courses of this patient group [27].

Results

Before operation the average age of 100 patients (50 males and 50 females) was 58 years: 55 tumors were located in the right hemisphere, 40 tumors were located in the left hemisphere, and the other 5 tumors were "butterfly gliomas." In 23 cases we found infiltration of the brainstem. Concerning the extent of operation, the tumors of 35 patients were macroscopically totally removed (21 tumors were located in the right and 14 tumors in the left hemisphere); in 64 cases there was a subtotal resection of the tumor. A biopsy was performed in only one patient. The lobar localization of the tumor highly influenced the extent of the operation. Because of the existing possibility of lobectomy, the rates of macroscopically total tumor resections were high above the average in the temporal and occipital regions (temporal only in the nondominant hemisphere). Histological examination revealed in 63 cases malignant WHO grade IV gliomas (50 glioblastomas, 12 WHO grade IV astrocytomas, and 1 WHO grade IV oligodendroglioma) and 37 malignant WHO grade III–IV astrocytomas. Additional radiation therapy was performed and completed in 70 patients. In ten chemotherapy followed as a supplementary procedure. Resection of recurrent tumor was done in 33 patients. The postoperative survival time found in 84 of the 100 operated patients was an average of 332 days, roughly 11 months. The postoperative survival rates after 6, 12, 24, and 36 months

[1] Neurochirurgische Klinik der Ruhr-Universität Bochum, Knappschaftskrankenhaus, In der Schornau 23, W–4630 Bochum 7, FRG.

Advances in Neurosurgery, Vol. 20
K. Piscol, M. Klinger, M. Brock (Eds.)

Table 1. Prognostic factors for malignant glioma of the brain

Favorable prognostic factors	Survival time (days)
Localization	
Temporal	406
Occipital	391
Nondominant cerebral hemisphere	358
Before operation	
Consciousness undisturbed	364
Little neurological deficit	
Operative therapy	
Total resection of the tumor	554
Adjuvant radiation therapy	456
Operation in case of recurrent glioma	443
Unfavorable prognostic factors	
Localization	
Parietal	120
Infiltration of the brainstem	143
Dominant cerebral hemisphere	314
Before operation	
Lack of consciousness	185
Severe neurological deficit	
Operative therapy	
Subtotal resection of tumor	202
Absence of adjuvant radiation therapy	31
Average survival time:	332

amounted to 55%, 32%, 12%, and 7%. There was a wide variation of the survival time depending on the existence of favorable and unfavorable prognostic factors, evaluating topical, individual, and therapeutic factors of prognosis (Table 1). The most important factor was the *extent of primary operation*. In 1987 five patients were alive with a postoperative recurrence-free survival time of more than 3 years whom we called long-term survivors (Table 2). Our endeavors to update the outcome of these patients provided no further information about patients No. 1 and No. 2. In March 1991 patient No. 3 died in our hospital after operation of a late recurrent glioblastoma, more than 9 years after the first operation. Up to this date (May 1991) patients No. 4 and No. 5 are recurrence-free and healthy without neurological deficits. Thus, for more than 8 years after the operation, two of these five long-term survivors are still alive. This is in contrast to the common opinion of a usually short survival time (about 1 year) in the case of glioblastoma. A neuropathological second look was done by another investigator, independently from the first opinion, in four of the five histological specimens of the long-term survivors to avoid a false estimation concerning the histological malignancy of our long-term survivors. This

Table 2. Long-term survivors of operated malignant glioma of the brain (date: May 1991)

No.	Age (years)	Sex	Localization	Neuropathological diagnosis [WHO] (second look)	Survival time
1	18	M	Right par.-occ.	None (first look: giant cell glioblastoma [WHO IV])	(10/87 > 4 years) ?
2	71	M	Right par.-occ.	Glioblastoma multiforme [WHO IV]	(10/87 > 3 years) ?
3	12	F	Right temp.-par.	Anaplastic oligodendroglioma [WHO III]	> 9 years
4	30	F	Left temp.-occ.	Anaplastic ependymoma [WHO III]	> 8 years
5	56	F	Right frontal	Glioblastoma multiforme [WHO IV]	> 8 years

neuropathological second look resulted in two WHO grade IV glioblastomas and two WHO grade III gliomas (one anaplastic oligodendroglioma and one anaplastic ependymoma).

In the following, a brief description is given of the two healthy patients who to date are with certainty recurrence-free. At time of operation in May 1982, the female patient No. 4 was 30 years old. She had a macroscopically total resection of the left temporo-occipital tumor without additional resection of brain tissue. After the operation the patient was irradiated. The neuropathological second look showed an anaplastic WHO grade III ependymoma. To date the woman – on whom a cranial computer tomogram was done yearly – has remained recurrence-free without neurological failures for the last 9 years.

At time of operation in February 1983, the female patient Nr. 5 was 56 years old. The right frontal tumor was macroscopically totally removed by additional resection of brain tissue. She also received postoperative radiation therapy. The neuropathological second look confirmed a WHO grade IV glioblastoma. Two cranial computer tomograms showed the right frontal resection cavity unchanged from 1989 to 1990 (Figs. 1 and 2). All slices of hitherto existing cranial computed tomograms showed no tumor recurrence. This female patient is observed regularly too. To date – more than 8 years after the operation – she is free of tumor recurrence, complaints, and neurological deficits.

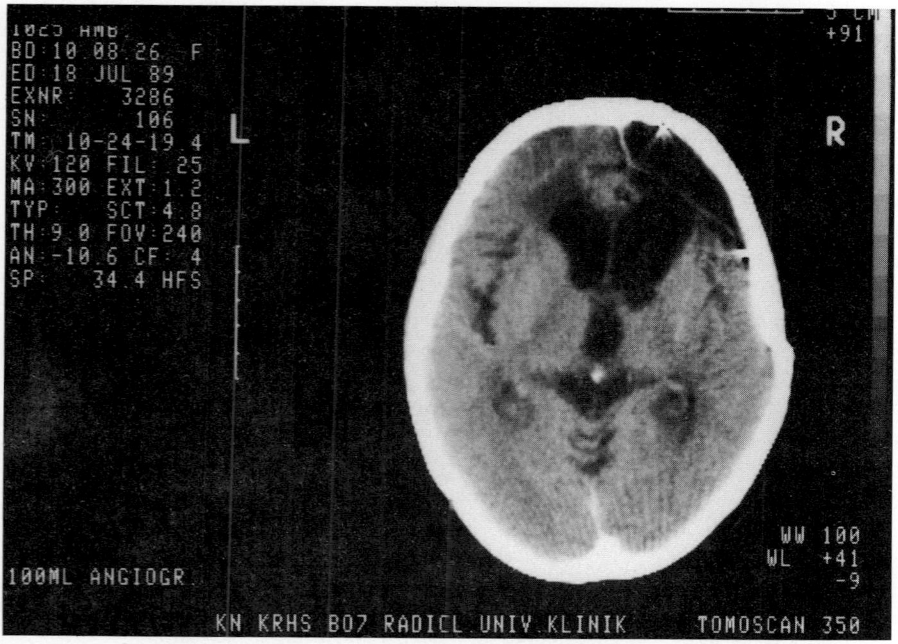

Fig. 1. Long-term survivor No. 5 (CCT in July 1989). To date more than 8 years after operation of a right frontal glioblastoma, the patient is free of tumor recurrence, complaints, and neurological failures

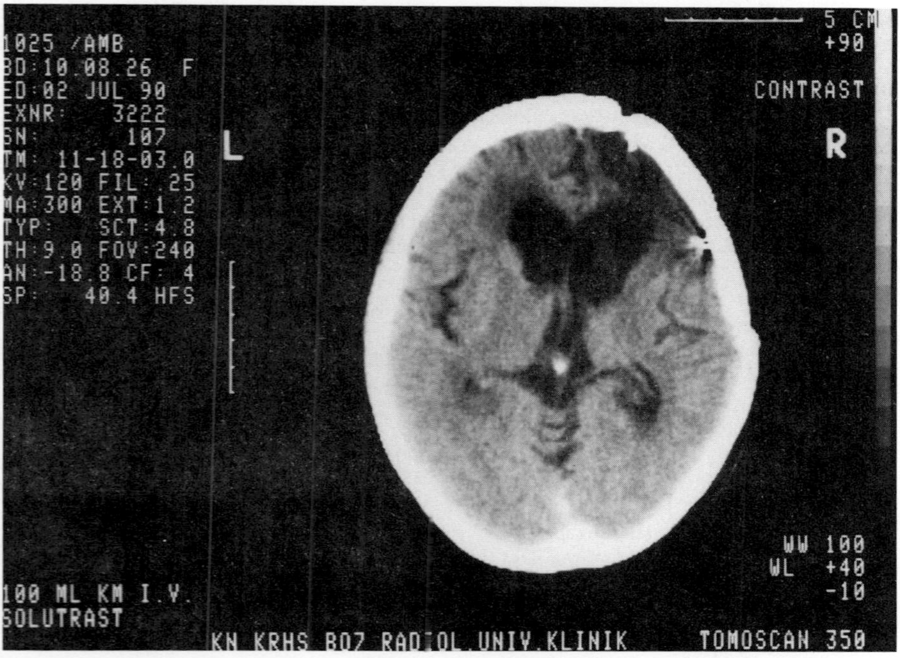

Fig. 2. Long-term survivor No. 5 (CCT in July 1990). One year later (see Fig. 1) the resection cavity is unchanged without sign of tumor recurrence

Summary and Conclusions

To date, in the treatment of malignant gliomas of the brain, neither chemotherapy nor other new therapeutic strategies – for example, treatment with hyperthermia or immunotherapy – have presented a real alternative to the traditionally common treatment of radical resection [1, 3, 8, 10, 11, 18, 19, 24, 26, 28–30]. A combination of extended tumor resection and postoperative irradiation has existed for 50 years unchanged [9, 22, 23, 25].

Our own results show that poor prognosis of malignant gliomas cannot be assumed in every individual case. The long-term survivors of our own patient group rather show the possibility of longer than average postoperative survival times (more than 8 years) and that in rare cases of malignant gliomas and glioblastomas real recurrence-free cures may occur.

References

1. Alexander JT, Saris SC, Oldfield EH (1989) The effect of interleukin-2 on the blood-brain barrier in the 9L gliosarcoma rat model. J Neurosurg 70:92–96
2. Bailey P, Cushing H (1926) Tumors of the glioma group. Lippincott, Philadelphia, pp 421–449
3. Barba D, Saris SC, Holder C, Rosenberg SA, Oldfield EH (1989) Intratumoral LAK cell and interleukin-2 therapy of human gliomas. J Neurosurg 70:175–182
4. Bauer B, Adrian G (1983) Kombinationsbehandlung maligner Hirntumoren. Ergebnisse erster Erfahrungen. Psychiatr Neurol Med Psychol (Leipzig) 35:566–573
5. Bennett AH, Godlee RJ (1884) Case of cerebral tumour. Lancet II:1090
6. Bucy PC (1985) Historical article: Glioblastomas: by K.G. McKenzie. Surg Neurol 24:589–590
7. Fischer J, Kostron H (1983) Glioblastoma multiforme. Postoperative Therapie. ZFA (Stuttgart) 59:232–233
8. Fischer DK, Chen TL, Narayan RK (1988) Immunological and biochemical strategies for the identification of brain tumor-associated antigens. J Neurosurg 68:165–180
9. Frankel SA, German WJ (1958) Glioblastoma multiforme: Review of 219 cases with regard to natural history, pathology, diagnostic methods, treatment. J Neurosurg 15:489–503
10. Greenberg HS, Chandler WF, Diaz RF, Ensminger WD, Junck L, Page MA, Gebarski SS, McKeever P, Hood TW, Stetson PL, Litchter AS, Tankanow R (1988) Intra-arterial bromodeoxyuridine radiosensitization and radiation in treatment of malignant astrocytomas. J Neurosurg 69:500–505
11. Heppner F (1986) The glioblastoma multiforme: a lifelong challenge to the neurosurgeon. Neurochirurgia (Stuttg) 29:9–14
12. Hochberg FH, Pruitt AA (1980) Assumptions in the radiotherapy of glioblastoma. Neurology 30:907–911
13. Jellinger K, Volc D, Prodreka I, Grisold W, Flament H, Vollmer R, Weiß R (1981) Ergebnisse der Kombinationsbehandlung maligner Gliome. Nervenarzt 52:41–50
14. Kelly KA, Kirkwood JM, Kapp DS (1984) Glioblastoma multiforme: pathology, natural history and treatment. Cancer Treat Rev 11:1–26
15. Kornblith PL, Walker M (1988) Chemotherapy for malignant gliomas. J Neurosurg 68:1–17

16. Kristiansen K, Hagen S, Kollevold T, Torvik A, Holme I, Nesbakken R, Hatlevoll R, Lindgren M, Brun A, Lindgren S, Notter G, Andersen AP, Elgen K (1981) Combined modality therapy of operated astrocytomas grade 3 and 4. Confirmation of the value of postoperative irradiation and lack of potentation of Bleomycin on survival time: a prospective multicenter trial of the Scandinavian Glioblastoma Study Group. Cancer 47:649–652
17. Leibel SA, Sheline GE (1987) Radiation therapy for neoplasms of the brain. J Neurosurg 66:1–22
18. Mahaley MS, Bertsch L, Cush S, Gillespie GY (1988) Systemic gamma-interferon therapy for recurrent gliomas. J Neurosurg 69:826–829
19. Mahaley MS, Hipp SW, Dropcho EJ, Bertsch L, Cush S, Tirey T, Gillespie GY (1989) Intracarotid cisplatin chemotherapy for recurrent gliomas. J Neurosurg 70:371–378
20. McKenzie KG (1936) Glioblastoma: A point of view concerning treatment. Arch Neurol Psychiatry 36:542–546
21. Müller H, Brock M, Ernst H (1985) Long-term survival and recurrence-free interval in combined surgical, radio- and chemotherapy of malignant brain gliomas. Clin Neurol Neurosurg 87:167–171
22. Neumann J (1983) Zur Prognose des Glioblastoma multiforme heute. Nervenarzt 54:191–193
23. Roth J, Elvidge A (1960) Glioblastoma multiforme: A clinical survey. J Neurosurg 17:736–750
24. Salcman M, Samaras GM (1983) Interstitial microwave hyperthermia for brain tumors. Results of a phase-1 clinical trial. J Neurooncol 1:225–236
25. Tönnis W, Walter W (1959) Das Glioblastoma multiforme. Bericht über 2611 Fälle. Acta Neurochirurgia (Wien) [Suppl] 1:40–62
26. Vaquero J, Martinez R, Barbolla L, de Haro J, de Oya S, Coca S, Ramiro J (1987) Intrathecal injection of autologous leucocytes in glioblastoma: Circulatory dynamics within the subarachnoid space and clinical results. Acta Neurochir (Wien) 89:37–42
27. Victor S (1990) Topik und Verlaufsformen maligner hirneigener Tumoren unter vergleichender Analyse der Tumorhistologie und des computertomographischen Befundes. Dissertation, Universitätsklinik Bochum
28. Walker MD, Alexander E, Hunt WE, McCarty CS, Mahaley MS, Mealey J, Norrell HA, Owens G, Ransohoff J, Wilson CB, Gehan EA, Strike TA (1987) Evaluation of BCNU and/or radiotherapy in the treatment of anaplastic gliomas. A cooperative clinical trial. J Neurosurg 49:333–343
29. Walker MD, Green SB, Byar DP, Alexander E Jr, Bathdorf U, Brooks WH, Hunt WE, Maccarty CS, Mahaley MS Jr, Mealey J, Owens G, Ransohoff J, Robertson JT, Shapiro WR, Smith KR Jr, Wilson CB, Strike TA (1980) Randomized comparisons of radiotherapy and nitrosoureas for the treatment of malignant glioma after surgery. N Engl J Med 303:1323–1329
30. Wen HL, Dahele JS (1984) Invasive microwave hyperthermia for treatment of glioma. Chin Med J [Engl] 97:813–818

Microsurgery of Malignant Gliomas of the Temporal Lobes: Cognitive Deficits Depend on the Extent of Lost Tissue

M. Peper[1], B. Wowra[2], E. Irle[3], and S. Kunze[2]

Introduction

The neuropsychological evaluation of neurosurgical treatment methods has a long tradition. The treatment for genuine epilepsy, or infantile hemiplegia, for example, has shown that even complete removals of one temporal lobe or one hemisphere may be followed by surprisingly little psychological deficit, provided that the contralateral hemisphere has an entirely normal function [6, 9]. However, in most of these cases, the brain had a lifelong opportunity to adapt to the disease, a fact completely missing in patients with malignant gliomas. Today, the neurosurgical treatment of malignant tumors is performed less radically than earlier: The availability and continuous improvement of radiation therapy and chemotherapy enables the neurosurgeon to extirpate gliomas within the solid tumor margins. However, radiotherapy may cause dementia in long-term survivors with glioblastoma [5]. Therefore, it still seems justified to decide about the extent of the neurosurgical approach on the basis of the assumed psychological importance of the region under treatment and the costs and benefits of its radical extirpation.

The continuous improvement of neuropsychological diagnostic techniques, especially computer-assisted techniques, makes it difficult to judge certain brain regions any longer as "silent." Besides the most salient deficits of motor performance and language, the detection of even subtle deficits of attention, cognition, memory, and perception is now within the scope of routine neuropsychological diagnostic processes. The same is increasingly true for affective and personality changes, which previously have been often misjudged as a reaction to instead of as a product of brain injury (for an overview of these topics, see [1]). The functions of the right hemisphere have been especially elucidated, leading to the opinion that the right hemisphere is heavily involved in attentional, perceptional, visuospatial cognitive, and affective behavior [8, 11]. Although more subtle deficits of these behavioral domains are likely to escape clinical routine examination, no one would doubt the importance of such deficits for the reorganization of the patient's daily life.

The goal of the present study was to investigate in a subsample of tumor patients from the neurosurgical department of the University of Heidelberg, having

[1] Psychologisches Institut der Universität, Niemensstr. 10, W–7800 Freiburg, FRG.
[2] Neurochirurgische Universitätsklinik, Im Neuenheimer Feld 400, W–6900 Heidelberg, FRG.
[3] Psychiatrische Universitätsklinik, Von-Siebold-Str. 5, W–3400 Göttingen, FRG.

Advances in Neurosurgery, Vol. 20
K. Piscol, M. Klinger, M. Brock (Eds.)

Table 1. Summary of the personal and medical data of all subjects

	LTG	RTG
Glioma grading		
Grade I/II (N)	4	9
Grade III/IV (N)	17	28
Total number of subjects	21	37
Age (years)[a]	49 (10)	50 (9)
Sex (male/female)	10/11	19/18
Lesion volumes		
Preoperative tumor volume[a, b]	43 (26)	67 (46)
Preoperative hypodensity volume[a, b, c]	31 (26)	38 (37)
Preoperative total lesion volume[a, b]	74 (41)	105 (51)
Postoperative total lesion volume[a, b]	59 (32)	72 (32)

LTG, group with left temporal tumors; RTG, group with right temporal tumors
[a] Means (and standard deviations) are given.
[b] The volume is expressed in cm^3.
[c] Zone of tumor infiltration and edema.

undergone neuropsychological follow-up examination, the relationship between the extent of tissue loss and postoperative behavior. Our results show that lesions of the right temporal lobe are associated to different, but similarly strong behavioral impairments as lesions of the left temporal lobe, and that the deficits following both left- or right-sided lesions increase with lesion size.

Methods

Subjects

Fifty-eight subjects were drawn from a population of 263 patients with cortical brain tumors, having undergone microsurgical treatment and follow-up evaluation between 1986 and 1991 at the neurosurgical department of the University of Heidelberg. All subjects had gliomas of the left ($n=21$) or right ($n=37$) temporal lobe. The personal and medical data of all subjects are summarized in Table 1.

Lesion Assessment

All tumors were diagnosed histologically. Tumor-related lesion volumes were estimated with the pre- and postoperative CT scans according to the standard procedure followed in this department [13]. The localization of the tumors was done using preoperative NMR scans. Only tumors covering temporal lobe structures completely or predominantly were considered in this report.

Neuropsychological Tests

The testing took place 1 week preoperatively, 1–2 weeks postoperatively, and was further repeated 5–9 months postoperatively (the data of 15 subjects are presently available for this assessment). For all three assessments, parallel forms of the respective tests were used. General intellectual abilities were tested with a shortened version of the Wechsler Adult Intelligence Scale (WAIS). Concentration and psychomotor speed were tested with the Stroop test and the trail making test. Possible receptive language disturbances were examined with the Token test. Special emphasis was laid on the assessment of memory functions. Verbal long-term memory was examined with a paired associate learning paradigm. Visual memory functions were assessed with the Benton Visual Retention test and a perceptual learning paradigm (Gollin's test). Short-term memory was assessed with the subtests "digit span" and "visual memory span" of the Wechsler Memory Scale (WMS-R). For a detailed description of all tests, see [7].

Results

Anatomical Findings

The tumor-related lesion volumes are described in Table 1. The glioma grading was significantly correlated with the pre- and postoperative total lesion volumes as well as the preoperative edema (hypodensity) volume (Spearman rank correlations; $P < 0.05$). Right-sided tumors were preoperatively significantly larger than left-sided tumors (Mann-Whitney U test; $P < 0.05$). The total lesion volumes of high-grade gliomas (grade III–IV) were significantly reduced from pre- to directly postoperatively as well as from directly postoperatively to long (5–9 months) postoperatively (Wilcoxon tests; $P < 0.05$), leading to a substantial release from intracranial pressure in these patients.

Neuropsychological Findings

Both left- and right-sided lesioned subjects were strongly impaired in their overall behavioral performance pre- and directly postoperatively (cf. Table 2). Behavioral deficits occurred not only in those tasks sensitive to damage of the lesioned hemisphere, but also in tasks sensitive to damage of the nonlesioned hemisphere. However, right-sided lesioned subjects showed stronger deficits in the tasks of visual attention and memory, and visuomotor construction, and left-sided lesioned subjects showed stronger deficits in the tasks of verbal memory and attention and verbal abstraction. Significant differences between left- and right-sided lesioned subjects emerged in the paired associate learning, Stroop test, Benton test, trail making test, and performance IQ ($P < 0.05$). At the time of the third examination (5–9 months postoperatively), subjects with low-grade gliomas showed significantly

Table 2. Psychological performances of all subjects

	LTG						RTG					
	G I/II			G III/IV			G I/II			G III/IV		
	T1	T2	T3	T1	T2	T3	T1	T2	T3	T1	T2	T3
Verbal IQ	10	–	70	10	–	10	12	–	24	30	–	5
Performance IQ	33	63	73	17	15	17	15	15	4	16	13	16
Paired associate learning	0	0	0	0	0	0	10	2	36	10	8	0
Stroop test: color naming	17	3	0	2	0	0	5	0	20	10	10	0
Benton test	23	35	81	2	1	0	2	4	3	2	1	3

The values represent percentiles derived from 41 normal control subjects matched for age and education to the tumor subjects. The value 10, for example, means that the average performance of the tumor subjects is similar to the performance of the lower 10% of the control subjects. LTG, group with left temporal tumors; RTG, group with right temporal tumors; G I/II, glioma grade I or II; G III/IV, glioma grade III or IV; T1, preoperative examination; T2, postoperative (1–2 weeks) examination; T3, postoperative (5–9 months) examination.

improved behavioral performances in the tasks sensitive to damage of the nonlesioned hemisphere, whereas subjects with high-grade gliomas deteriorated in most tasks under measurement ($P < 0.05$). However, the behavioral recovery of subjects with low-grade gliomas at this time was far from complete (cf. Table 2). Correlation and regression analyses showed that pre- and directly postoperatively for both hemispheres significant relationships between lesion extent and behavioral deficits existed. These relationships occurred for those tasks sensitive to damage of the respective hemisphere and were equally strong for either right-sided or left-sided lesions (cf. Figs. 1 and 2).

Discussion

Our results show that for both right- and left-sided tumors of the temporal lobe, the postoperative total lesion volume is correlated with the amount of behavioral deficits. Thus, it may be suggested that only little or no tissue around the solid tumor can be resected without provoking severe behavioral impairments in the patient.

Still, a decision about the therapy of an individual patient is difficult to obtain. First, it must be kept in mind that the extent of tumor removal has been shown to be of prognostic significance [10]. Extensive radiotherapy may also cause a dismal therapeutic outcome [5], probably surpassing the negative effects produced

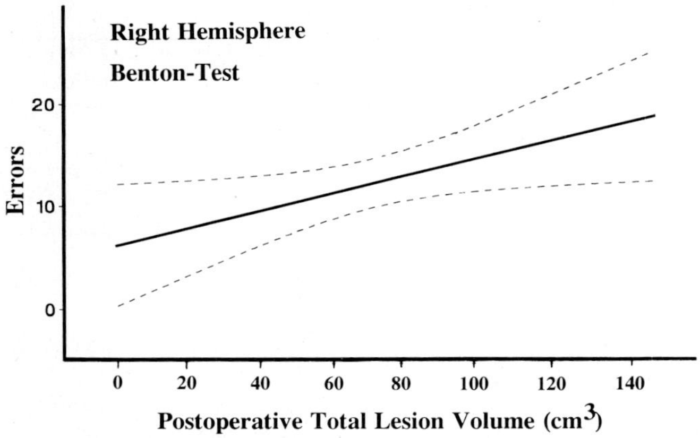

Fig. 1. Results of the Benton test in subjects with right-sided lesions. A linear regression with 95% confidence intervals is shown with the postoperative total lesion volume as independent and the errors performed as dependent variable ($r_s = 0.46$; $r^2 = 0.21$; $b = 0.08$; $P < 0.03$)

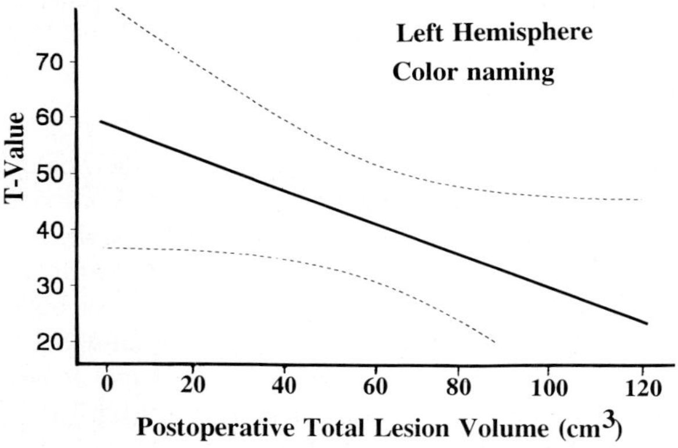

Fig. 2. Results of the Stroop subtest "color naming" in subjects with left-sided lesions. A linear regression with 95% confidence intervals is shown with the postoperative total lesion volume as independent and the age-corrected T values as dependent variable (a high T value means good performance) ($r_s = -0.56$; $r^2 = 0.32$; $b = -0.3$; $P < 0.06$)

by radical tumor extirpation. Second, the individual psychological characteristics of a patient must be considered [6]. Whereas most of our subjects with high-grade gliomas, as well as those reported by others [2–4], had a very poor behavioral outcome, there are few cases in our sample with a favorable outcome despite enormous residual lesions. The behavioral recovery of these patients seemed to depend on strong motivation and social support. Cognitive rehabilitation procedures may also substantially improve behavioral recovery, as was shown for a patient who underwent a radical right temporal lobe resection to remove a grade II–III astrocytoma

[12]. However, even in the case of an intelligent and motivated patient, a radical resection should be carefully thought over, as our data indicate that the behavioral losses of intelligent patients are, compared with their premorbid intellectual functioning, in general stronger than those of average ones.

Conclusions

Malignant gliomas of the left and right temporal lobe lead to markea cognitive deficits, which increase with lesion size. Therefore, tumors of *both* temporal lobes should be generally resected anatomically exactly, i.e., within the solid tumor limits.

However, other therapeutic, as well as psychological factors may lead to behavioral deterioration of a patient as well. The therapeutic strategy, thus resembling the passage of Scylla and Charybdis, should therefore be entirely adjusted to the individual patient.

References

1. Boller F, Grafman J (eds) Handbook of neuropsychology, vols 1–4. Elsevier, Amsterdam
2. Cavazzuti V, Winston K, Baker R, Welch K (1980) Psychological changes following surgery for tumors in the temporal lobe. J Neurosurg 53:618–626
3. Hochberg FH, Slotnick B (1980) Neuropsychological impairment in astrocytoma survivors. Neurology 30:172–177
4. Hom J, Reitan RM (1984) Neuropsychological correlates of rapidly vs slowly growing intrinsic cerebral neoplasms. J Clin Neuropsychol 6:309–324
5. Imperato JP, Paleologos NA, Vick NA (1990) Effects of treatment on long-term survivors with malignant astrocytomas. Ann Neurol 28:818–822
6. Irle E (1987) Lesion size and recovery of function: some new perspectives. Brain Res Rev 12:307–320
7. Lezak M (1983) Neuropsychological assessment, 2nd edn. Oxford University Press, New York
8. Mesulam MM (ed) (1985) Principles of behavioral neurology. Davis, Philadelphia
9. Milner B (1975) Psychological aspects of focal epilepsy and its neurosurgical management. In: Purpura DP, Penry DK, Walter RD (eds) Advances in neurology, vol 8. Raven Press, New York, pp 299–321
10. Murovic J, Turowski K, Wilson CB et al. (1986) Computerized tomography in the prognosis of malignant cerebral gliomas. J Neurosurg 65:799–806
11. Peper M, Irle E, Wowra B (1990) Perzeptuelle und konzeptuelle Verarbeitung affektiver Information bei Patienten mit cerebralen Tumoren. In: Frey D (Hrsg) Bericht über den 37. Kongreß der Deutschen Gesellschaft für Psychologie. Hogrefe, Göttingen, S 445
12. Rao SM, Bieliauskas LA (1983) Cognitive rehabilitation two and one-half years post right temporal lobectomy. J Clin Neuropsychol 5:313–320
13. Wowra B, Irle E, Peper M et al. (1989) Evaluation of lesion volumes in neuro-oncology: Basic data for carrier-mediated chemotherapy. Reg Cancer Treat 2:178–183

Multiple Primary and Multiple Recurrent Gliomas

G. Hildebrandt[1], I. Reuter[1], J. C. Tonn[2], and K. Roosen[1]

Introduction

The phenomenon of multiple cerebral gliomas has been the subject of many reviews for nearly 100 years [4]. However, their nomenclature, incidence, and implications for therapy are still a matter of debate [1, 5, 14]. The objectives of this retrospective clinical study were to outline conditions and patterns of multiple cerebral glioma growth in treated and untreated patients, to evaluate whether diagnostic or therapeutic strategies eventually have to be modified in patients presenting with these nonfocal tumors, and to propose a simplified nomenclature for the clinician in such cases.

Patients and Methods

The study covered the period from January 1985 to June 1990. During that time, 311 patients with an initial diagnosis of supratentorial glioma underwent partial or radical tumor removal. A subgroup received adjuvant therapy including whole-brain radiation of 40 Gy with focal tumor boost of 20 Gy alone or in combination with chemotherapy (intra-arterial ACNU or intravenous BCNU). High-resolution contrast-enhanced CT or T1/T2-weighted MRI studies were performed before treatment and periodically during the follow-up. Histological classification was based upon conventional neuropathological procedures. CT studies in the early postoperative period and the intraoperative reports served to outline the extent of tumor removal.

To classify the different tumor growth patterns, the following terms for nonfocal disease in untreated patients were used: multiple primary gliomas, gliomatosis cerebri, single widespread glioma, and primary leptomeningeal gliomatosis [3, 7, 8, 10]. In treated patients, recurrent or progressing disease was termed local or hemispheric spread (which denotes extension by centrifugal growth along white matter tracts compromising at least two neighboring lobes) and multiple (affecting both hemispheres with or without local meningeal/ependymal spread or metastasis by the CSF). Patients with underlying disease, such as neurofibromatosis, were excluded from the study.

---

1 Neurochirurgische Universitätsklinik, Joseph-Stelzmann-Str. 9, W–5000 Köln 41, FRG.
2 Neurochirurgische Klinik, Justus-Liebig-Universität Gießen, Klinikstr. 29, W–6300 Gießen, FRG.

Advances in Neurosurgery, Vol. 20
K. Piscol, M. Klinger, M. Brock (Eds.)

Table 1. Recurrent gliomas ($n = 65$ patients)

	Local	Hemispheric	Multiple
Frequency	46/65	8/65	11/65
Age (mean ± SEM)	49 ± 2	48 ± 2	51 ± 4
Females/males	20/26	3/ 5	2/ 9
Radical surgery	35/46	5/ 8	7/11
Radiation	22/46	2/ 8	6/11
Chemotherapy	21/46	0/ 8	0/11
2nd operation	23/46	6/ 8	6/11
Recurrence-free interval (weeks)	53 ± 9	22 ± 6	42 ± 17
Time interval 1st operation recurrence			
Weeks	54 ± 9	24 ± 6	61 ± 25
Min–max	1–276	12–64	12–296
Infiltration of corpus callosum	6/45	1/ 8	4/11
Necrosis	31	4	8
Classification of original tumor			
Astrocytoma	16		4
Oligodendroglioma	12	2	3
Glioblastoma	18	2	4
WHO grade			
II	7	1	3
II–III	4	2	0
III	9	3	4
III–IV	7	1	1
IV	19	1	3

Results

According to neurodiagnostic studies, one 38-year-old male patient out of 311 was found to have multiple primary gliomas (distinct bilateral foci of oligodendroglioma WHO grade II–III). Sixty-five patients (65 CT and 38 MRI examinations) were identified who had progressing or recurring tumor growth: local (group A, $n = 46$), hemispheric spread (group B, $n = 8$), and multiple foci (group C, $n = 11$). No potential prognostic indicator to predict the pattern of recurrence could be found (Table 1) because age, Karnofsky index (data not shown), the extent of initial tumor removal, amount of consecutive therapy, the frequency of different histological findings, and grading, and the original tumor localization (data not shown) were comparable in all subgroups. Only in group C was a preponderance of males and an increased rate of necrosis found during neuropathological examination of the original tumor material. In the same group, an insignificant tendency for an increased time interval between the initial operative procedure and recurrence of disease was observed (Table 1). Table 2 outlines the different morphological data according to CT/MRI findings in group C. It shows the predominance of the subarachnoid and parenchymal (mostly at the subcortical level) tumor dissemination, which did not imply

Table 2. CT/MRI pattern of multiple recurrent glioma growth ($n = 11$ patients)

		Mode of spread		
Patient	WHO grade	Intraventricular/ subependymal	Subarachnoid	Subcortical/ parenchymal
L., H.	II	–	–	+
E., H.	II	+	–	+
Z., H.	II	–	+	+
A., K.	III	–	+	–
H., J.	III	–	+	+
R., R.	III	–	–	+
U., H.	III	–	+	–
R., O.	III–IV	–	+	–
B., G.	IV	–	+	+
J., M.	IV	+	+	+
M., K.H.	IV	+	–	+

infiltration of the corpus callosum per se in the majority of cases (Table 1, Fig. 1). Only a minority of the reoperated patients showed further tumor dedifferentiation (group A, 7/23; B, 2/6; C, 2/6), whereas multiple recurrences of originally low malignant gliomas were related with the development of anaplastic features.

Discussion

In spite of several shortcomings of this retrospective study, such as patient loss for follow-up and the possible underestimation of microscopically connected multiple tumor foci by neurodiagnostic examinations [9], several conclusions may be drawn from our observations. Multiple recurrent gliomas are more frequent, at least ten-fold, than multiple primary gliomas and may thus differ in their origin. The former do not seem to be the consequence of metachronous lesions related to an increased survival time (development of distinct tumor foci separated by time [15]). They are rather the result of CSF dissemination with or without parenchymal reinvasion [12] possibly induced by the operative procedure.

Two autopsy series disclosed a 77% incidence of ventricular and subarachnoid seeding of neuroectodermal tumors [11] and a 21% rate of meningeal gliomatosis in patients with malignant gliomas [16] after surgical and adjuvant therapy, whereas Bernard et al. [1] found only a 6% incidence of primary multiple gliomas in postmortem celloidin-embedded whole brain sections of patients without treatment. For such cases malignant transformation is assumed, which affects a single clone of cells very early in embryogenesis, with the affected progeny subsequently migrating

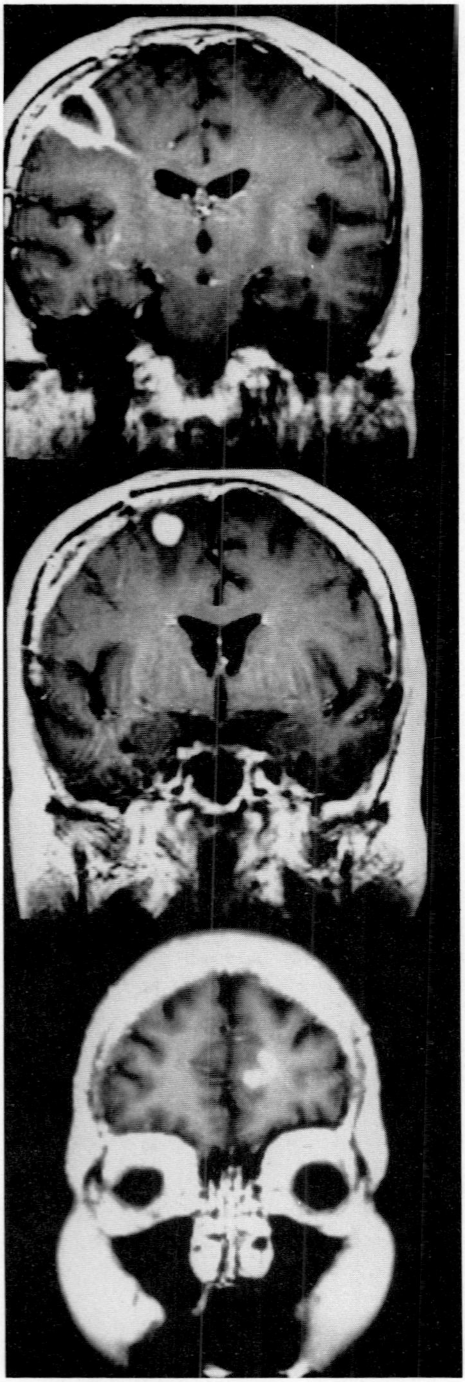

Fig. 1. Illustrative case report. The figure outlines the contrast-enhanced MRI findings of a 60-year-old female patient who underwent radical surgery for an oligodendroglioma WHO grade III in the right frontal lobe 12 weeks before. She received conventional radiotherapy of 60 Gy. The *upper panel* shows local tumor recurrence with centrifugal spread along white matter tracts directed toward the corpus callosum. The *lower panel* represents another ipsilateral focus at the subcortical level and possibly subarachnoid/subdural extension over both convexities. The *third MRI image* discloses additional tumor satellite formation within the frontal lobe of the contralateral hemisphere (T1-weighted spin-echo sequences, coronal view, obtained after gadolinium injection)

into the entire central nervous system [8, 13] or an active locomotion and spread of subclones via white matter tracts arising from a glioma at one site [14].

Because issues such as false negative results of CSF cytology, risk of tumor cell shedding by operative contamination, and tumor cell viability within the CSF compartment are still a matter of debate [2, 6], we propose to reevaluate the patterns of recurrent tumor growth, the incidence of CSF tumor cell dispersion, the value of repeated spinal MRI studies during follow-up, and the possible role of intrathecal chemotherapy in glioma studies of the future.

References

1. Barnard RO, Geddes JF (1987) The incidence of multifocal cerebral gliomas. Cancer 60:1519–1531
2. Batzdorf U, Gold V (1974) Dispersion of central nervous system tumors. J Neurosurg 41:691–698
3. Budka H, Podreka I, Reisner TH, Zeller K (1980) Diagnostic and pathomorphological aspects of glioma multiplicity. Neurosurg Rev 3:233–241
4. Choucair AK, Levin VA, Gutin PH, Davis RL, Silver P, Edwards HSP, Wilson CB (1986) Development of multiple lesions during radiation therapy and chemotherapy in patients with gliomas. J Neurosurg 65:645–658
5. Hildebrandt G, Tonn JC, Rap ZM, Reiner J, Schachenmayr W, Zierski J, Agnoli L (1988) Multifokale, multilokuläre, multiple oder multizentrische Gliome? Nervenarzt 59:539–544
6. Johnson DL, Schwarz S (1987) Intracranial metastases from malignant spinal-cord astrocytoma. J Neurosurg 66:612–652
7. Kitahara M, Katakura R, Wada T, Namiki T, Suzuki J (1985) Diffuse form of primary leptomeningeal gliomatosis. J Neurosurg 63:283–287
8. Louis DN (1990) Case records of the Massachusetts General Hospital. Case 26-1990. N Engl J Med 322:1866–1878
9. Nasher HC, Gerhard L, Reinhardt V, Nau HE, Bamberg H (1981) Diffuse and multicentric brain tumors – correlation of histological, clinical and CT appearance. Acta Neuropathol (Suppl) 7:101–104
10. Nevin S (1938) Gliomatosis cerebri. Brain 61:170–191
11. Nishio S, Korosue K, Tateishi J, Fukui M, Kitamura K (1982) Ventricular and subarachnoid seeding of intracranial tumors of neuroectodermal origin – a study of 26 consecutive autopsy cases with reference to focal ependymal defect. Clin Neuropathol 1:81–91
12. Onda K, Tanaka R, Takahasi H, Takeda N, Ikutu F (1990) Symptomatic cerebrospinal fluid dissemination of cerebral glioblastoma. Neuroradiology 31:146–150
13. Russel DS, Rubinstein LJ (1990) Pathology of the nervous system, 5th edn. Williams & Wilkins, Baltimore, pp 412–448
14. Scherer HJ (1940) The forms of growth in gliomas and their practical significance. Brain 63:1–35
15. Van Tassel P, Lee Y-Y, Brunner JM (1988) Synchronous and metachronous malignant gliomas. AJNR 9:725–732
16. Yung WA, Horten BC, Shapiro R (1980) Meningeal gliomatosis: a review of 12 cases. Ann Neurol 8:605–608

Relationship Between the Recurrence of Intracranial Ependymomas and the Grade of Malignancy

R.-I. Ernestus[1], R. Schröder[2], and N. Klug[1]

Introduction

The histogenetic classification of ependymomas among primary brain neoplasms was controversially discussed for a long time [4, 5, 8, 18–20, 22, 24, 26, 27]. Their origin from ependymal cells, which arise directly from the neural tube [4, 6, 13, 25], however, justifies their classification as gliomas in the group of neuroepithelial tumors [27, 28]. As previously reported, prognosis of ependymomas predominantly depends on their grade of malignancy based on histomorphological features of anaplasia [10–12]. In the present series we have studied whether recurrent tumor growth – as known from other gliomas – is determined by the grade of malignancy.

Material and Methods

Between 1951 and 1990, a total of 127 patients with intracranial ependymomas – subependymomas excluded – underwent operation at the Department of Neurosurgery, University of Cologne, FRG. Distribution of tumor localization and age is given in Table 1. Follow-up was reviewed in 83 patients who survived surgery of the primary tumor for more than 30 days. Median follow-up was 44 months (range 1 month to 34.4 years). Survival rates were calculated by the method of Kaplan and Meier [17].

In all cases histological grading was reevaluated following the proposal of the World Health Organization (WHO) in 1976 [27, 28]: 88 ependymomas were classified as grade II and 39 as grade III. In comparison to other slowly proliferating tumors such as pilocytic astrocytoma or subependymoma, we could not assign any ependymoma to grade I. The highest grade of malignancy – grade IV – is equivalent to glioblastoma multiforme histologically as well as clinically.

[1] Neurochirurgische Universitätsklinik, Joseph-Stelzmann-Str. 9, W–5000 Köln 41, FRG.
[2] Institut für Pathologie, Laboratorium für Neuropathologie, Universität Köln, Joseph-Stelzmann-Str. 9, W–5000 Köln 41, FRG.

Advances in Neurosurgery, Vol. 20
K. Piscol, M. Klinger, M. Brock (Eds.)

Table 1. Intracranial ependymomas 1951–1990 ($n = 127$): localization, age, and histological grading (WHO 1976 [27, 28])

	Supratentorial		Infratentorial		Total
	< 10 years	≥ 10 years	< 10 years	≥ 10 years	
Grade II	11	31	19	27	88
Grade III	18	11	6	4	39

Table 2. Rate of local recurrences in intracranial ependymomas

	Supratentorial		Infratentorial		Total
	< 10 years	≥ 10 years	< 10 years	≥ 10 years	
Grade II	62.5% (5/8)	31.8% (7/22)	55.6% (5/9)	33.3% (5/15)	40.7% (22/54)
Grade III	56.3% (9/16)	44.4% (4/9)	50.0% (1/2)	50.0% (1/2)	51.7% (15/29)

Numbers in parentheses indicate number of local recurrences ($n = 37$) vs number of all patients with intracranial ependymomas who survived operation of the primary tumor for more than 30 days ($n = 83$).

Table 3. Interval between therapy of the primary tumor and diagnosis of recurrence

Interval (years)	Grade II			Grade III		
	OP	OP + RT	%	OP	OP + RT	%
< 1	• • •	•	46		• • • • •	87
1– 2	• • •	• • •		• • •	• • • • • •	
2– 3	•			•		
3– 4	• •		18			13
4– 5	•				•	
5–10	• •	• • •				
10–15		•	36			0
15–20		• •				
Median (range)	34 months (4–236 months)			16 months (4–53 months)		

OP, operation; RT, radiation therapy.

Results

Local recurrences occurred in 37 of 83 patients who had survived primary surgery for more than 30 days. Thus, the total rate of recurrence was 45%. It was independent of tumor localization, but it tended to increase with rising malignancy (Table 2). In children the rate of relapse was highest (59%), almost independent of the histological grading.

The median interval between the initial operation and the diagnosis of recurrence was 34 months (range 4–236 months) for grade II, but only 16 months (range 4–53 months) for grade III ependymomas (Table 3). Of 15 grade III recurrences (87%), 13 became apparent within 2 years after primary surgery. In these malignant tumors, additional postoperative radiation therapy could not prevent early relapse. Late recurrences were observed exclusively in the group of low-grade ependymomas. Six out of those eight patients who developed recurrences more than 5 years following initial therapy had received irradiation after the primary operation. Thus, in contrast to malignant ependymomas, radiation therapy delayed new tumor growth in more benign tumors.

Histological examination was possible after repeated surgery in 21 cases and post mortem in one additional case. Eight recurrences were classified as grade II and 14 tumors as grade III. An increase in anaplasia from grade II to grade III was observed in six patients.

Prognosis of recurrences was poor, irrespective of their histological grading (Fig. 1). It could only be improved by repeated surgical intervention. Median survival from the time of diagnosis of recurrence was 14 months with operation (range 0–> 154 months), but only 4 months without operation (range–96 months). The 5-year survival after diagnosis of relapse was 20% (four patients) for surgical and 13% (two patients) for nonsurgical treatment, respectively.

Twelve of 19 patients (63%) who had survived the recurrent operation relapsed again; 10 of these 12 recurrences were observed in the group of grade III ependymomas. With one exception, the third tumor manifested itself within 2 years after operation of the second tumor. The median interval between the first and the second recurrence was only 8 months (range 2–27 months) as compared with 18 months (range 4–236 months) between the primary tumor and the first relapse. With repeated recurrences, in consequence, the time in between markedly decreased.

Discussion

Intracranial ependymomas are prone to develop local recurrences. The rate of relapse in 450 ependymomas reported in the literature is 40% [10, 11]. It ranges from 19% [7] to 80% [9]. Frequency of recurrences is comparable in supratentorial (47%) and in infratentorial ependymomas (42%), but it increases with rising malignancy (low-grade 42%, high-grade 52%) [10].

The interval from therapy of the primary tumor to diagnosis of local recurrence decreases with higher malignancy [1, 7, 15, 23]. Early recurrences are particu-

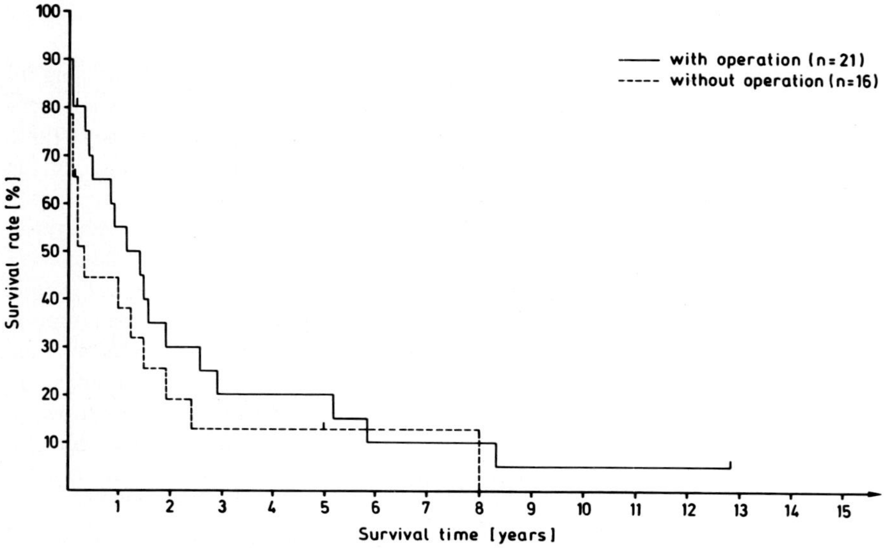

Fig. 1. Survival after diagnosis of recurrence with or without operation (calculation of survival rates according to the method of Kaplan and Meier [17])

larly found in infratentorial ependymomas of childhood [16] and in supratentorial hemispheric tumors of adolescence [26]. Our observation of late recurrences in the group of irradiated grade II ependymomas with manifestation more than 5 years after initial operation suggests that new tumor growth can be delayed but not prevented by additional postoperative radiation therapy [10–12, 21].

Prognosis of recurrent ependymomas is rather poor. Mean survival of 7 months reported by Hahn et al. [14] corresponds to survival in the present series. As known from other tumors of the glioma group, an increase in anaplasia from the primary to the recurrent tumor is not rare [1, 2]. Dedifferentiation can proceed so that the tumor finally reaches the grade of glioblastoma multiforme [3]. Due to often small and not necessarily representative tumor samples, a microscopic increase of malignancy does not reflect the biological growth patterns in all cases. Nevertheless, the growth rate of ependymomas seems to accelerate with rising number of relapses.

In conclusion, the clinicopathological characteristics of recurrent ependymomas are predominantly determined by the grade of malignancy. They are similar to those of other neuroepithelial tumors and, in consequence, underline the classification of ependymomas as gliomas.

References

1. Afra D, Müller W, Slowik F, Wilcke O, Budka H, Turoczy L (1983) Supratentorial lobar ependymomas: Reports on the grading and survival periods in 80 cases, including 46 recurrences. Acta Neurochir (Wien) 69:243–251
2. Arendt A, Senitz D (1972) Histologische Kriterien zur biologischen Wertigkeit beim Ependymom. Arch Geschwulstforsch 40:44–50
3. Bachmann DS, Ostrow PT (1978) Fatal long-term sequela following radiation "cure" for ependymoma. Ann Neurol 4:319–321
4. Bailey P (1924) A study of tumors arising from ependymal cells. Arch Neurol Psychiatry (Chicago) 11:1–27
5. Bailey P (1927) Further remarks concerning tumors of the glioma group. Bull Johns Hopk Hosp 40:354–389
6. Centeno RS, Lee AA, Winter J, Barba D (1986) Supratentorial ependymomas. Neuroimaging and clinicopathological correlation. J Neurosurg 64:209–215
7. Chin HW, Maruyama Y, Markesbery W, Young AB (1982) Intracranial ependymoma: Results of radiotherapy at the University of Kentucky. Cancer 49:2276–2280
8. Del Rio Hortega P (1932) Estructura y systematisacion de los gliomas y paragliomas. Arch Esp Oncol 2:411–677
9. Enzmann DR, Norman D, Levin VA, Wilson CB, Newton TH (1978) Computed tomography in the follow-up of medulloblastomas and ependymomas. Radioalogy 128:57–63
10. Ernestus R-I (1989) Klinik und Prognose der intrakraniellen Ependymome. Lang, Frankfurt/M Bern New York Paris
11. Ernestus R-I, Wilcke O, Schröder R (1989) Intracranial ependymomas: Prognostic aspects. Neurosurg Rev 12:157–163
12. Ernestus R-I, Wilcke O, Schröder R (1991) Supratentorial ependymomas in childhood: Clinicopathological findings and prognosis. Acta Neurochir (Wien)
13. Goutelle A, Fischer G (1977) Les épendymomes intracrâniens et intrarachidiens. Monographies des Périodiques Masson No 11. 27e Congrès de la Société de Neuro-chirurgie de langue française, Nice 24–25 Mai 1977. Masson, Paris New York Barcelone Milan
14. Hahn FJY, Schapiro RL, Okawara S-H (1975) Supratentorial ependymoma. Neuroradiology 10:5–13
15. Hanakita J, Handa H (1984) Clinical features and CT scan findings of supratentorial ependymomas and ependymoblastomas. No Shinkei Geka 12:253–260
16. Ilgren EB, Stiller CA, Hughes JT, Silberman D, Steckel N, Kaye A (1984) Ependymomas: A clinical and pathologic study. Part II – Survival features. Clin Neuropathol 3:122–127
17. Kaplan EL, Meier P (1958) Nonparametric estimation from incomplete observations. J Am Statist Assoc 53:457–481
18. Kernohan JW, Fletcher-Kernohan EM (1935) Ependymomas: A study of 109 cases. Proc Assoc Res Nerv Ment Dis (Baltimore) 16:182–209
19. Kernohan JW, Mabon RF, Svien HJ, Adson AW (1949) A simplified classification of the gliomas. Proc Staff Meet Mayo Clin 24:71–75
20. Mabon RF, Svien HJ, Kernohan JW, McK Craig W (1949) Ependymomas. Proc Staff Meet Mayo Clin 24:65–71
21. Mørk SJ, Løken AC (1977) Ependymoma: A follow-up study of 101 cases. Cancer 40:907–915
22. Ringertz N (1950) "Grading" of gliomas. Acta Pathol Microbiol Scand 27:51–64
23. Ringertz N, Reymond A (1949) Ependymomas and choroid plexus papillomas. J Neuropathol Exp Neurol 8:355–380
24. Roussy G, Oberling C (1932) Histologic classification of tumors of the central nervous system. Arch Neurol Psychiatry (Chicago) 27:1281–1289
25. Rubinstein LJ (1972) Tumors of the central nervous system. In: Atlas of tumor pathology, 2nd ser, fasc 6. Armed Forces Institute of Pathology, Washington DC

26. Zülch KJ (1950) Fortschritte auf dem Gebiet der Morphologie und Biologie der Hirngeschwülste unter besonderer Berücksichtigung der Klassifikation. Fortschr Neurol Psychiatr 18:513–538
27. Zülch KJ (1981) Historical development of the classification of brain tumours and the new proposal of the World Health Organization (WHO). Neurosurg Rev 4:123–127
28. Zülch KJ (1986) Brain tumors. Their biology and pathology, 3rd completely revised edn. Springer, Berlin Heidelberg New York Tokyo

Prognostic and Biological Significance of Gross Residual Tumor Following Extirpation of High-Grade Gliomas: Clinical Study Based on Early Postoperative MR Imaging

F. K. Albert[1], M. Forsting[2], G. Schackert[1], J. Hamer[1], J. Hampl[1], H. H. Steiner[1], B. Wowra[1], K. Sartor[2], and S. Kunze[1]

Introduction

In malignant gliomas, the patient's fate is determined by the extremely high rate of local recurrence, which occurs within 1 year after operation in nearly all cases [6, 9, 11]. For decades, the view has generally been accepted that regrowth mainly arises from microscopic remnants, inevitably left behind during surgery beyond the macroscopic boundaries of the tumor, in consequence of its invasive and ill-defined spreading [3, 5, 6].

In the overwhelming majority of studies that address the role of surgery in the management of high-grade gliomas, the degree of tumor removal accomplished is solely based on the neurosurgeon's intraoperative perception [5, 13]. Despite representing one of the most fundamental prerequisites for the comparison of different treatment modalities, there is a lack of systematic efforts to evaluate the primary residual gross tumor immediately after surgery by using modern neuroimmaging [1, 5, 13].

Among the few available CT-based studies there is no consistency in the methods of assessing residual tumor or in the timing that avoids the well-known postoperative "benign" enhancement. First, Cairncross and co-workers [4] and Jeffries et al. [8] could demonstrate that prior to the 5th postoperative day, enhancement reflects residual glioma only, thus minimizing interpretative difficulties caused by postsurgical repair artifacts. To our knowledge, comparable studies using magnetic resonance imaging have not been published until now, with the exception of preliminary reports by Sze et al. [12] and by ourselves [7].

In the following, we will report the results of a prospective study, started in March 1989, in which we used contrast-enhanced CT and MRI to monitor 60 patients after extirpation of a high-grade glioma.

The first objective of our study was to determine the role of MR in evaluating residual tumor during the immediate postoperative period. By comparing MRI and CT, we additionally were able to assess the capacities of both methods for clinical use. Second, by performing consecutive MRI examinations and by monitoring the

[1] Neurochirurgische Universitätsklinik, Im Neuenheimer Feld 400, W-6900 Heidelberg, FRG.
[2] Neuroradiologische Universitätsklinik, Im Neuenheimer Feld 400, W-6900 Heidelberg, FRG.

Advances in Neurosurgery, Vol. 20
K. Piscol, M. Klinger, M. Brock (Eds.)

patients' clinical courses, we tried to establish the significance of gross residual tumor which already has been proved to be an important prognostic factor in malignant gliomas [1, 2, 10, 13].

Material and Methods

In March 1989, we started a prospective clinical study, in which we used contrast-enhanced early postoperative neuroimaging (EPNI) to establish gross residual tumor following extirpation of a high-grade glioma. Until now, the study has comprised more than 80 patients. The findings of the first 60 cases will be evaluated in the following. The histological classification was: glioblastoma in 57 cases and anaplastic astrocytoma (III) in 3 cases. Nine tumors were regrowths. Early postoperative MR (EPMR) was performed in all patients; early postoperative CT (EPCT) could be obtained in 35 of them only. In MRI, pre- and postcontrast scans were performed on a 1.0 Tesla Picker Vista unit using 0.1–0.2 mmol/kg gadolinium-DTPA i.v. (T1-weighted images; TR, 600 s; TE, 20 ms). For CT, we also used pre- and postcontrast scans (100 ml Iohexol i.v.). Prior to the imaging, the surgeon had tried to achieve gross total resection of the tumor burden in all suitable cases, as assessed by intra-operative perception, always with the aid of an operating microscope. The EPNI was performed as soon as possible after surgery, usually between day 1 and 4. Follow-up scans were obtained at the end of the 2nd postoperative week, after 4–6 weeks, and then every 1–3 months consecutively, usually until substantial clinical deterioration or death.

Postoperative radiotherapy was performed in all cases according to the usual guidelines, with the exception of seven patients with a recurrent glioblastoma and six patients who refused to be irradiated. Chemotherapy was not given.

Results

As to the first objective of our study, we can summarize the role of early postoperative MR imaging in patients operated on for a malignant glioma, as shown in Table 1. These findings were in accordance with those reported by Cairncross et al.

Table 1. The role of early postoperative MR imaging in patients operated on for a malignant glioma

Gadolinium-enhanced MRI, when performed during day 1 to 3 following extirpation of a preoperatively enhancing glioma, is a valuable method for evaluating the amount of solid residual tumor.
With a variable onset, usually beginning on the 4th to 6th postoperative day, a nonspecific benign enhancement caused by postsurgical artifacts impedes the interpretation of the scans for several weeks.

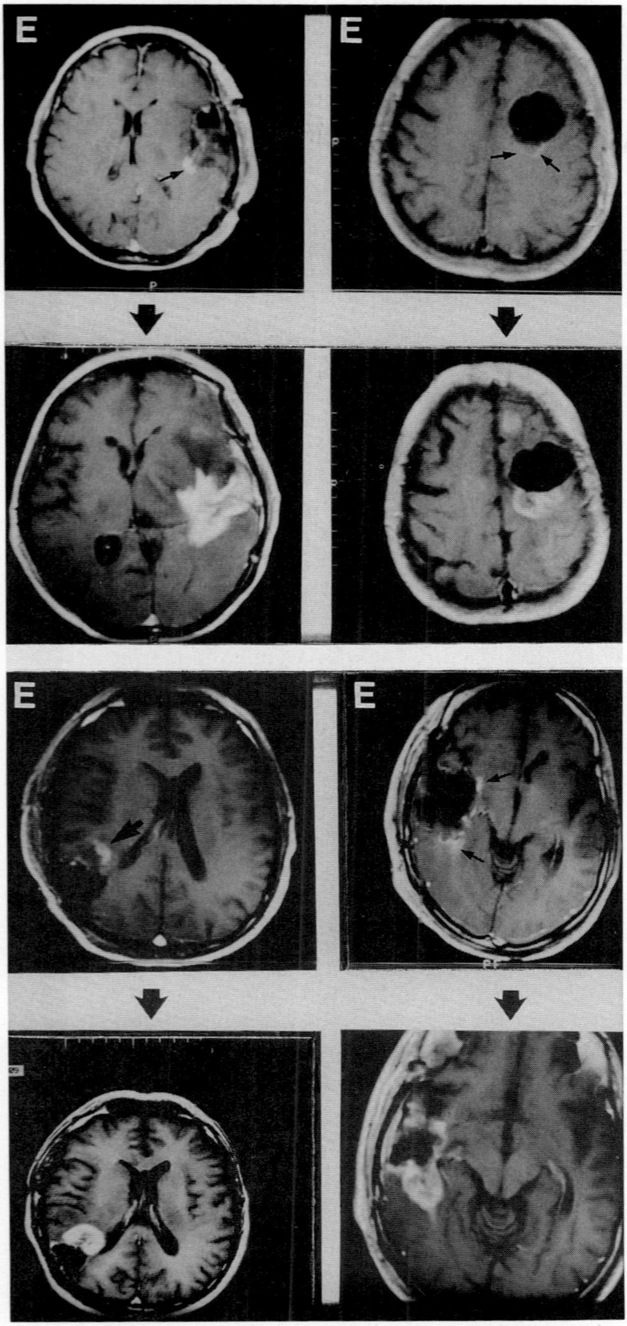

Fig. 1. Four cases illustrating the outgrowth of later tumor progression from the site of enhancement in early postoperative Gd MR. (*E*, early postoperative Gd MR; → enhancement of residual tumor)

[4]. However, by comparing both MRI and CT, we were able to assess that MRI is largely superior to CT regarding sensitivity and specificity of enhancement. For further details, we refer to our previous communication on this issue [7].

In view of this experience, in the following we only deal with results obtained by MRI. Of the 60 patients, EPMR unveiled significant enhancement in 75%, clearly delineating residual tumor in the majority of cases. In nine patients (15%), any enhancement was absent with certainty.

The EPMR findings were equivocal in 10%, in which interpretation was made difficult due to discrete enhancement only, or on account of an early methemoglobin artifact.

In two cases with early postoperative deaths, histological examination was obtained, which revealed close correlation of enhanced area to gross residual tumor. In all other cases, we had to observe the patients' further clinical courses to investigate the significance of EPMR-assessed findings.

To make our results more valid, we further confine the evaluation to those 39 patients who could be observed for more than 12 months.

In all cases but one, the enhanced area in the EPMR scan represented the site of later tumor progression, i.e., the site of outgrowth of the so-called recurrence (Fig. 1).

In general, there was an obvious dependency of regrowth characterisitics on whether radiotherapy was performed or was not: following irradiation, several EPMR-revealed tumor remnants exhibited a stable state, or even a temporary regression for a few months, whereas nearly all nonirradiated patients suffered a rapid deterioration within a significantly shorter period.

Nevertheless, the in situ progression of the primary residual tumor in both groups frequently showed distinct interindividual variabilities, presumably in consequence of differences in radioresistance, or in the individual biological behavior. It was very impressive how exactly these characteristics could be depicted by consecutive MR scans!

There was an overall close interrelation between the detection as well as the absence of any enhancement in EPMR and the patients' further clinical courses: of the group of 28 patients who had revealed significant enhancement in EPMR, nearly 90% ($n = 25$) died within 15 months. The median survival time in these cases was 9 months. Two patients developed clinically apparent regrowth; in another patient, tumor progression could be diagnosed only in Gd MR. The rate of progressive disease in this group was 100%.

On the other hand, in the small group of cases without EPMR enhancement, the rate of progressive disease was 50%. Until now, no regrowth has been observed in three patients (all of them grade IV gliomas!), also radiologically confirmed, covering an observation period of 13, 16, and 18 months, respectively. Two patients have suffered a local regrowth; one patient died from a multicentric recurrent glioblastoma of the contralateral hemisphere.

All five patients with primary equivocal enhancement died; their median time of survival was 54 weeks as opposed to 37 weeks in the group with significant enhancement.

Our results suggest that the patient's clinical course within the first 15 months following extirpation of a malignant glioma is greatly influenced by the fact of gross residual tumor left behind during surgery. This is in contradiction to the view of many authors who have come to the conclusion that the type of operation (radical or subtotal) is not of major concern [1, 13]. Interestingly, in most of these investigations the assessment of tumor removal accomplished is based on the neurosurgeon's intraoperative perception alone. We therefore evaluated the reliability of the surgeons' estimation in our cases, concerning the completeness of gross tumor extirpation achieved, compared with the corresponding MR findings. Tables 2 and 3 clearly document the wide margins of error the neurosurgeon is subject to during operation (Fig. 2). It also demonstrates that the evaluation of gross residual tumor as a prognostic factor in glioma surgery particularly depends on the way in which it is assessed.

Table 2. Assessment of the completeness of gross tumor extirpation: estimation of the neurosurgeon vs EPMR findings

Residual tumor	Neurosurgeon		EPMR	
	%	*n*	%	*n*
Yes	21	12	76	44
?	8	5	7	4
No	71	41	17	10

Table 3. Completeness of gross tumor extirpation: affects on median survival time

Residual Tumor	Median survival time (weeks)
According to the neurosurgeon's estimation	
Yes	33
?	43
No	38
According to EPMR	
Yes	34
?	53
No	> 61

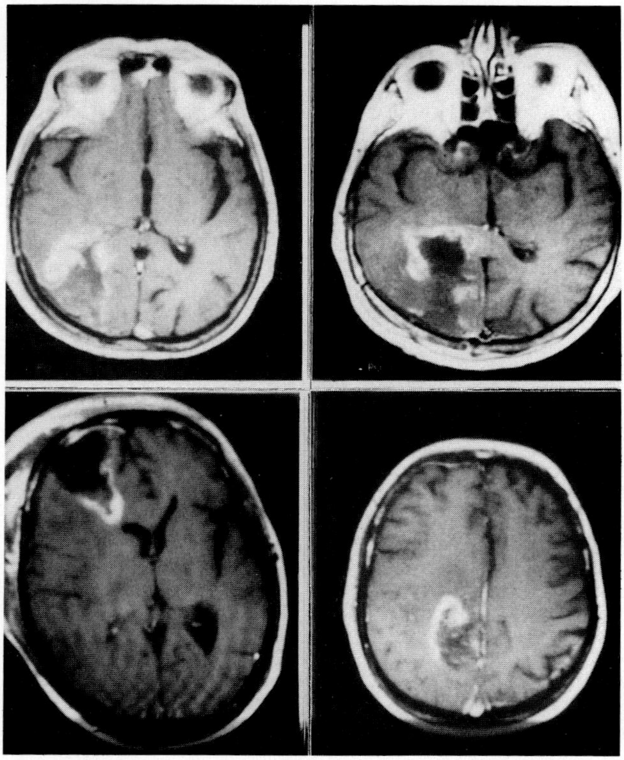

Fig. 2. Four cases of substantial residual tumor enhancement in early postoperative Gd MR. As the neurosurgeon had stated in each case; *"complete removal of all visible tumor was achieved"* at the end of the operation

Conclusions

Gadolinium-enhanced MRI, when performed during day 1 to 3 following extirpation of a preoperatively enhancing high-grade glioma, is a valuable method for assessing solid residual tumor.

In a high percentage, regrowth in glioblastoma occurring within the 1st year after operation originates from significantly enhancing remnants, already detectable in the early postoperative Gd MR.

The neurosurgeon's intraoperative ability to estimate the degree of tumor removal achieved is very limited. This may have led to misjudgment of gross residual tumor as not being a decisive prognostic factor in the past.

Early postoperative gadolinium-enhanced MRI may serve as an essential baseline examination at the beginning of and during any other therapy following surgery in glioblastoma. Furthermore, consecutive MR imaging represents a sensitive in situ monitoring of the treated or untreated residual tumor, thereby providing a basis for correlative neuro-oncological research.

References

1. Ammirati M, Vick N, Liao Y, Ciric I, Mikhael M (1987) Effect of the extent of surgical resection on survival and quality of life in patients with supratentorial glioblastomas and anaplastic astrocytomas. Neurosurgery 21:201–206
2. Andreou J, George AE, Wise A et al. (1983) CT prognostic criteria of survival after malignant glioma surgery. Am J Neuroradiol 4:488–490
3. Burger PC, Heinz ER, Shibata T, Kleihues P (1988) Topographic anatomy and CT correlations in the untreated glioblastoma multiforme. J Neurosurg 68:698–704
4. Cairncross JG, Pexman JHW, Rathbone MP, DelMaestro RF (1985) Postoperative contrast enhancement in patients with brain tumor. Ann Neurol 17:570–572
5. Ciric I, Vick NA, Mikhael MA, Cozzens J, Eller T, Walsh A (1990) Aggressive surgery for malignant supratentorial gliomas. Clin Neurosurg 36:375–383
6. Cohadon F (1990) Indications for surgery in the management of gliomas. In: Symon L, Calliauw L, Cohadon F et al. (eds) Advances and technical standards in neurosurgery, vol 17. Springer, Wien New York
7. Forsting M, Albert FK, Sartor K, Kunze S (1991) Early postoperative CT and MRI in glioblastoma. Neuroradiology [Suppl] 33:25–27
8. Jeffries BF, Kishore PRS, Singh KS, Ghatak NR, Krempa J (1981) Contrast enhancement in the postoperative brain. Radiology 139:409–413
9. Mineura K (1988) Statistical considerations of therapeutic results in glioblastoma. In: Suzuki J (ed) Treatment of glioma. Springer, Tokyo Berlin Heidelberg
10. Murovic J, Turowski K, Wilson CB, Hoshino T, Levin V (1986) Computerized tomography in the prognosis of malignant cerebral gliomas. J Neurosurg 65:799–806
11. Salcman M (1980) Survival in glioblastoma: Historical perspective. Neurosurgery 7:435–439
12. Sze G, Bravo S, Krol G, Zimmerman RD (1988) Postoperative enhancement: Gd-DTPA in a clinical series and an animal model. Radiology [Suppl] 169:70
13. Wood JR, Green SB, Shapiro WR (1988) The prognostic importance of tumor size in malignant gliomas: A computed tomographic scan study by the Brain Tumor Cooperative Group. J Clin Oncol 6:338–343

Malignancy-Dependent Formation of Cysteinyl-Leukotrienes in Human Brain Tumor Tissues and Its Detection in Urine

M. Winking[1], G. Lausberg[1], and T. Simmet[2]

Leukotrienes (LT) are biologically highly active compounds which can be synthesized from arachidonic acid via the 5-lipoxygenase pathway of polyunsaturated fatty acid metabolism. The unstable epoxide LTA_4 can be converted to LTC_4 by addition of glutathione at C-6. The peptic cleavage of glutamic acid and glycine from the peptide side chain leads to the formation of LTD_4 and LTE_4 [5].

There is now considerable evidence that cysteinyl-leukotrienes might be involved in a number of pathophysiological states of the CNS [4, 8]. In previous studies it has been shown already that brain tissue has the capacity to produce cysteinyl-leukotrienes [2, 3, 6, 8]. Recently, we have demonstrated biosynthesis of cysteinyl-leukotrienes in human brain tumors.

The brain tumor tissue was obtained from patients who underwent craniotomy for therapeutic reasons. This study was approved by the Ethics Committee of the Ruhr University.

The stimulation of the resected astrocytoma tumor tissue resulted in an increased release of cysteinyl-leukotrienes depending on the malignancy of the tumor. Brain tumors with higher malignancy such as WHO grade III and IV astrocytoma were found to release very large amounts of cysteinyl-leukotrienes even under basal conditions [7, 9]. Considering that LTE_4 is the main metabolite of cysteinyl-leukotrienes in man, we have studied the urinary LTE_4 excretion in patients with malignant grade III and IV astrocytomas. We were particularly interested in the question of whether cysteinyl-leukotrienes might be related to the formation of perifocal edema in patients suffering from such tumors.

Urine from patients with brain tumors of higher malignancy corresponding to grade III and IV astrocytoma was collected preoperatively as well as 7 and 14 days after operation. Using the reverse phase high-performance liquid chromatography (HPLC) in combination with a specific radioimmunoassay, we determined the urinary LTE_4 excretion.

The urinary excretion of LTE_4 in patients with grade IV astrocytoma was calculated by the Wilcoxon matched-pair signed-rank statistics and was found to be significantly higher ($P < 0.05$) than in patients with grade III astrocytoma.

Seven days after operation, the mean reduction of the urinary LTE_4 excretion was about 87%. Fourteen days after operation, the mean value of urinary LTE_4 excretion

[1] Neurochirurgische Klinik der Ruhr-Universität Bochum, Knappschaftskrankenhaus, In der Schornau 23–25, W-4630 Bochum 7, FRG.
[2] Abteilung für Pharmakologie und Toxikologie der Ruhr-Universitäts Bochum, Knappschaftskrankenhaus, In der Schornau 23–25, W-4630 Bochum 7, FRG.

Advances in Neurosurgery, Vol. 20
K. Piscol, M. Klinger, M. Brock (Eds.)

was 92% lower than the preoperative excretion. Fourteen days after operation, two patients of this group showed values similar to those prior to operation. In their CCT scans large tumor recurrences could already be detected. It has been suggested that the peritumoral edema found in such patients might possibly be the result of the synthesis of cysteinyl-leukotrienes by the tumor tissues [1, 9].

Therefore, in this study we have determined the tumor surrounding edema as well as the tumor volume by computer-assisted planimetric measurement in the CCT scan.

In patients with grade III astrocytoma, a significant correlation could be detected between the urinary LTE_4 excretion corrected for the tumor volume and the peritumoral edema. In patients with grade IV astrocytoma, however, this correlation could not be established. We believe that this apparent inconsistency can be explained by the fact that except for one patient all grade III astrocytomas had a solid structure of the tissue. In contrast, however, in patients with grade IV astrocytoma, all tumors had a cystic configuration. In addition, angiography suggesting significant variation in tumor vascularization, which might result in a variable diffusion of cysteinyl-leukotrienes into the circulation, in patients with grade IV astrocytoma exhibited a tumor blush of different intensity. In patients with grade III astrocytoma, except for one single case, a tumor blush could not be observed.

From the data presented, we conclude that malignant astrocytomas trigger a malignancy-dependent formation of cysteinyl-leukotrienes which can be detected in the patients urine and which in solid astrocytomas appears to be related to the perifocal edema.

References

1. Black KL, Hoff JT, McGillincuddy JE, Gebarski SS (1986) Increased leukotriene C_4 and vasogenic edema surrounding brain tumors in humans. Ann Neurol 19:592–595
2. Dembinska-Kiec A, Simmet Th, Peskar BA (1984) Formation of leukotriene C_4-like material by rat brain tissue. Eur J Pharmacol 99:57–62
3. Lindgren JA, Hökfelt T, Dahlen SE, Patrono C, Samuelson B (1984) Leukotrienes in the rat central nervous system. Proc Natl Acad Sci USA 81:6212–6216
4. Moskowitz MA, Kiwak KJ, Hekimian K, Levine L (1984) Synthesis of compounds with properties of leukotrienes C_4 and D_4 in gerbil brain after ischemia and reperfusion. Science 224:886–889
5. Samuelsson B, Dahlen SE, Lindgren JA, Rouzer CA, Serhan CN (1987) Leukotrienes and lipoxins: Structures, biosynthesis and biological effects. Science 237:1171–1176
6. Simmet Th, Luck W, Delank WK, Peskar BA (1988) Formation of cysteinyl-leukotrienes by human brain tissue. Brain Res 456:344–349
7. Simmet Th, Luck W, Winking M, Delank WK, Peskar BA (1989) Formation of cysteinyl-leukotrienes by human intracranial tumors. New Trends Lipid Mediators Res 3:166–170
8. Simmet Th, Peskar BA (1990) Lipoxygenase products of polyunsaturated fatty acid metabolism in the central nervous system: Biosynthesis and putative functions. Pharmacological Research 22:667–681
9. Simmet Th, Luck W, Winking M, Delank WK, Peskar BA (1990) Identification and characterization of cysteinyl-leukotriene formation in tissue slices from human intracranial tumors: Evidence for their biosynthesis under in vivo conditions. J Neurochem 54:2091–2099

Immunohistochemical Expression of Epidermal Growth Factor Receptor in Human Gliomas

J. Behnke, J. Bayer, H. Ludwig, and B. Rama[1]

Introduction

In the search for more specific tumor antigens, epidermal growth factor receptor (EGFR) mediated mechanisms have been found to play an important role for growth of malignancies. EGFR is a transmembrane mitogenic glycoprotein of 170 K. Besides the increased expression in human cervical, ovarian and vulval carcinomas [3], and human sarcomas [4] EGFR was found to be increased in human brain tumors [5].

In the following, human gliomas were examined for expression of EGFR by means of binding the monoclonal antibody (Mab) 425, which binds to the external domain of EGFR [6].

Methods

Tests for sensitivity were performed on 113 gliomas and 13 recurrences with Mab 425 on frozen sections and using the avidin-biotin-immunoperoxidase method [2]. As listed in Table 1, 126 gliomas were obtained after surgical resection. The tumor material was immediately frozen after resection in isopentane cooled in liquid nitrogen and then kept at –80°C until the tissues were cut into 10-μm-thick sections at –20°C on a cryostat. The sections were fixed in 4°C cold acetone for 5 min and kept at –20°C overnight up to 5 days. For immunohistochemistry with the Mab 425 the three-stage avidin-biotin-immunoperoxidase method was applied. 3-Amino-9-ethylcarbazole was used as chromogen and counterstaining was done with Gill's hematoxylin. The slides were mounted in Mowiol. The slides were checked for Mab 425 binding cells that were defined as EGFR positive. These data were related to histopathological grading of the glioma and clinical course of the patient.

Results

Of all gliomas tested, 63% had some tumor cells binding Mab 425. Mab 425 did not bind to endothelial cells nor to endothelial proliferations within the tumors. The

---

[1] Neurochirurgische Universitätsklinik, Robert-Koch-Str. 40, W–3400 Göttingen, FRG.

Advances in Neurosurgery, Vol. 20
K. Piscol, M. Klinger, M. Brock (Eds.)

Table 1. Gliomas examined and the number binding Mab 425

Gliomas	Total	EGFR positive
Glioblastomas, astrocytomas (IV), oliglodendrogliomas (IV) including 8 recurrences	62	51
Astrocytomas (III) including 3 recurrences	17	12
Oligodendrogliomas (III) including 1 recurrence	13	10
Astrocytomas (I, II)	18	1
Oligodendrogliomas (I, II)	4	1
Ependymomas (I, II) including 1 recurrence	9	3
Ependymoma (III, IV)	3	1

highest incidence of EGFR-positive tumors was found in the glioblastoma group with 82%.

A positive correlation between the histopathological malignancy grade and the EGFR expression occurred in three respects:

1. As shown in Table 1, the incidence of EGFR-positive tumors increased from grade I/II astrocytomas and grade I/II oligodendrogliomas, grade III astrocytomas, and grade III oligodendrogliomas up to the glioblastoma group. The same correlation was seen.
2. For the proportion of positive tumor cells within the tumors and
3. For the intensity of immunohistochemical staining of single cells.

In recurrences the expression of EGFR decreased compared with the primary tumor. In the glioblastoma group only one recurrence showed a more intense staining within the tumor; one had the same staining pattern, but five of the eight recurrences had an decreased expression of EGFR, and three of them did not bind the Mab 425 at all. In the group of grade III astrocytomas, all three recurrences had a decreased binding of Mab 425 within the tumors, and one of them did not express EGFR in contrast to the primary tumor. The only recurrence in the group of grade III oligodendrogliomas had the same staining pattern as the primary tumor.

In the glioblastoma group, the above-mentioned correlation between malignancy and EGFR expression lost validity. In a group of 13 patients with recurrence within 3 months after surgical resection, two tumors did not express the EGFR at all. In the remaining 11 positive recurrences, only half of the tumors expressed EGFR in a high proportion of tumor cells. In contrast, within a group of 17 patients relapsing after more than 3 months, all tumors strongly bound Mab 425 on a high proportion of their tumor cells. The intensity of EGFR expression showed a similar pattern. Early recurrences had lower EGFR expression.

Discussion

In gliomas expression of EGFR can be defined as a parameter of malignant behavior. In contrast, rapidly recurring glioblastomas show a decreased expression of EGFR compared with other glioblastomas.

In this context, it is important that Mab 425 binds to the external domain of EGFR which is often lost in the gene product of amplified and rearranged EGFR genes [1]. In these highly malignant glioblastomas, the EGFR cannot be functional because with loss of the external domain the EGF binding site is also lost. These circumstances might give some insights into the EGFR- and EGF-dependent and independent mechanisms controlling tumor growth.

The ability of Mab 425 to block EGF binding [7] raises the possibility of its use as an antagonist in blocking the growth of EGF-dependent tumors. The high binding of Mab 425 on the tumor cells of nearly 80% of malignant gliomas tested confirmed that Mab 425 is a likely candidate for an "adjuvant rational therapy" of malignant gliomas.

References

1. Bigner SH, Vogelstein B (1990) Cytogenetics and molecular genetics of malignant gliomas and medulloblastomas. Brain Pathology 1:12–292
2. Guesdon JL, Ternynck T, Avrameas S (1979) The use of avidin-biotin interaction in immunoenzymatic techniques. J Histochem Cytochem 27:1131–1139
3. Gullick WJ, Marsden JJ, Whittle N, Ward B, Babrow L, Waterfield MD (1986) Expression of epidermal growth factor receptors on human cervical, ovarian, and vulval carcinomas. Cancer Res 46:285–292
4. Gusterson B, Cowley G, McIlhinney J, Ozanne B, Fisher C, Reeves B (1985) Evidence for increased epidermal growth factor receptors on human sarcomas. Int J Cancer 36:689–693
5. Libermann TA, Razon N, Bartal AD, Yarden Y, Schlessinger J, Sareq H (1984) Expression of epidermal growth factor receptors in human brain tumors. Cancer Res 44:753–760
6. Murthy U, Basu A, Rodeck U, Herlyn M, Ross AH, Das M (1987) Binding of an antagonistic monoclonal antibody to an intact and fragmented EGF-receptor polypeptide. Arch Biochem Biophys 252:549–560

Winning Poster and Lecture Presentations

Pituitary Microcirculation Measured by Laser Doppler Flowmetry: Physiological and Clinical Aspects

R. Steinmeier, A. Dötterl, and R. Fahlbusch[1]

Introduction

There is considerable controversy concerning the vascular supply and angioarchitecture of the anterior pituitary lobe (AL). Following the innovative studies of Wislocki and King [28] and Green and Harris [9], the concept of a dominant portal blood supply to the AL has been generally accepted and has led to significant progress in neuroendocrinological scientific work and understanding of hypothalamic-pituitary interactions. Experimental studies in animals clearly demonstrated a completely different level of microcirculation between anterior and posterior (PL) pituitary lobe, the latter exhibiting values exceeding the highest found in any other region of the brain [4, 7, 8, 12, 13, 15, 21, 22, 26, 27].

For technical reasons, it has hitherto not been possible to study pituitary microflow in humans. With the recent development of laser Doppler flowmetry (LDF), very small probes can now also be applied in man [1, 2, 17–20, 25]. Although the theoretical background of this new method remains controversial and the values received do not – or only with restrictions – allow calibration in physical units (ml/100 g tissue per min), the validity of LDF in cerebral tissue has been proven by many studies which showed a linear and strong correlation to standard physiological methods of microcirculatory measurement [5, 6, 10, 11, 16, 23].

Since extremely different microflow values betwen AL and PL are described in animals, LDF offers the unique possibility for objective real-time identification of different histological tissues in man during surgery. In addition, computational methods applied to the LDF signals allow a system analytical approach for the understanding of interdependency between different systemic physiological parameters and pituitary microflow.

Materials and Methods

Laser Doppler Flowmetry and Data Acquisition

LDF was performed by TSI's Laserflo blood perfusion monitor (BPM 403 A; TSI Inc., St. Paul, USA) with a standard 0.8-mm-diameter needle probe (type P-433–3).

[1] Neurochirurgische Klinik der Universität Erlangen-Nürnberg, Schwabachanlage 6, W–8520 Erlangen, FRG.

Advances in Neurosurgery, Vol. 20
K. Piscol, M. Klinger, M. Brock (Eds.)

The illuminated tissue volume is about 1 mm^3. Three values are given simultaneously: mean velocity of RBCs (kHz, ranging from 0 to 8), the fractional volume of the RBCs (arbitrary units, ranging from 0 to 1.6), and microflow, calculated as the product of velocity and volume ("flux", ranging from 0 to 400). For detailed technical information, extensive literature is available [1–3, 14, 17–20, 25].

A specially designed data acquisition program was developed (programmed by Ullrich Sigwanz and Klaus Appelbaum) to simultaneously record all LDF values (time constant 0.2 s), the electrocardiogram (ECG), arterial blood pressure (aBP), end-expiratory pCO_2, central venous pressure (CVP), and ventilation pressure (VP) using a 16-channel analog-to-digital converter (DT2814, Data Translation, Inc., Marlboro, USA), with an A/D converter throughput of 25 kHz, and a sampling rate of 300/s (ISI 3.3 ms).

Intraoperative Protocol

A standardized neuroanesthetical procedure with barbiturate pretreatment, oral intubation, and isoflurane/N_2O/fentanyl/relaxant administration was performed. End-expiratory pCO_2 was adjusted to approximately 35 mmHg.

Transsphenoidal microsurgical resection of the adenomas was carried out via a standard transsphenoidal approach. Usually flowing removal of the adenoma, the anterior and posterior lobes were identified, and whenever possible, measurements were taken from the adenoma plus the anterior and posterior lobe. Only when the anterior and/or posterior lobe could be clearly identified before or after tumor removal, the needle probe was carefully placed on the surface of that area and the measurement performed. Taking advantage of the long nasal speculum, no fixation of the probe was necessary.

Patients

Between January 1990 and May 1991, all patients ($n = 92$) who underwent primary transsphenoidal microsurgery for intra-/supra-/parasellar adenomas were included in this series, irrespective of the endocrinological activity of pharmacological pretreatment (bromocriptine, octreotide) in cases of prolactinoma or acromegaly. Fifty-two of this total group were systematically analyzed (Tables 1 and 2).

Statistical and Computational Methods

For an offline-controlled artifact-free 15-s time interval, mean values of microflow, velocity, and volume were calculated which are assumed to estimate the trend of this interval in the individual case.

These individual mean values were pooled into two groups (AL and PL), and mean values, standard error of the mean (SEM), standard deviation (SD), and the

Table 1. Pooled nonpusatile LDF data (microflow, velocity, and volume) for anterior and posterior pituitary lobe (n = 52 patients)

	Anterior lobe (n = 48)				Posterior lobe (n = 36)				P
	Mean	± SEM	SD	Median	Mean	± SEM	SD	Median	
Microflow (flux)	27.4	2.7	18.7	21.9	177.7	12.7	76.1	158.7	< 0.001
Velocity (kHz)	0.81	0.12	0.79	0.68	4.35	0.27	1.59	3.9	< 0.001
Volume	0.73	0.06	0.42	0.62	0.79	0.07	0.44	0.63	NS

Table 2. Interpeak latencies for ECG-triggered averaged pulsatile LDF data (n = 44 patients)

	Anterior lobe (n = 33)				Posterior lobe (n = 25)				P
	Mean	± SEM	SD	Median	Mean	± SEM	SD	Median	
Cardiac cycle (ms)	856.5	25.3	171.5	843	862.8	27.0	162.1	882	NS
ECG aBP (ms)	310.8	7.5	47.8	307	318.1	8.9	50.6	316.5	NS
EDG microflow (ms)	515.5	16.2	91.7	521	483.4	28.6	143.2	503	NS
ECG velocity (ms)	664.5	28.7	162.5	638	524.0	16.5	82.6	513	< 0.01
ECG volume (ms)	419.3	16.9	97.1	403	328.7	32.9	164.7	277	< 0.001

median were calculated for each group. This approach allows determination of mean LDF data denoted as "nonpulsatile LDF data" (for results, see Table 1).

One of the outstanding features of LDF is its ability to detect pulsatile microflow patterns which are assumed to be generated by other pulsatile physiological parameters, i.e., blood pressure or ventilation. To analyze the effect of any of these parameters on pituitary microflow, an average response computing procedure ("signal averaging") was applied to the original data to transform LDF signals and evoke the underlying coherent part [24]. The averaging procedure results in a new signal, and the pulsatile pattern of this evoked new signal is assumed to derive mainly from the physiological parameter taken as the trigger signal (i.e., blood pressure, ventilation).

Three physiological parameters are thought to influence pituitary microcirculation: arterial blood pressure (aBP), central venous pressure (CVP), and ventilation pressure (VP).

The R peak of the ECG as a clear-cut time marker of the cardiac cycle was taken as the internal physiological trigger for the analysis of influence of aBP and CVP on pituitary microcirculation, and the offline-triggered sweep duration was set at 2 s. Averaging of 30 cardiac cycles was sufficient to achieve stable transformed signals with clearly defined peaks (Figs. 1–4). The interpeak latencies between the R peak of the ECG, maximum peak of aBP, and maximum peaks of LDF signals were systematically determined after this transformation in all cases. The first positive peak of microflow, velocity, and volume following the aBP peak was used for analysis, and LDF signals transformed by signal averaging and analyzed as to their time domain are denoted as "pulsatile LDF data" (for results, see Table 2). The influence of the CVP (Fig. 3) and VP (Fig. 4) was analyzed in a sample of these cases.

Results

Nonpulsatile LDF Signals

Significant differences for the nonpulsatile LDF signals were found between the anterior and posterior lobe (Table 1). Mean AL microflow and velocity were 27.4 $\pm$ 2.7 flux and 0.81 $\pm$ 0.12 kHz, while mean PL microflow and velocity were 177.7 $\pm$ 12.7 flux and 4.35 $\pm$ 0.27 kHz. No difference was found between LDF fractional volume in the anterior (0.73 $\pm$ 0.08) and posterior lobes (0.77 $\pm$ 0.07).

Pulsatile Pattern of LDF Signals

All LDF signals (microflow, velocity, and volume) exhibit pulsatile fluctuations. The major part of these fluctuations can obviously be attributed to blood pressure pulsatility (Fig. 2). In addition, other factors such as CVP (Fig. 3) and VP (Fig.

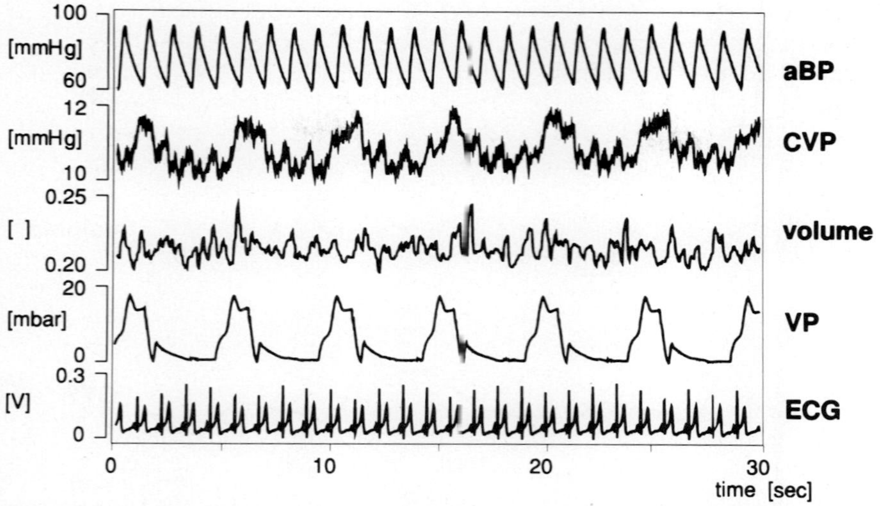

Fig. 1. Original curves of systemic physiological parameters (ECG, aBP, CVP, VP) and the LDF signal volume measured in the anterior pituitary lobe over a period of 30 s (patient with endocrinologically inactive adenoma)

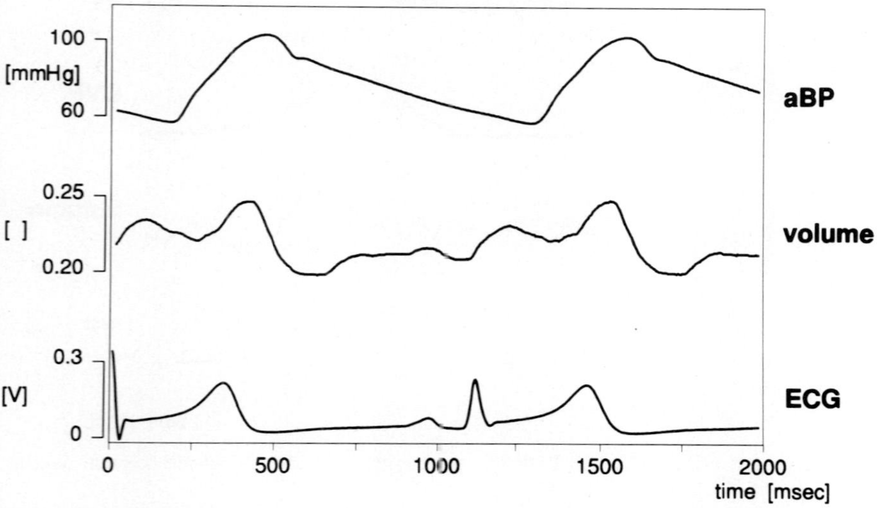

Fig. 2. Averaged aBP and LDF volume triggered by the R peak of the ECG (same original data as Fig. 1). Heart-cycle-dependent changes of the LDF signal can clearly be evaluated

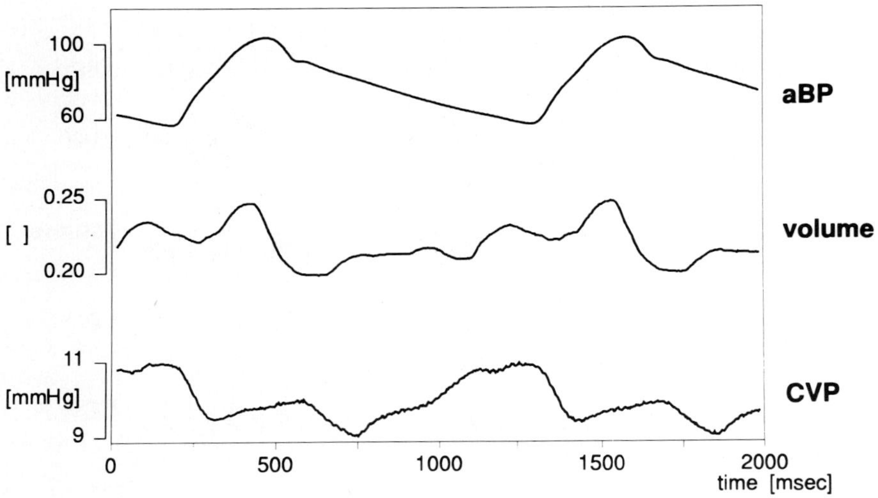

Fig. 3. Averaged aBP, CVP, and LDF volume triggered by ECG (same original data as Fig. 1). Parts of the LDF signal are obviously evoked by CVP

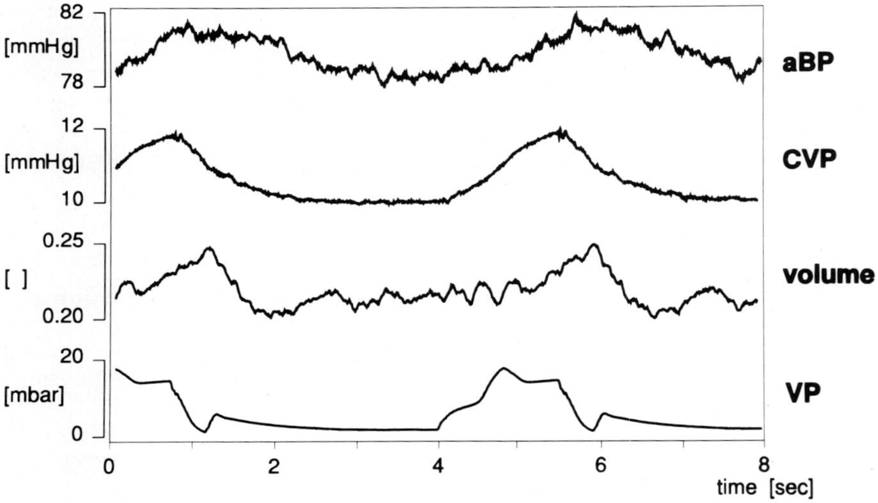

Fig. 4. Averaged aBP, CVP, and LDF volume triggered by the VP (same original data as Fig. 1)

4) influence these pulsatile variations, especially the LDF volume signal. Pulsatile LDF signal patterns are seen in both AL and PL, and amplitude increase depending on the mean value of each LDF signal.

A systematic analysis (Table 2) of mean time delay in the cardiac cycle between the R peak of the ECG (trigger of the averaging process) and the first peak of

LDF signals following the peak of aBP reveals a significant difference for anterior and posterior lobes concerning LDF velocity and volume. In the posterior lobe, peaks of LDF velocity and volume showed a mean time delay of 531.0 ± 13.5 ms and 355.8 ± 33.8 ms, respectively: in the anterior lobe, velocity and volume peaks were markedly delayed ($P < 0.001$), showing a mean maximum peak at 679.6 ± 29.5 ms and 436.1 ± 15.2 ms, respectively.

Discussion

Mean (nonpulsatile) LDF data differ largely and significantly between anterior and posterior lobes and reliably allow identification of the different tissue types in the individual case.

Averaging of LDF signals tiggered by systemic physiological parameters appears to be extremely useful for a system physiological approach and the understanding of different pituitary microflow patterns (wave-form analysis). A wide range of innovative microvascular research regarding functional coherence between blood pressure, central venous pressure, ventilation pressure, and LDF velocity, volume, and microflow can be managed by this technique taking advantage of the simultaneous measurement of all these parameters by one device.

Mean velocity of RBCs and microflow in tissue is governed by the law of Poiseuille, depending mainly on aBP and vascular arteriolar resistance. The time domain of the flow, volume, and pressure pulse in tissue has been rarely analyzed, but in general an increasing time delay of pulses depending on the vascular length, mass, and viscosity of fluid, and elasticity of the wall (vascular resistance) is generally accepted. Dispersion of waves and the averaging procedure itself might give incorrect results in the analysis of the maximum LDF peaks. Hence, the absolute values should be interpreted carefully, but we think that analysis of different patterns (the chronological order of the 3 LDF peak maxima) seems applicable. The mean time differences of the velocity and volume pulse waves between the AL and PL cannot be ascribed to the different vascular distance from the heart since this parameter is virtually identical. Hence, the time delay must be due to a large difference in the elastance of microvessels or largely differing vascular resistance between the two lobes, and this resistance is assumed to be connected in series. These differing system properties would exhibit an attenuating effect on the velocity and volume signal of the AL. This functional physiological model corresponds with the anatomical findings of a portal vascular supply to the AL.

References

1. Bonner R, Nossal R (1981) Model for laser Doppler measurements of blood flow in tissue. Applied Optics 20:2097–2107
2. Bonner RF, Clem TR, Bowen PD, Bowman RL (1981) Laser-Doppler continuous real-time monitor of pulsatile and mean blood flow in tissue microcirculation. In: Chen SH,

Schu B, Nossal R (eds) Scattering techniques applied to supramolecular and nonequilibrium systems. Plenum Press, New York, pp 685–701
3. Borgos JA (1990) LDV blood flowmeter. In: Shepherd AP, Öberg PÅ (eds) Laser-Doppler blood flowmetry. Kluwer Academic Publishers, Boston, pp 73–92
4. David MA, Csernay L, László FA, Kovács K (1965) Hypohysial blood flow in rats after destruction of the pituitary stalk. Endocrinology 77:183–187
5. DiResta GR, Kiel JW, Riedel GL, Kaplan P, Shepherd AP (1987) Hybrid blood flow probe for simultaneous H_2 clearance and laser-Doppler velocimetry. Am J Physiol 253 (Gastrointest Liver Physiol 16):G573–G581
6. Eyre JA, Essex TJH, Flecknell PA, Bartholomew PH, Sinclair JI (1988) A comparison of measurements of cerebral blood flow in the rabbit using laser Doppler spectroscopy and radionuclide labelled microspheres. Clin Phys Physiol Meas 9:65–74
7. Goldmann H (1961) Endocrine gland blood flow in the unanesthetized, unrestrained rat. J Appl Physiol 16:762–764
8. Goldmann H (1963) Effect of acute stress on the pituitary gland: endocrine gland blood flow. Endocrinology 72:588–591
9. Green JD, Harris GW (1947) The neurovascular link between the neurohypophysis and adenohypophysis. J Endocrinol 5:136–146
10. Haberl RL, Heizer ML, Marmarou A, Ellis EF (1989) Laser-Doppler assessment of brain microcirculation: effect of systemic alterations. Am J Physiol 256 (Heart Circ Physiol 25):H1247–H1254
11. Haberl RL, Heizer ML, Ellis EF (1985) Laser-Doppler assessment of brain microcirculation: effect of local alterations. Am J Physiol 256 (Heart Circ Physiol 25):H1255–H1260
12. Hanley DF, Wilson DA, Feldman MA, Traystman RJ (1988) Peripheral chemoreceptor control of neurohypophysial blood flow. Am J Physiol 254 (Heart Circ Physiol 23):H742–H750
13. Kemeny AA, Jakubowski JA, Jefferson AA, Paztor E (1985) Blood flow and autoregulation in rat pituitary gland. J Neurosurg 63:116–119
14. Leclercq TA, Grisoli F (1983) Arterial blood supply of the normal human pituitary gland. An anatomical study. J Neurosurg 58:678–681
15. Lichardus B, Albrecht I, Ponec J, Linhart L (1977) Water deprivation for 24 hours increases selectively blood flow in posterior pituitary of conscious rats. Endocrinol Exp 11:99–104
16. Lindsberg PJ, O'Neill JT, Paakkari IA, Hallenbeck JM, Feuerstein G (1989) Validation of laser-Doppler velocimetry in measurement of spinal cord blood flow. Am J Physiol 257 (Heart Circ Physiol 26):H674–H680
17. Nilsson GE (1984) Signal processor for laser Doppler tissue flowmeters. Med Biol Eng Comput 22:343–348
18. Nilsson GE, Tenland T, Öberg PA (1980) A new instrument for continuous measurement of tissue blood flow by light beating spectroscopy. IEEE Trans Biomed Eng 27:12–19
19. Nilsson GE, Tenland T, Öberg PA (1980) Evaluation of a laser Doppler flowmeter for measurement of tissue blood flow. IEEE Trans Biomed Eng 27:597–604
20. Nilsson GE, Salerud EG, Tenland T, Öberg PA (1982) Laser-Doppler tissue blood-flow measurements. In: Sattelle DB, Lee WI, Ware BR (eds) Biomedical applications of laser light scattering. Elsevier Biomedical Press, New York, pp 335–348
21. Page RB, Funsch DJ, Brennan RW, Hernandez MJ (1981) Regional neurohypophyseal blood flow and its control in adult sheep. Am J Physiol 241 (Regulatory Integrative Comp Physiol 10):R36–R43
22. Porter JC, Hines MFM, Smith KR, Repass RL, Smith AJK (1967) Quantitative evaluation of local blood flow of the adenohypophysis in rats. Endocrinology 80:583–598

23. Skarphedinsson JO, Hårding H, Thorén P, Hässle AB (1988) Repeated measurements of cerebral blood flow in rats. Comparisons between the hydrogen clearance method and laser Doppler flowmetry. Acta Physiol Scand 134:133–142
24. Steinmeier R, Fahlbusch R, Powers AD, Dötterl A, Buchfelder M (1991) Pituitary microcirculation: Physiological aspects and clinical implications. A laser Doppler flow study during transsphenoidal adenomectomy. Neurosurgery 29:47–54
25. Stern MD (1975) In vivo evaluation of microcirculation by coherent light scattering. Nature 254:56–58
26. Takaoda Y, White RJ, Billiar RB, Little BA (1977) Regional arterial blood flow in the primate pituitary gland. Surg Forum 28:464–466
27. Vella LM, Hanley DF, Wilson DA, Traystman RJ (1989) Peripheral baroreceptor control of neurohypophysial blood flow during hemorrhage. Am J Physiol 257 (Heart Circ Physiol 26):H1498–H1506
28. Wislocki GB, King LS (1936) The permeability of the hypophysis and hypothalamus to vital dyes, with a study of the hypophyseal vascular supply. Am J Anat 58:421–472

Can Motor Evoked Potentials Contribute to the Indication for Surgery in Cervical Spondylotic Disease?

B. Meyer[1], J. Zentner[2], and C. Ozdoba[3]

Summary

Motor evoked potentials (MEP) were recorded in a total of 62 patients with proven or suspected cervical spondylotic myelopathy. In all cases MEP were elicited both by electrical and magnetoelectric stimulation of the motor cortex. Peripheral conduction time was determined by electrical stimulation of the lumbar nerve roots. It was the aim of this study to find out whether there is a correlation between clinical, radiological, and electrophysiological findings and whether MEP can influence the indication for surgery in cases in which clinical examination results are ambiguous. We found pathological MEP in all patients showing clinical evidence of myelopathy. Regardless of the clinical status, there were also pathological MEP in all cases with radiological evidence of myelomalacia or myelon impairment and in 50% of the cases with borderline signs of myelon impairment. Moreover, we observed abnormal MEP in 25% of the patients without clinical or radiological signs of myelopathy. Our results allow the following conclusions:

1. Clinical and radiological evidence of cervical myelopathy is always accompanied by pathological MEP.
2. In patients whose clinical examination results are ambiguous but show radiological evidence of myelon impairment, the indication for surgery may therefore be corroborated by pathological MEP indicating spinal cord lesion.
3. In subclinical cases with radiological borderline myelon impairment, electrophysiological follow-up examinations may provide useful information in addition to clinical findings to detect neurological deterioration early and subsequently refer such patients to surgery.

Introduction

Transcranial electrical and magnetoelectric stimulation of the motor cortex and recording the electromyographic responses (motor evoked potentials, MEP) allow noninvasive electrophysiological assessment of the descending pathways [3, 8]. As

[1] Neurochirurgische Klinik der Städtischen Kliniken, Klinikum Kalkweg, Zu den Rehwiesen 9, W-4100 Duisburg, FRG.
[2] Neurochirurgische Universitätsklinik, Sigmund-Freud-Str. 24, W-5300 Bonn, FRG.
[3] Neuroradiologische Universitätsklinik, W-7400 Tübingen, FRG.

Advances in Neurosurgery, Vol. 20
K. Piscol, M. Klinger, M. Brock (Eds.)

has been shown previously both in animal experiments as well as in humans, MEP have proven to be a sensitive electrophysiological tool for detecting lesions along the spinal cord even in the subclinical condition [1, 4, 5, 7, 9, 10]. As there is still some controversy regarding the indication for surgery in cervical spondylotic disease, this study was designed to clarify whether MEP can provide additional information, especially in cases in which clinical and radiological findings are ambiguous. To achieve this goal, we correlated MEP with radiological and clinical results in 62 patients with suspected or proven cervical myelopathy.

Patients and Methods

A total of 62 patients (41 males, 21 females) aged from 27 to 73 years (mean age 57 years) were included in this study. All were admitted for evaluation of cervical spine syndrome and examined clinically with respect to local cervical, radicular, and myelopathic symptoms. Radiological findings were categorized as follows: (a) evidence of myelomalacia encompassed cases with intramedullar hyperintensity on T2-weighted MRI or intramedullar contrast depot on delayed myelo-CT; (b) evidence of myelon impairment was indicated by oval deformation of the myelon on myelo-CT or complete stop of the contrast medium on myelography; (c) borderline signs of myelon impairment included incomplete stop of contrast medium on myelography or consumption of ventral subarachnoid space on myelo-CT [2, 6]. Based on these criteria the patients were categorized into three groups: group I encompassed patients with clinical and radiological evidence of myelopathy. Patients in group II had radiological but no clinical evidence of myelon impairment. Group III consisted of patients without clinical myelopathic signs and with no or only borderline radiological myelon impairment.

In all 62 patients MEP were elicited by electrical and magnetoelectric stimulation of the motor leg area. The peripheral conduction time was determined by electrical stimulation of the lumbar nerve roots. Electrical stimulation was performed with voltage constant condenser discharges using a Digitimer D 180, which delivers a maximum output of 750 V with a time constant of 50 or 100 μs. For central stimulation, the anode was placed over the bregma and the cathode 6 cm behind it on the midline. The lumbar nerve roots were stimulated by positioning the anode at the intervertebral space of D11-12 and the cathode one segment below, each on the midline. Magnetoelectric excitation of the motor leg area was achieved by positioning the coil over Fz with the current running clockwise for activation of the right side and counterclockwise for the left side (Magstim 200, 1.5 T).

Electromyographic responses were recorded from the anterior tibial muscle using EMG electrodes in a belly/tendon-fashion. While electrically evoked responses were recorded with the target muscle at rest, magnetoelectrically elicited potentials were facilitated by voluntary contraction of the target muscle with about 10% of the maximum muscle strength. This was controlled by audio-EMG. Stimulus strength was gradually increased until a clear EMG response was obtained, or the absence of any response was documented despite a maximum stimulus strength as tolerated by the individual patient. The time base was 100 ms with a gain ranging from 100 μV to 1 mV per division. Filter settings ranged from 20 Hz to 3 kHz. Only single stimuli were applied with a time interval of 3–5 s. At least three potentials were obtained from each recording site. The central motor conduction time (CMCT) was determined by subtraction of the peripheral latency from the total latency (electrophysiological system Compact 4, Nicolet).

We decided upon the following criteria for pathological MEP changes: absence of any response on one or both sides, CMCT cortex-D12 $>$ 14 ms (electrical stimulation) or $>$ 16.3 ms (magnetoelectric stimulation). These limits for acceptable CMCT result from our normative data (including 2.5 SD) obtained from 50 healthy volunteers. Based on these criteria, MEP were correlated with the clinical and radiological findings in our 62 patients.

Results

Thirty-two patients belonged to group I. Thirteen patients had sensory and 19 motor signs of cervical myelopathy. Fifteen of them showed radiological evidence of myelomalacia and 17 of myelon impairment. Eleven of the 18 patients of group II had radicular and 7 local symptoms. Radiological findings indicated myelomalacia in 3 patients and myelon impairment in the remaining 15 cases. In group III consisting of 12 patients, 5 had radicular and 7 had local symptoms. Six of them showed either borderline myelon impairment or were inconspicuous radiologically (Table 1).

Comparing MEP with the three different radiological categories regardless of clinical findings, we obtained the following results. In category 1 with evidence of myelomalacia ($n = 18$) we observed pathological MEP in all cases. This was

Table 1. Results of MEP in the three groups of patients as categorized according to clinical and radiological findings

Patient group	Clinical examination		Radiological findings		Pathological MEP
I	Myelopathy		Myelopathy		
(n = 32)	sensory	n = 13	myelomalacia	n = 15	100%
	motor	n = 19	myelon impairment	n = 17	
II	Local/radicular symptoms		Myelopathy		
(n = 18)	local	n = 7	myelomalacia	n = 3	100%
	radicular	n = 11	myelon impairment	n = 15	
	Local/radicular symptoms		Borderline/inconspicuous		
III	local	n = 7	borderline	n = 6	50%
(n = 12)	radicular	n = 5	inconspicuous	n = 6	25%

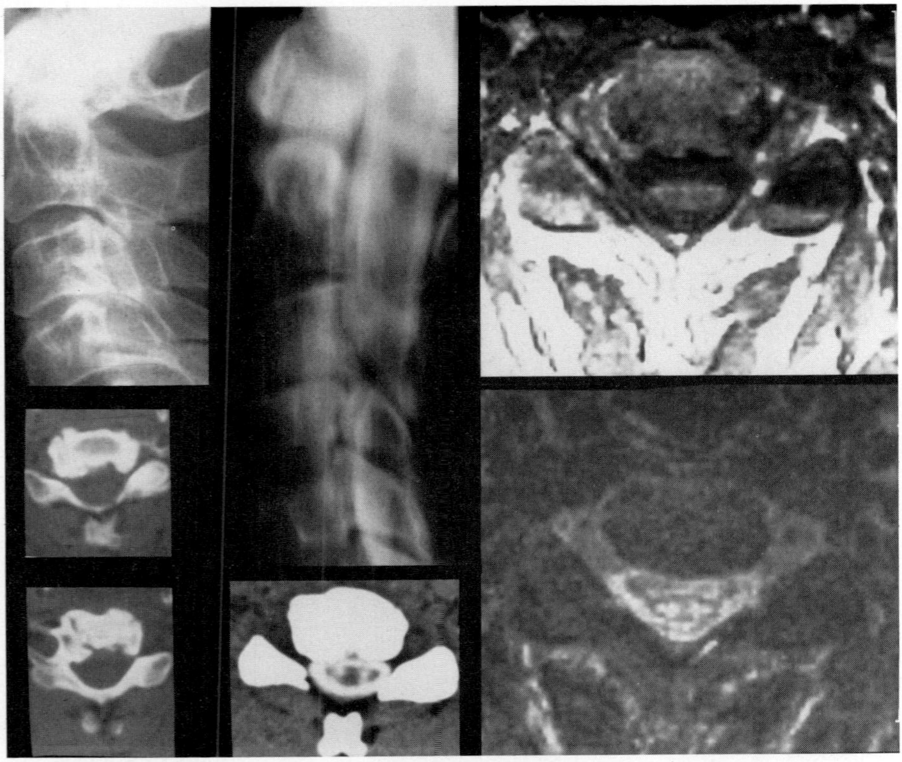

Fig. 1. A 62-year-old patient with radiological evidence of myelomalacia. Conventional X-rays and CT show a hard disc at C3-4. Myelography demonstrates incomplete stop of the contrast medium at C3-4. Myelo-CT and MRI show intramedullar contrast depots and intramedullary hyperintensities, respectively. MEP were pathological in every case of this category

also true for category 2 with evidence of myelon impairment ($n=32$). In category 3 ($n=6$) with borderline radiological signs MEP were abnormal in 50% of the patients. Figures 1–3 show typical examples.

Discussion

Cervical spondylosis is a frequent disease in elderly patients. Consensus exists about the indication for surgery in patients demonstrating myelopathy or severe radicular deficits when the lesion has been confirmed by radiological studies. However, there is still controversy about the indication for surgery in patients with only minor radicular and/or local symptoms, but with gait disturbance which, however, cannot be unequivocally related to myelopathy and may also result from other

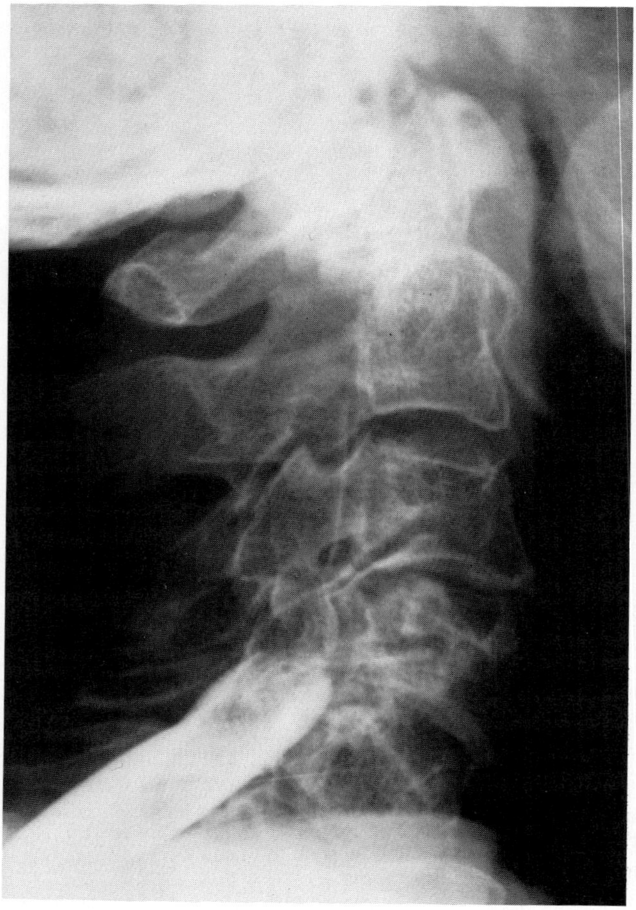

Fig. 2. Radiological evidence of myelon impairment as demonstrated by complete stop of the contrast medium on myelography at C4-5. MEP were pathological in every case of this category

disorders. Therefore, it was the aim of our work to find out whether the electrophysiological assessment of the descending pathways by means of MEP might provide additional information with respect to the indication for surgical treatment in these cases. To achieve this goal, MEP findings were correlated with the clinical and radiological results of our 62 patients.

Our results clearly show that clinically evident cervical spondylotic myelopathy is always accompanied by pathological changes in MEP. Thus, MEP are sensitive for detection of clinically evident spinal cord lesions. According to our experience, MEP are also able to indicate subclinical lesions of the descending pathways [10]. Therefore, MEP can provide useful information in patients in whom clinical examination is not conclusive for myelopathy and may support the indication for surgery in these cases. This is especially true when there is radiological evidence

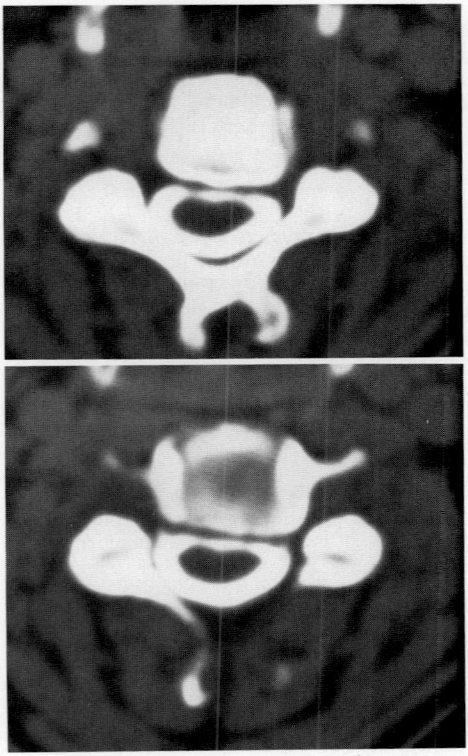

Fig. 3. Borderline signs of myelon impairment with consumption of the ventral subarachnoid space on myelo-CT. There were pathological MEP in 50% of the patients belonging to this category

of myelon involvement (myelomalacia or myelon impairment). According to our results, all of these patients had electrophysiological signs of myelopathy.

In cases in which ambiguous results are obtained by clinical examination and in which radiological studies show only borderline myelon impairment, follow-up examinations with MEP may provide useful information to realize neurological deterioration of spinal cord function at an early stage. Consequently, such patients can be referred to surgical treatment at the opportune time.

In conclusion, it is not our intention to state that motor evoked potential studies are necessary in every patient with a cervical spondylotic disease or that MEP findings alone may justify a decision for surgical treatment. What we want to say is that MEP may be helpful for making a decision for either surgical or conservative treatment in special cases in addition to clinical and radiological studies.

References

1. Abbruzzese G, Dall'Agata D, Morena M, Simonetti S, Spadavechia L, Severi P, Andriolio GC, Favale E (1988) Electrical stimulation of the motor tracts in cervial spondylosis. J Neurol Neurosurg Psychiat 51:796–802
2. Al-Mefty O, Harkey LH, Middleton TH, Smith RR, Fox JL (1988) Myelopathic spondylotic lesions demonstrated by magnetic resonance imaging. J Neurosurg 68:217–222
3. Barker AT, Jalinous R, Freeston IL (1985) Non-invasive magnetic stimulation of the human motor cortex. Lancet I:1106–1107
4. Cushick JF (1987) Monitoring of cervical spondylatic myelopathy. Spine 13:877–880
5. Fehlings MG, Tator CH, Linden RD, Piper IR (1987) Motor evoked potentials recorded from normal and spinal cord injured rats. Neurosurgery 20:125–130
6. Larsson EM, Holtas S, Cronquist S, Brandt L (1989) Comparison of myelography, CT myelography and magnetic resonance imaging in cervical spondylosis and disc herniation. Pre- and postoperative findings. Acta Radiol 30:233–239
7. Levy WJ (1987) Clinical experience with motor and cerebellar evoked potential monitoring. Neurosurgery 20:169–182
8. Merton PA, Morton HB (1980) Stimulation of the cerebral cortex in the intact human subject. Nature 285:227
9. Patil AA, Nagaray MP, Mehta R (1985) Cortically evoked motor action potentials in spinal cord injury research. Neurosurgery 16:473–476
10. Zentner J, Rieder G (1990) Diagnostic significance of motor evoked potentials in space-occupying lesions of the brainstem and spinal cord. Eur Arch Psychiatr Neurol Sci 239:285–289

Is the Hunt and Hess Scale Outdated?

A. Aschoff[1], J. Hampl[1], E. Hund[2], J. Raety[1], W. Hacke[2], and S. Kunze[1]

In 1968, Hunt and Hess published a modified version of the five-grade Botterell classification [1, 3]. This was based on a retrospective study of only 275 patients over a 12-year period. Most patients had been admitted in the second week or later after bleeding, when the clinical state has usually stabilized. The most recent technical diagnostic aids such as computer tomography (CT), transcranial Doppler, and evoked potentials were not available.

Their intention was not to inaugurate a new descriptive grading system, but to "present a method for the evaluation of risk and selection of the optimal time for surgical intervention"[3]. Today, such an intention would be classified as an "expert system."

This modified Botterell scale has become the most-cited paper in the literature on aneurysm. In spite of some disadvantages and 36 concurrent scales [5] the Hunt and Hess score is still the most popular (Table 1).

In the 1980s, 78% of our patients were admitted in the first week, 54% even within the first 24 h, after subarachnoid hemorrhage. During this period the majority of patients pass through significant changes of vigilance and neurological status, sometimes repeatedly.

Table 1. Thirty-seven neurological scores for subarachnoid hemorrhage: a selection of the main developments

Botterell et al. (1956)	
Nishioka (1966)	
Hunt and Hess (1968)	
Hunt and Kosnick (1974)	Jennett and Teasdale (1974)
Nibbelink (1977)	
COP Studie I, Sahs (1982)	
Yasargil (1984)	
Sano and Tamura (1985)	
COOP Studie II, Jagger and Kassell (1989/90)	
World Federation of Neurological Surgeons, Drake (1988)	

[1] Neurochirurgische Universitätsklinik, Im Neuenheimer Feld 400, W–6900 Heidelberg, FRG.
[2] Neurologische Universitätsklinik, Im Neuenheimer Feld 400, W–6900 Heidelberg, FRG.

Advances in Neurosurgery, Vol. 20
K. Piscol, M. Klinger, M. Brock (Eds.)

Table 2. Variability of aneurysm scores

Grade	Percentage	Author(s)
I	4.7–62.5	Symon (1979) , Suzuki (1979) [14, 13]
II	17.1–48	Sano (1978), Sengupta (1986) [10, 12]
III	12.1–37.6	Sano (1978), Hunt and Hess (1977) [10, 4]
IV	4.4–22	Yasargil (1980), Symon (1979) [16, 14]
V	0.0–10.8	Kempe (1979), Hunt and Hess (1977) [8, 4]

Additional handicaps for grading are postictal state, analgesic-sedative drugs, intubation, and ventilation. Criteria such as age and serious systemic diseases which are included, but not specified clearly, in the appendix to the original Hunt and Hess score were used arbitrarily. In addition, the use of CT or other apparative diagnostic findings is popular, but not standardized. A secondary phenomenon like early hydrocephalus, which is readily treatable and itself irrelevant to outcome, may also influence the actual grading.

In 600 aneurysm patients admitted between 1983 and 1991 we reevaluated retrospectively the Hunt and Hess scores. Over the same period, we also found 40% discordances between the gradings of the admitting examiner and the authors of discharge reports.

On the 13-point Glasgow Coma Scale, Teasdale observed a complete convergence of examiners in 53% of cases, and when the respective next gradings were included to make it more comparable to the Hunt and Hess score with only five points 88% convergence was found [15].

Statistically, we might expect the Hunt and Hess scores I–III to show a comparable distribution. In reality, we found a variability in grade I from 4.7% to 62.5%, in grade II from 17.1% to 48%, and in grade III from 12.1% to 37.6% (Table 2). The poor-grade patients show similar differences, but selection factors of admission policy are, of course, acting here.

In a study conducted by Lindsay, 15 patients with subarachnoid hemorrhage were scored by 13 independent examiners [9]: full interrater reliability was found in only 27% of the Hunt and Hess scores. Six of fifteen patients had been given three different gradings, and two had even been given four different gradings. Lindsay used the kappa index for interrater reliability, where 0 means a random distribution and +1 full congruence. An adequate scale should have a kappa of 0.8, or better 0.9.

Lindsay observed a kappa of the Hunt and Hess scale of only 0.43. Even the external reference examiners reached only 0.58. Grade III, which is especially important for decision-making, had a kappa of only 0.31. The lowest concordance was found when the Hunt and Hess score included systemic diseases: the kappa of 0.09 found was very close to a random distribution.

In clinical practice we can observe a number of different uses of Hunt and Hess grading:

1. For *retrospective evaluation* in scientific papers
2. As a *prognostic index* during treatment
3. As a short and unpretentious *descriptive term* for bedside information
4. As a *flexible term for "clinical policy,"* e.g., for better acceptance in patient transferral procedures.
5. As a pliant scale for use in *inter-hospital competition.* It has, for instance, proven possible to "clean up" poor statistics by shifting grade III to IV, thus masking relatively poor results.
6. Finally, a very important use is the *function of a "latent expert system":* In most hospitals the grading procedure is identical with operative decision making.

The grading is therefore not a descriptive problem, but the decision for or against a high-risk operation, above all in the borderline grades III and IV. De facto, the empirical "expert system" of a neurosurgeon takes into account not only the clinical status, but also CT, Doppler, angiographic, and electrophysiological findings. For *verbalization* of this complex decision, however, a Hunt and Hess score adapted to the needs of the situation is used.

This "decisional-terminological dissociation" often neglects the classical definitions, but is usually helpful for the patient. Obviously, these different needs and uses must result in a terminological disaster, and because of this the Hunt and Hess score is not sufficiently reliable for use in scientific research.

More recent variants of neurological rating of subarachnoid hemorrhage have implemented the Glasgow Coma Scale and have a better interrater reliability (e.g., the scales of Sano and Tamura [11], of the Cooperative Study Group [5–7], or of the World Federation of Neurological Surgeons [2]). However, they remain inadequate for patients under analgesic sedation or ventilation, and a *single* grading of patients with permanent changes of vigilance and neurological status in the first days produces unreliable results and may well obscure the clinical dynamics.

We propose the following procedure:

Temporarily, we may use the Hunt and Hess scale or one of the subsequently developed versions [2]. Nevertheless, the selected version must be used consistently.

Taking the Apgar scale as a model, it should be obligatory to *repeat* the grading at *standardized time intervals,* to make transparent the clinical dynamics (e.g., at 1 h, 24 h, 48 h and 1 week after bleeding). As in the proven TNM system in oncology, we might note time periods without examination using the index X, postoperative grades with a P, and so on (e.g., 4-2-2-2p; see Tables 3, 4).

As in the TNM system, we might supplement the purely clinical-neurological scales with an abbreviation system for essential apparative findings. Subarachnoid, intracerebral, and intraventricular hemorrhage, hydrocephalus, vasospasm, and disturbed evoked potentials could be scaled 1–4, or with 0 if absent (unknown = x; see Tables 3, 4).

Table 3. Supplements of a scale for subarachnoid hemorrhage using indices (analogous to the TNM system)

S	Subarachnoid hemorrhage (SAH)
S0	Absent, clear CSF on lumbar puncture (LP)
S1	Bloody LP, not visible in CT
S2	Moderate SAH, regional in 1–2 cisterns
S3	Significant SAH, bilateral, 3 or more cisterns
S4	Severe SAH
rS	Recurrent bleeding (rS1–4), (r2,3,...)
I	Intracerebral hematoma
I0	Absent
I1	Small hematoma, diameter < 10 mm
I2	Minor intracerebral hematoma (11–23 mm)
I3	Significant hematoma (26–40 mm)
I4	Massive space-occupying bleeding (> 40 mm)
V	Ventricular bleeding
V0	Absent
V1	Minimal (e.g., in cornua posteriora)
V2	Minor/regional ventricular bleeding
V3	Significant, in multiple ventricles
V4	Hemorrhagic tamponade
H	Hydrocephalus
H0	Absent
H1	Ventricles plump, third ventricle oval
H2	Moderate hydrocephalus
H3	Significant hydrocephalus
H4	Massive hydrocephalus
Sp	Vasospasm (SpX, TCD not available)
Sp0	Normal velocity, normal angiography
Sp1	TCD: Moderate acceleration (80–120 cm/s[a]), angiography normal
Sp2	TCD: 120–160 cm/s[a]. Angio: Visible spasms
Sp3	TCD: More than 160 cm/s[a]. Angio: Significant vasospasms; passager neurological deficits
Sp4	Secondary (not clip-associated) infarctions, irreversible deficits
E	Electrophysiology (EX, not available)
E0	Normal electrophysiological findings
E1	Moderately pathological
E2	Significantly pathological
E3	Severely pathological
E4	Secondarily absent
R	Risks of age, general diseases (R 1–4)

CSF, cerebrospinal fluid; CT, computed tomography; LP, lumbar puncture; SAH, subarachnoid hemorrhage; TCD, transcranial Doppler.

[a] Flow velocity in A. cerebri media.

Table 4. Neurological scoring at standardized time intervals

1	1 h after subarachnoid bleeding
2	24 h after SAH
3	48 h after SAH
4	8 days after SAH
Indices:	
x	Not known
p	Postoperative
r	Recurrent bleeding
36 h, 5d, 2w	"Atypical" time interval
Examples:	
H&H	4-3-2-3p
H&H	3-2-4p-3p
H&H	3-1-5r-4r
H&H	x-2-2p-2p
H&H	x-x-x-3(2w)
ACoA	3-2-2p-2p S2 I2 V2 H2 Sp2 E2 R2
MCA	5-4p-3p-3p S2 I4 V0 H0 Sp2 E4 R2
ACI	2-1p-3p-4p S3 I1 V1 H1 Sp4 E3 R2

Such an addition would have the same information that a meticulous referral report includes and would therefore not take up much time. The supplemented grading could reduce the danger of overpromoting the scale to the level of an expert system.

On the basis of the traditional Botterell-Hess system, the problems of a valid and reliable scale are not to be solved, even if the Glasgow Coma Scale is integrated. We must, therefore, seek a completely new scale using more recent statistical methods.

Conclusions

1. For bedside communication the Hunt and Hess score is acceptable.
2. For scientific research, especially for comparisons, the reliability is unsufficient.
3. As an expert system, the Hunt and Hess scale is completely inadequate. This de facto expert system should not be forced into a bed Procrusteans. A historical scale from the 1950s is helpful neither for communication of a grading nor for rational and transparent decision making.

References

1. Botterell EHJ, Lougheed WM, Scott JW et al. (1956) Hypothermia, and interruption of carotid and vertebral circulation, in the surgical management of intracranial aneurysms. J Neurosurg 13:1–42

2. Drake CG, Hunt WE, Kassell N, Pertuiset B, Sano K, Teasdale G, DeVilliers JC (1988) Report of World Federation of Neurological Surgeons committee on a universal subarachnoid hemorrhage grading scale. J Neurosurg 68:985–986
3. Hunt WE, Hess RM (1968) Surgical risk as related to time of intervention in the repair of intracranial aneurysms. J Neurosurg 28:14–20
4. Hunt WE, Miller CA (1977) The results of early operation for aneurysm. Clin Neurosurg 234:208–215
5. Jagger J, Torner JC, Kassell NF (1989) Neurologic assessment of subarachnoid hemorrhage in a large patient series. Surg Neurol 32:327–333
6. Kassell NF, Torner JC, Haley C, Jane JA, Adams HP, Kongable GL et al. (1990) The international cooperative study on the timing of aneurysm surgery. Part I: Overall management results. J Neurosurg 73:18–36
7. Kassell NF, Torner JC, Jane JA, Haley C, Adams HP et al. (1990) The international cooperative study on the timing of aneurysm surgery. Part II: Surgical results. J Neurosurg 73:37–47
8. Kempe LG (1979) Technical aspects. In: Pia HW, Langmaid C, Zierski J (eds) Cerebral aneurysms. Springer, Berlin Heidelberg New York, pp 260–265
9. Lindsay KW, Teasdale G, Knill-Jones RP, Murray L (1982) Observer variability in grading patients with subarachnoid hemorrhage. J Neurosurg 56:628–633
10. Sano K, Saito I (1978) Timing and indication of surgery for ruptured intracranial aneurysms with regard to cerebral vasospasm. Acta Neurochir (Wien) 41:49–60
11. Sano K, Tamura A (1985) A proposal for grading of subarachnoid hemorrhage due to aneurysm rupture. In: Auer LM (ed) Timing of aneurysm surgery. Walter de Gruyter, New York, pp 3–7
12. Sengupta RP, McAllister VL (1986) Subarachnoid haemorrhage. Springer, Berlin Heidelberg New York Tokyo, pp 237–267
13. Suzuki J (1979) Cerebral aneurysms. Neuron, Tokyo
14. Symon L (1979) Material of Institute of Neurology, London. In: Pia HW, Langmaid C, Zierski J (eds) Cerebral aneurysms. Springer, Berlin Heidelberg New York, p 433
15. Teasdale G, Knill-Jones R, Van der Sande J (1978) Observer variability in assessing impaired consciousness and coma. J Neurol Neurosurg Psychiatry 41:603–610
16. Yasargil MG, Fox JL (1984) The microsurgical approach to intracranial aneurysms. Surg Neurol 3:7–14

Monocyte Killing of Malignant Brain Tumor Cells

M. Kirsch and G. Schackert[1]

Abstract

In vitro and in vivo experiments with human peripheral blood monocytes activated by biological response modifiers (BRM) show enhanced tumoricidal activity against extracerebral tumors whereas normal cells stay unharmed.

The purpose of our study was to investigate whether stimulation of human monocytes leads to tumoricidal activity against malignant brain tumors. Therefore, peripheral blood monocytes from healthy donors were isolated by density separation and adherence. After an incubation period of 24 h with BRMs, such as gamma and beta interferon (IFN-γ-β), tumor necrosis factor-alpha (TNFα), lipopolysaccharide (LPS), and muramyl dipeptide (MDP), the monocytes were mixed with [^{3}H]methylthymidine-labeled target cells to provide an effector:target cell ratio of 20:1.

Activated monocytes were tested against seven different glioblastoma cell lines, one metastasis cell line, and one melanoma cell line. High cytotoxicity rates were found after activation with IFN-β and TNFα. The combination of IFN-β with TNFα decreased monocyte cytotoxicity when compared with single agents, whereas the combination of IFN-β with IFN-γ or TNFα with IFN-γ enhanced monocyte tumoricidal activity. We conclude that activated monocytes kill malignant brain tumor cells in vitro. Activation of tumoricidal properties of monocytes may offer new strategies in brain tumor immunotherapy.

Introduction

The prognosis of patients with glioblastoma is still fatal. Standard treatment with surgery and radiation, and in addition chemotherapy, does not prolong survival time beyond 18 months.

The brain has no lymphatic system and is characterized by a lack of immunogenicity. Furthermore, entry of high-molecular drugs and proteins into the parenchyma is restricted by the blood-brain barrier. The brain is known to be a partially immunologically privileged site (for review, [7]). However, the central nervous system has complex relations with the immune system, and in many cases

[1] Neurochirurgische Universitätsklinik, Im Neuenheimer Feld 400, W–6900 Heidelberg, FRG.

Advances in Neurosurgery, Vol. 20
K. Piscol, M. Klinger, M. Brock (Eds.)

brain tumor growth is associated with a depression of cellular immunity [1, 6, 8]. To date, clinical trials with immunomodulators (TNF, IFN-β), lymphokine-activated killer cells (LAK), and tumor-infiltrating killer cells (TIL) did not show significant improvement or cure (for review, see [11, 12]). Therefore, we chose a new biological approach for immunotherapy: the monocyte-macrophage activation.

In vitro and in vivo experiments with activated human peripheral blood monocytes against extracerebral tumors demonstrate enhanced tumoricidal activity [2, 5], whereas normal cells stay unharmed [3]. The monocytes can be activated with biological response modifiers (BRM). Activated monocytes release interleukin-1 (IL-1) and TNFα. Monocytes immigrate into the tumor site. Previous investigators could demonstrate that malignant brain tumors are infiltrated by numerous macrophages. Immunohistochemical studies revealed that these macrophages do not express IL-1 or TNFα [9].

The purpose of our study was the activation of monocytes against malignant glioma cells in vitro. Furthermore, we determined the most effective single agents and combinations of BRMs for stimulation of monocytes.

Materials and Methods

Target Cells

Seven human glioblastoma cell lines (HeRo, T508, T739, T829, T1026, T1083, T1115), one human brain metastasis cell line of a bronchial adenocarcinoma (T1020), as well as one human melanoma cell line (A375-P), which served as control, were used as target cells. All cell lines were free of mycoplasma. Cell cultures were maintained on plastic in BME and 10% heat-inactivated FCS and incubated in 5% CO_2 and 95% air at 37°C.

Isolation and Activation of Human Blood Monocytes

All reagents were free of endotoxin as measured by Limulus-Amebocyte-Lysate assay (Pyroquant, Walldorf; sensitivity < 0.06 ng LPS/ml). Mononuclear cells were isolated from peripheral blood of healthy donors by centrifugation at 400 g for 30 min on Ficoll and at 1000 g for 20 min on 54% Percoll. Monocytes were obtained with a purity of 65%–85% (as determined by Hemacolor and peroxidase staining). They were allowed to adhere to tissue microtiter plates at a concentration of 2×10^5 cells/200 μl per well for 2 h at 37°C in 5% CO_2 atmosphere. The wells were rinsed three times with medium at 37°C to remove nonadherent cells. The remaining cells (purity $> 97\%$ monocytes) were incubated in medium alone, in medium containing 1 μg lipopolysaccharide (LPS) with 10 U IFN-γ or several BRMs, such as human recombinant IFN-γ and IFN-β (Bioferon, Laupheim), human recombinant TNFα (Boehringer, Mannheim), LPS from *E. coli* 0111:B4, and *N*-acetyl-muramyl-Dalanyl-*D*-isoglutamine (MDP; Sigma, Deisenhofen). After 24 h the monocytes were washed four times to remove the BRMs.

Monocyte Cytotoxicity Assay

Target cells in their exponential growth phase were incubated with the appropriate supplemented BME medium containing 1 μCi [^{3}H]methylthymidine/ml for 24 h. The cells were washed twice and incubated for an additional hour at 37°C, washed again, and incubated on ice to remove labeled DNA precursors. The cells were harvested by short-time trypsination and washed twice. Labeled cells were resuspended in endotoxin-free medium (RPMI 1640 and suppl.). The cells were plated into microtiter plates providing a monocyte:tumor cell ratio of 20:1. The cells were incubated for 24 h, washed, and incubated for an additional 48 h. Adherent, viable cells were lysed with 0.1 *N* NaOH. The radioactivity of the lysate was measured in a beta counter.

The cytotoxic activity of the monocytes was calculated as follows:

$$\% \text{ Cytotoxicity} = \frac{100 \times (M_{DPM} - A_{DPM})}{M_{DPM}}$$

(M_{DPM} = DPM target cells alone; A_{DPM} = DPM target cells and monocytes)

Statistical Analysis

All data represent means of triplicates of three independent experiments. The statistical significance was determined by Student's two-tailed *t* test.

Results and Discussion

To evaluate the question of whether monocytes are able to kill glioblastoma cell lines, we established the above-described assay to measure monocyte tumor cytotoxicity (MTC). As glioblastoma cell line we used the HeRo cell line. The A375-P melanoma cell line is well-known in monocyte assays and served as control. The killing mechanism of activated monocytes requires close cell to cell contact [4] and is a time-dependent process [2]. It has been described earlier that glioma cells are less sensitive in short-time assays [10]. Therefore, we determined in our first experiments the time for MTC on glioma cells. Target cell lysis of A375-P and HeRo cells by activated monocytes began after 16 h of cocultivation and nearly reached its maximum after 72 h of cocultivation, as shown in Fig. 1. Only activated monocytes (here: LPS with IFN-γ) were able to kill target cells. Nonactivated monocytes did not show MTC rates exceeding 12%. Another determinant is the relative number of effector cells to target cells. We found an effector:target radio

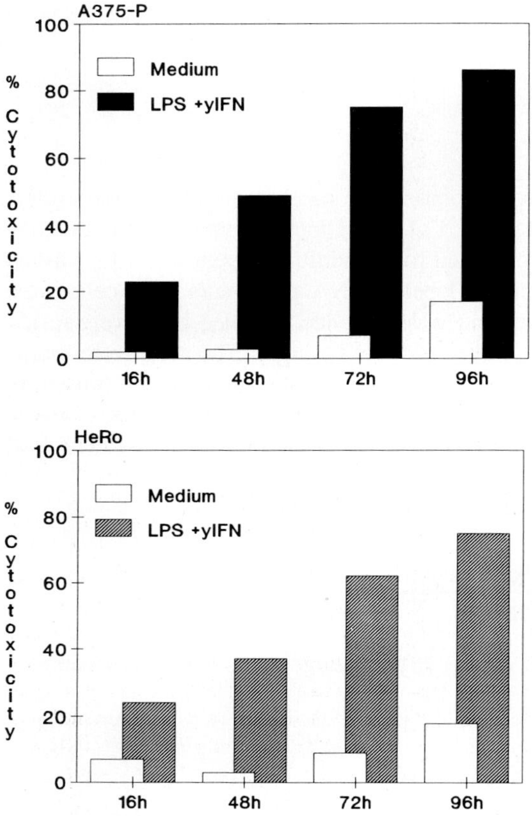

Fig. 1. Cytotoxicity of activated monocytes depending on the time of cocultivation. Monocytes were incubated in medium alone or medium containing 1 μg LPS with 10 IFN-γ/ml for 24 h. [^{3}H]methyl-thymidine-labeled A375-P or HeRo cells were added. The cells were washed and lysed after different times of cocultivation. The differences between stimulated and non-stimulated monocytes are significant with $P \leq 0.01$ for the incubation period of 16 h and with ≤ 0.001 for > 16 h

dependent killing of A375-P and HeRo cells by activated monocytes (Fig. 2). The 20:1 ratio was chosen for the following assays since it showed the highest increase in MTC.

Different BRMs were used to stimulate monocytes. The activation with 1 μg LPS + 10 U IFN-γ/ml served as positive control, as negative control medium alone. We used seven glioblastoma cell lines and one brain metastasis cell line. A representative part of our results is shown in Table 1 and Fig. 3.

To examine dose-dependent effects, we stimulated monocytes with one agent in different concentrations. After activation with IFN-γ, IFN-β, and TNFα, dose-dependent MTC was observed. IFN-β and TNFα yielded high MTC rates. To enhance MTC we examined the effect of the combination of different BRMs. The combinations IFN-β with MDP, IFN-β with TNFα, and MDP with TNFα (data not shown) did not result in enhancement of MTC. Nearly all effects were lower than the effects of single agents. However, a significant increase was measured using the combinations of IFN-γ with IFN-β, IFN-γ with MDP, and IFN-γ with

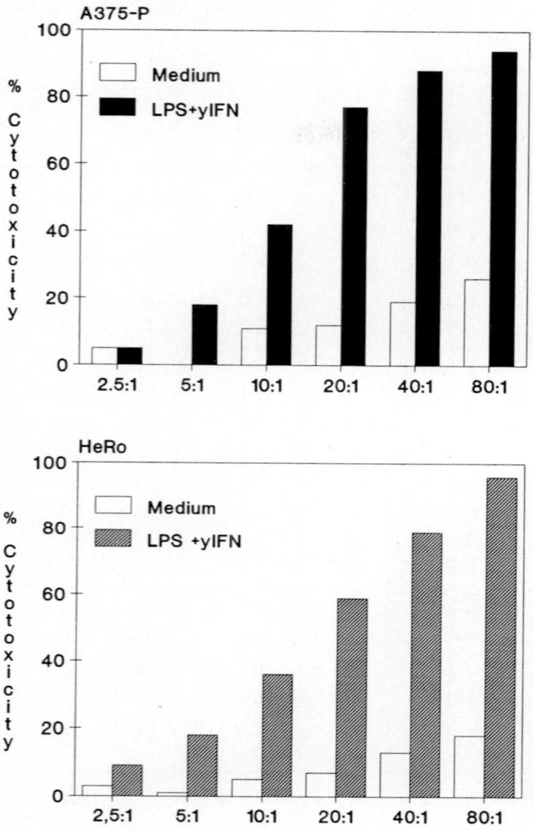

Fig. 2. Cytotoxicity of activated monocytes depending on the ratio of monocytes (effector) to A375-P and HeRo target cells. Different concentrations of monocytes (2.5×10^4, 5×10^4, 10×10^4, 20×10^4, 40×10^4, 80×10^4) were incubated in medium alone or medium containing 1 μg LPS with 10 U IFN-γ/ml for 24 h. 1×10^4 [^{3}H]methylthymidine-labeled A375-P or HeRo cells were added. The cells were washed and lysed after 72 h of cocultivation. The values between activated and nonactivated monocytes are significant with $P \leq 0.01$ for ratios 5:1 and 10:1 and with $P \leq 0.001$ for 20:1, 40:1, and 80:1

TNFα. MTC stimulated by IFN-γ with IFN-β and IFN-γ with TNFα showed dose dependency. All brain tumor cell lines demonstrated highest susceptibility either to IFN-γ with IFN-β or to IFN-γ with TNFα activated monocytes. The combinations of IFN-γ with MDP and IFN-γ with TNFα are already known to activate murine macrophages and human monocytes to the tumoricidal state [3, 13] and to inhibit spontaneous lung metastases of extracerebral cancers in mice.

Conclusions

We could demonstrate that unstimulated monocytes did not kill human glioblastoma cell lines. After incubation with LPS, IFN-γ, IFN-β, and TNFα cytotoxic effects of monocytes were dose dependent. The combination of activators led to a change of cytotoxicity rates: (a) IFN-γ in combination with other BRMs enhanced MTC; highest cytotoxicity rates were found using the combinations of IFN-γ with IFN-β

Table 1. Cytotoxicity of BRM-stimulated human peripheral blood monocytes against three glioblastoma cell lines (HeRo, T508, T739)

Cell line	HeRo	T508	T739
Stimulus/ml	% ± SD	% ± SD	% ± SD
Medium	5 ± 1.7	5 ± 5.0	6 ± 3.7
1 μg LPS	53 ± 2.9		
1 μg LPS + 10 U IFN-γ	62 ± 4.1	51 ± 5.1	45 ± 0.6
10000 U IFN-γ	39 ± 6.5	26 ± 1.6	26 ± 5.8
1000 U IFN-γ	17 ± 5.8	22 ± 2.2	13 ± 1.3
100 U IFN-γ	7.6 ± 5.1	3.4 ± 4.1	7 ± 4.0
10000 U IFN-β	60 ± 8.7	42 ± 6.6	51 ± 7.8
1000 U IFN-β	46 ± 5	36 ± 3.6	45 ± 4.6
100 U IFN-β	20 ± 1.5	11 ± 2.3	13 ± 0.6
10000 U TNF	74	65	54
1000 U TNF	73 ± 0.4	60 ± 5.9	51 ± 3.3
100 U TNF	47 ± 4.7	35 ± 2.4	29 ± 4.2
10 U TNF	14 ± 0.5	11 ± 7.7	5 ± 3.0
1000 U IFN-γ + 1000 U TNF	77 ± 2.5	64 ± 5.5	58 ± 11
100 U IFN-γ + 100 U TNF	63 ± 7.0	36 ± 3.6	51 ± 7.6
1000 U IFN-γ + 1000 U IFN-β	66 ± 4.4	46 ± 3.6	58 ± 7.6
100 U IFN-γ + 100 U IFN-β	46 ± 1.0	25 ± 4.9	42 ± 5.0
1000 U IFN-γ + 100 ng MDP	33 ± 1.6	28 ± 2.6	24 ± 8.9

Monocytes were incubated with the BRMs (LPS = 1 μg LPS + 10 U IFN-γ/ml; IFN-γ = 1000 U IFN-γ/ml; IFN-β = 1000 U IFN-β/ml; MDP = 100 ng MDP/ml; TNF = 1000 U TNFα/ml) for 24 h. 1×10^4 [^{3}H]methylthymidine-labeled target cells were added. The cells were washed and lysed after 72 h of cocultivation.

and TNF-γ with TNF; (b) other combinations were mainly less effective. Monocyte killing varied between different cell lines. However, the patterns of activation were comparable. The tumoricidal effects of monocytes provide a new model for immunotherapy against brain tumors, especially malignant gliomas. Further investigations to study monocyte tumoricidal properties as well as in vivo studies are under way.

References

1. Brooks WH, Caldwell HD, Mortara RH (1974) Immune responses in patients with gliomas. Surg Neurol 2:419–423
2. Bucana C, Hoyer LC, Hobbs B, Breesman S, McDaniel M, Hanna MG Jr (1976) Morphological evidence for the translocation of lysosomal organells from cytotoxic macrophages into the cytoplasm of tumor target cells. Cancer Res 36:4444–4458

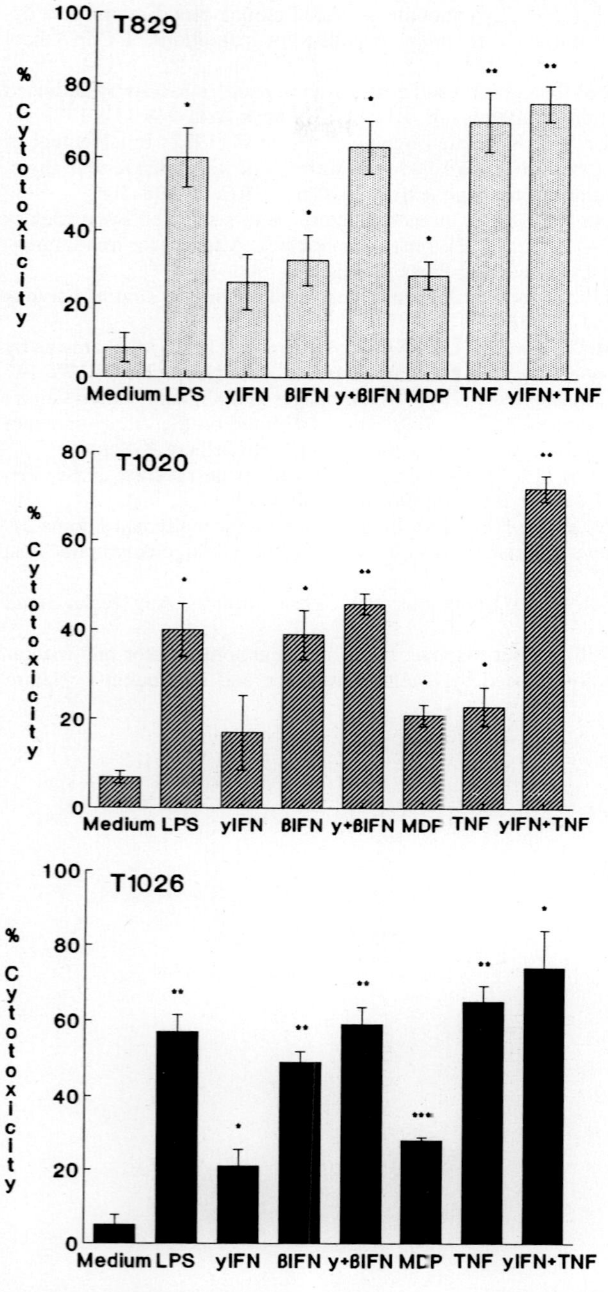

Fig. 3. Cytotoxicity of BRM-stimulated human peripheral blood monocytes against the glioblastoma cell lines T829 and T1026 and the metastasis cell line T1020. Monocytes were incubated in RPMI 1640 medium with or without BRMs for 24 h. 1×10^4 [^{3}H]methylthymidine-labeled target cells were added. The cells were washed and lysed after 72 h of cocultivation

3. Fidler IJ, Kleinermann ES (1984) Lymphokine-activated human blood monocytes destroy tumor cells but not normal cells under cocultivation conditions. J Clin Oncol 2:937–943
4. Fidler IJ, Schroett AJ (1988) Recognition and destruction of neoplastic cells by activated macrophages: discrimination of altered self. Biochim Biophys Acta 948:151–173
5. Fidler IJ, Barnes Z, Fogler WE, Kirsh R, Bugelski P, Poste G (1982) Involvement of macrophages in the eradication of established metastases following intravenous injection of liposomes containing macrophage activators. Cancer Res 42:496–501
6. Fontana A, Bodmer S, Frei K (1987) Immunoregulatory factors secreted by astrocytes and glioblastoma cells, 91–121. In: Pick E (ed) Lymphokines. A forum for immunoregulatory cell products, vol 14. Academic Press, San Diego
7. Fuchs HE, Bullard DE (1988) Immunology of transplantation in the central nervous system. Appl Neurophysiol 51:278–296
8. Gateley MK, Glaser M, McGarron RM, Dick SJ, Dick MD et al. (1982) Mechanisms by which human gliomas may escape cellular immune attack. Acta Neurochir 64:175–197
9. Hihn R, Kirsch M, Kist A, Schackert G (1990) Macrophages in malignant human tumors of brain origin does not express TNFα or Il-1. Paper presented on the 7th symposium "Sektion experimentelle Krebsforschung" on April 10–12, Heidelberg, Germany
10. Malter M, Süss R, Fischer H (1987) Natural cytotoxic cells from rat liver and spleen kill human glioma cells. J Cancer Res Clin Oncol 113:498–501
11. Merchant RE, Ellison MD, Young HF (1990) Immunotherapy for malignant glioma using human recombinant interleukin-2 (rIl-2) for and activated autologous lymphocytes. J Neuro Oncol 8:173–188
12. Sawamura Y, Tribolet N de (1990) Immunobiology of brain tumors. Adv Techn Stand Neurosurgery 17:3–502
13. Philip R, Epstein LB (1986) Tumor necrosis factor as immunomodulator and mediator of monocyte cytotoxicity induced by itself, γ-interferon and interleukin-1. Nature 323:86–89

Temporary Middle Cerebral Artery Clipping: Pathophysiological Investigation on the Effect of Mannitol and Nimodipine: A Model for Aneurysm Surgery

E. Rickels, M. R. Gaab, and H. E. Heissler[1]

Introduction

There are ethical and practical reasons to develop a model of reversible temporary focal ischemia in small animals especially to study the efficiency of drugs during aneurysm surgery in a sufficient number of animals. For ischemia caused by trapping cerebral arteries the decrease in extracellular calcium is an indicator for the cell damage. On the other hand, the increase in extracellular potassium shows the cell membrane leakage.

Material and Method

Male Sprague rats were anesthetized with xylazine (6 mg/kg body weight) and ketamine (100 mg/kg body weight) intraperitoneally. After skin incision the left zygomatic arch and the upper mandibular ramus were removed. A small lateral craniotomy was performed and the dura resected. The middle cerebral artery (MCA) was ligated where it crosses the inferior cerebral vein to prevent collateral blood flow. Then the MCA was separated from the arachnoid tissue proximally to the lentriculostriatal artery. Thus, a small clip can be placed near the origin of the MCA.

Heart rate and blood pressure were measured. The rCBF was estimated by laser Doppler flowmetry. The extracellular potassium and calcium concentrations were measured by ion-selective microelectrodes. The MCA was clipped for 1 h. After 1 h of reperfusion the brain was fixated and the volume of infarction was measured in serial sections. The randomized study was divided into three groups: control group ($n = 15$), nimodipine group ($n = 11$), and mannitol group ($n = 15$). The mannitol group was treated with 0.03 ml/min per kilogram body weight of 20% mannitol solution and the nimodipine group was given 30 μg/min per kilogram body weight. The treatment started 5 min before clipping the MCA.

[1] Neurochirurgische Klinik, Medizinische Hochschule Hannover, Konstanty-Gutschow-Str. 8, W–3000 Hannover 61, FRG.

Advances in Neurosurgery, Vol. 20
K. Piscol, M. Klinger, M. Brock (Eds.)

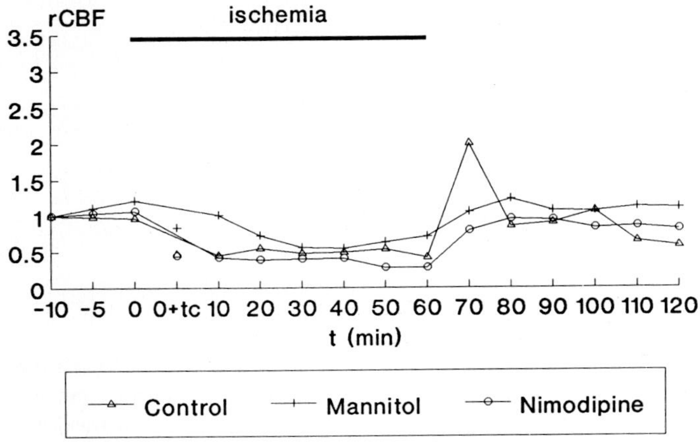

Fig. 1. Regional cerebral blood flow during ischemia and reperfusion

Results

Blood pressure and heart rate remained constant throughout the experiment in all animals. The rCBF showed a breakdown immediately after clipping the MCA. After removal of the clip, an initial hyperperfusion was followed by hypoperfusion in the control group. In contrast, there was an almost normal flow during the reperfusion time in the treatment groups (Fig. 1).

The extracellular postassium started at a level of 4 mmol/liter in all animals. The potassium rose up to 35 mmol/liter immediately after clipping and did not reach baseline values after reopening the MCA in the control and mannitol groups. Only in the nimodipine group was the increase in potassium slower. This can be demonstrated by the differential of the concentration changes over time (Fig. 2). All animals showed a decrease in extracellular calcium during ischemia, but returned to starting levels during reperfusion. In the mannitol group and especially in the nimodipine group, the animals started at a significantly higher level than in the control group and never reached critical values (Fig. 3). The infarction volumes ranged from 20% of total brain volume in controls to 15% in the nimodipine group. In the mannitol group, the infarction was only 11% of the whole brain (Fig. 4).

Discussion

A model of permanent focal ischemia in rats was established by Tamura et al. and modified by Bederson et al. We introduce a model of temporary focal ischemia in rats which allows the study of the pathophysiology caused by trapping during aneurysm surgery. The great pathological differences between general and focal ischemia are caused by the fact that general ischemia happens in a closed compartment while focal ischemia occurs in an area which still has an exchange of energy

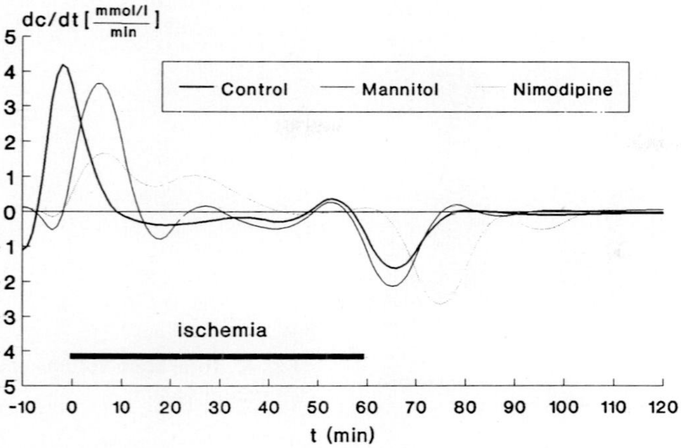

Fig. 2. Change in the differential of potassium concentration over time

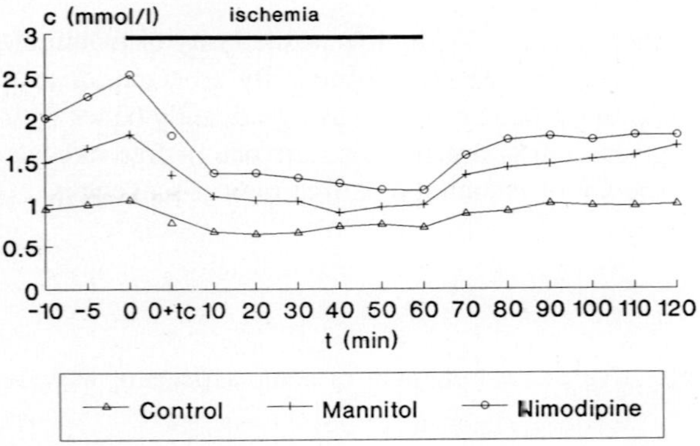

Fig. 3. Change in calcium concentration over time

and electrolytes to the surrounding area. Therefore, the results in focal ischemia are worse in comparison with general ischemia. Calcium influx in ischemic cells is regarded as one of the main reasons of cell damage. Calcium initiates the disaggregation of microtubuli and the metabolism of the arachidonic acid as well as the increase of free radicals [8]. Therefore, calcium antagonists promise to be an efficient treatment of ischemia. The breakdown of energy supply during ischemia is followed by depolarization of the plasma membrane indicated by an efflux of potassium [1, 3]. Nimodipine treatment is a way to stabilize the membrane for a short period. This might be the reason for the good results of nimodipine treatment in different animals models [4, 7, 11]. The postischemic hyperperfusion followed by a hypoperfusion caused by an intravasal coagulopathy [5] can be treated by mannitol and nimodipine. The infarct reduction in the mannitol-treated animals as

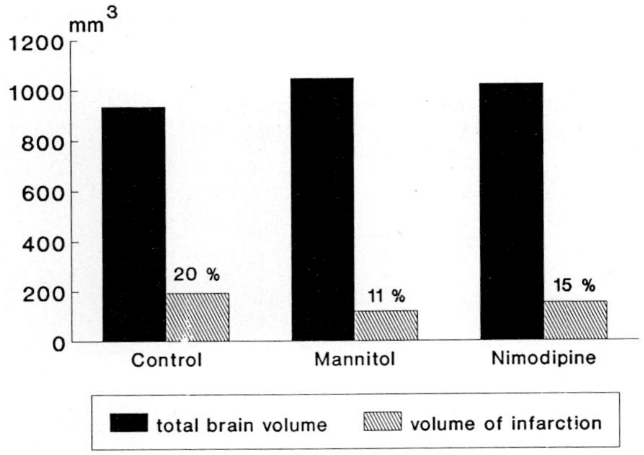

Fig. 4. Total brain volume and infarction volume

well as the better reperfusion cannot be explained by hyperosmolarity of mannitol. Magover et al. gave a glucose infusion of the same osmolarity as mannitol in a heart ischemia model. The function of the heart muscle was significantly better with mannitol. The experiments of Suzuki demonstrated the occurrence of free radicals in cerebral ischemia and the efficiency of mannitol as a free radical scavenger.

Conclusion

Mannitol and nimodipine are effective in the treatment of some aspects of temporary ischemia in the rat model.

References

1. Astrup J, Rehncrona S, Siesjö BK (1980) The increase in extracellular potassium concentration in the ischemic brain in relation to the preischemic functional activity and cerebral metabolic rate. Brain Res 199:161–174
2. Bederson JB, Pitts LH, Tsuij M, Nishimura MC, Davis RL, Bartkowski H (1986) Rat middle cerebral artery occlusion: Evaluation of the model and development of a neurologic examination. Stroke 17:472–476
3. Hansen AJ, Nedergaard M (1988) Brain ion homeostasis in cerebral ischemia. Neurochem Pathol 9:195–209
4. Harris RJ, Symon L, Branston NM (1982) Changes in extracellular calcium activity in cerebral ischemia and the influence of a calcium antagonist. Acta Neurochir 65:292–293
5. Hossmann K-A (1987) Experimentelle Grundlagen der Ischämietoleranz des Hirnes. Z Kardiol (Suppl 4) 76:47–66
6. Magovern SR Jr, Bolling SF, Casale AS (1984) The mechanism of mannitol in reducing ischemic injury: Hyperosmolarity or hydroxyl scavenger. Circulation (Suppl 1) 70:191–195

7. Meyer EB, Anderson RE, Yaksh TL Sundt TM (1986) Effect of nimodipine on intracellular brain pH cortical blood flow and EEG in experimental focal cerebral ischemia. J Neurosurg 64:617–626
8. Siesjö BK (1984) Cerebral circulation and brain metabolism. J Neurosurg 60:883–908
9. Suzuki J (1987) Treatment of cerebral infarction. Springer, Wien New York, pp 108–141
10. Tamura A, Graham DI, McCulloch J, Teasdale GM (1981) Focal cerebral ischemia in rat: 1. Description of technique and early neuropathological consequences following middle cerebral artery occlusion. J Cereb Blood Flow Metab 1:53–60
11. Wong CMW, Haley EC Jr (1990) Calcium antagonists: Stroke therapy coming of age. Stroke 21:495–501

Experimental Peripheral Nerve Regeneration: Interposition of Placenta-Amnion Membrane and Umbilical Cord Versus Autologous Transplantation

H. Müller, T. Dombert, and H. Arnold[1]

The macromolecule laminin, first described by R. Timpl in 1979 [11], has been shown to be the most potent neurite outgrowth promoting factor in cell culture experiments [2, 4] and in vivo [1, 6–8] known so far. In vivo, it occurs substrate-bound to basal lamina structures. The question arises whether the reported experimental findings have implications for future clinical nerve repair and regeneration.

We report here on a series of experiments where laminin-containing biosubstrates such as placenta-amnion membrane and umbilical cord were used to bridge defined gaps of transected rabbit peripheral nerves. The regeneration success was measured by electrophysiological and histological means and compared to autologous grafting as the supposed "standard" routine method.

Material and Methods

The tibial and peroneal nerves of 30 New Zealand White rabbits were transected microsurgically under general anesthesia. A 5-mm piece of nerve was removed, then replaced by a 10-mm long transplant, held in place by a few 10×0 atraumatic epineurial sutures. As transplants were used: an autologous piece of nerve from the animal's contralateral side ($n = 12$), homologous placenta-amnion membrane arranged longitudinally ($n = 12$), and homologous umbilical cord ($n = 6$). The homologous materials were all pretreated with ammonium hydroxide to reduce antigeneicity, according to the method described by Liotta et al. [3].

After 3 months (91 days), the animals were reanesthetized and evaluated by neurographic and evoked motor response measurements (data to be reported elsewhere). For histology, specimens from the center of the regenerated nerve, as well as from proximal and distal sites of the injured nerve, were cut and embedded in epon. Also, some uninjured normal nerves were sampled as controls. Semithin sections of all specimens were examined by light microscopy and evaluated with the aid of a Kontron Videoplan morphometric device.

[1] Neurochirurgische Klinik der Medizinischen Universität zu Lübeck, Ratzeburger Allee 160, W–2400 Lübeck 1, FRG.

Advances in Neurosurgery, Vol. 20
K. Piscol, M. Klinger, M. Brock (Eds.)

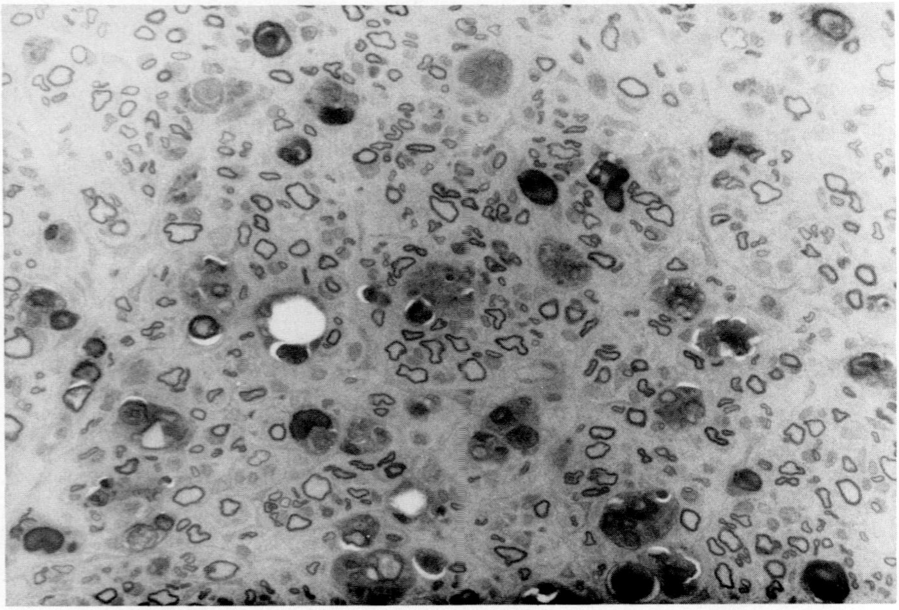

Fig. 1. Semithin section of autologous transplant: largely isomorphic axonal distribution besides myelin debris. Toluidine blue, ×400

Histological Results

Axonal regeneration was similar in both the examined peripheral nerves. Axons were distributed

- In a largely isomorphic pattern in autologous transplants (AT) (Fig. 1),
- More heterogenously and preferentially along remnants of basal lamina in placenta-amnion membrane grafts (rbAM) (Fig. 2),
- Throughout the connective tissue of umbilical cord (rbUC) structures (the so-called Wharton's substance) (Fig. 3).

Autologous transplants appeared to be surrounded by perineuriumlike circumferential cells, whereas in regenerated amnion membrane we could not observe any such structure forming a border to the surrounding wound. Furthermore, the amnion membrane as the outer layer of umbilical cord could not substitute for a perineurial sheath. As one consequence, this led to pronounced neuroma formation distal to the transplanted substrates in the latter groups.

Computer-aided morphometric analysis did not reveal statistically significant differences between the experimental groups in numeric terms. However, within the transplanted structure such an analysis could appear rather problematic when inhomogeneity of axonal distribution was encountered. Figure 4 shows, as an example, the caliber spectrum of myelinated fascicles in peroneal nerves distal to the

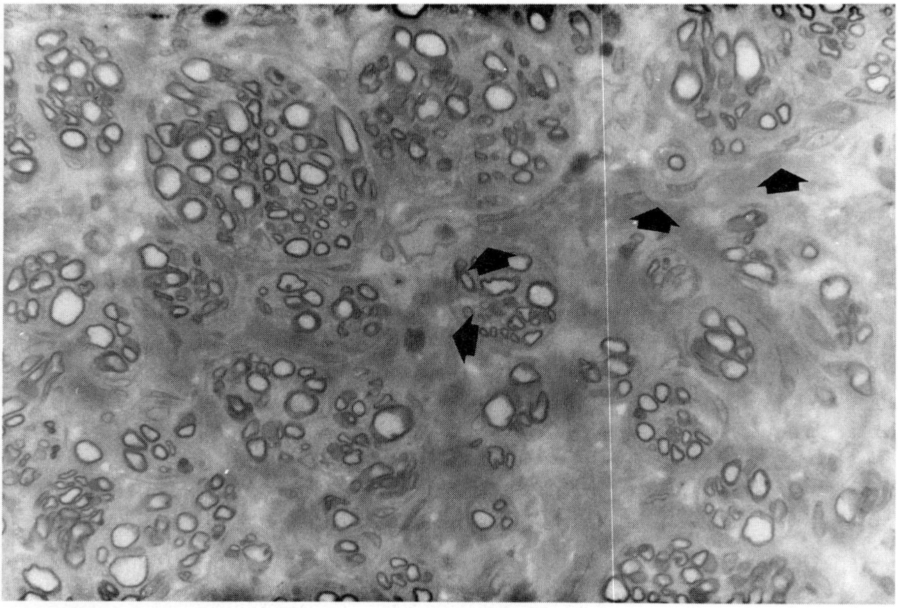

Fig. 2. Nerve regeneration through amnion membrane matrix: heterogeneously growing axons preferentially along remnants of basal lamina structures (*arrows*). ×400

transplantation site. The normally bimodal spectrum is shifted towards a unimodal distribution and smaller diameters. This can be considered a rather classical finding of numerous regeneration studies [5, 9, 10].

Conclusions

Laminin-containing biosubstrates of nonneural origin, e.g. amnion membrane and umbilical cord matrices, do promote axonal regeneration. When studied in an experimental paradigm like the rodent (rabbit) peripheral nerve transection and transplantation model, highly significant numerical differences of axonal regeneration parameters were observed when these matrices were compared to autologous nerve transplants. However, nerve transplants still appear to be slightly superior when histological features such as perineurial scarring or neuroma formation are considered.

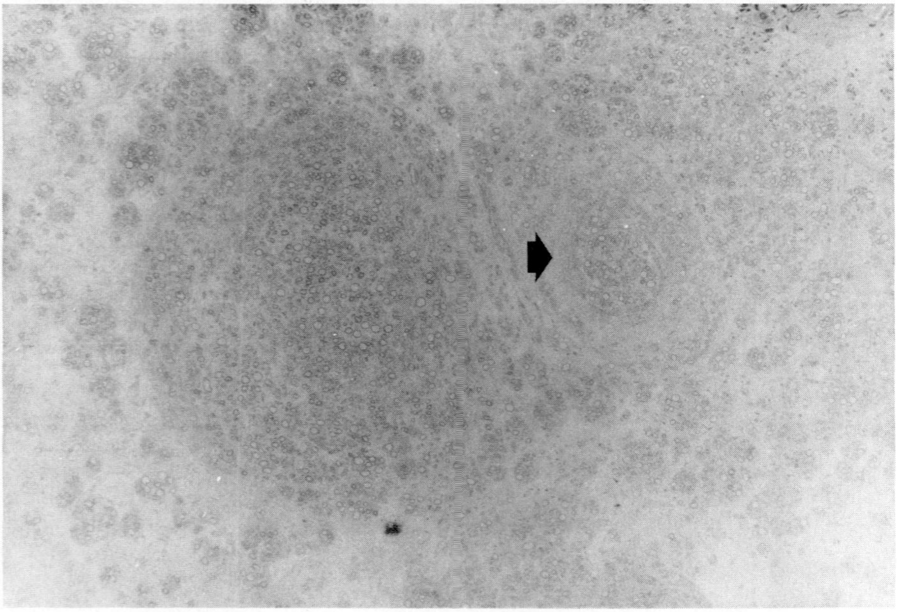

Fig. 3. Low magnification (×400) of umbilical cord graft to demonstrate regrowing axons throughout a central vessel (*see arrow*) and within Wahrton's substance

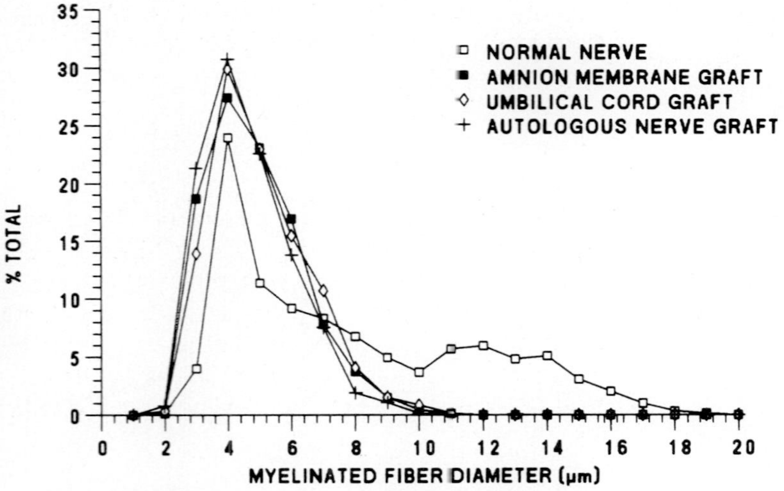

Fig. 4. Distribution of fiber diameters 2 mm distal to the graft (peroneal nerve)

References

1. Danielsen N, Müller H, Williams LR, Manthrope M, Davis GE, Varon S (1988) Rat amnion membrane matrix as a substratum for regenerating axons from peripheral and central neurons: Effects in a silicone chamber model. Dev Brain Res 39:39–50
2. Davis GE, Manthorpe M, Engvall E, Varon S (1985) Isolation and characterization of rat schwannoma neurite promoting factor: Evidence that the factor contains laminin. J Neurosci 5:2552–2571
3. Liotta LA, Lee CW, Morakis DJ (1980) New method for preparing large surfaces of intact human basement membrane for tumor invasion studies. Cancer Lett 11:141–142
4. Manthorpe M, Engvall E, Ruoslahti E, Longo FM, Davis GE, Varon S (1983) Laminin promotes neuritic regeneration from cultured peripheral and central neurons. J Cell Biol 97:1882–1890
5. Morris JH, Hudson AR, Weddel G (1972) A study of degeneration and regeneration in divided rat sciatic nerve based on electron microscopy. IV. Changes in fascicular microtopography, perineurium and fibroblasts. Z Zellforsch 124:165–203
6. Müller H (1988) Further evaluation of the effects of laminin, testosterone, ganglioside GM1, and catalase on early growth in rat nerve regeneration chambers. Exp Neurol 101:228–233
7. Müller H (1990) Biochemical manipulation of the microenvironment in experimental nerve regeneration chambers. In: Samii M (ed) Peripheral nerve lesions. Springer, Berlin Heidelberg New York Tokyo, pp 81–87
8. Müller H, Williams LR, Varon S (1986) Nerve regeneration chamber: Evaluation of exogenous agents applied by multiple injections. Brain Res 413:320–326
9. Müller H, Shibib K, Modrack M, Friedrich H (1987) Nerve regeneration in synthetic and autogenous interfascicular grafts: II. morphometric analysis. Exp Neurol 98:161–169
10. Ramon y Cajal S (1928) Degeneration and regeneration of the nervous system. Hafner Publications, New York
11. Timpl R, Rohde H, Robey PG, Rennard SI, Foidart J-M, Martin GR (1979) Laminin – a glycoprotein from basement membranes. J Biol Chem 254:9933–9937

Growth Characteristics and Proliferation Parameters of Invasive Pituitary Adenomas*

M. Buchfelder[1], R. Fahlbusch[1], E. F. Adams[1], M. Roth[2], and P. Thierauf[2]

Introduction

Pituitary adenomas arise from anterior pituitary cells and usually displace, rather than invade, the surrounding anatomical structures. We have considered pituitary adenomas as invasive if they have infiltrated or even perforated the normal anatomical confines of the pituitary gland, namely, the sella diaphragm, the basal dura, or the cavernous sinuses. Estimates of the incidence of invasion in pituitary adenomas have varied, particularly between those reported by neurosurgeons [4] and pathologists [10, 11]. Histological studies reveal invasion in up to 85% of adenomas. This incidence is much lower (up to 35%) in surgical series. Clinical observations do not indicate whether aggressive growth is the result of an increased proliferative potential of pituitary adenoma cells. We have therefore addressed this question by comparing invasive characteristics with laboratory assessments of proliferation parameters.

Patients and Methods

During the last 8 years, 1121 operations for pituitary adenomas were performed in the Department of Neurosurgery, University of Erlangen-Nürnberg. Among them were 1024 transsphenoidal and 97 transcranial operations. About 90% of the tumors were treated by transsphenoidal surgery. The following analysis of the invasive cases is based on this surgical material.

To determine how reliable our surgical impression on invasion is, we have performed biopsies of the basal dura which we in Erlangen call the endosteum during transsphenoidal surgery. In contrast to other authors [11], we have additionally performed immunohistological examinations of the dura specimens after obtaining conventionally stained sections in selected cases.

To obtain a biochemical estimate of the proliferative activity, the replication enzyme for DNA (α-DNA polymerase) was measured. This technique has been successfully applied to the study of proliferation in breast tumor tissue [3]. A total

---

* Supported by Johannes and Frieda Marohn Stiftung (Buch/90).

[1] Neurochirurgische Klinik der Universität Erlangen-Nürnberg, Schwabachanlage 6, W-8520 Erlangen, FRG.

[2] Pathologisches Institut der Universität Erlangen-Nürnberg, W-8520 Erlangen, FRG.

Advances in Neurosurgery, Vol. 20
K. Piscol, M. Klinger, M. Brock (Eds.)

of 81 tumors was assessed. Human pituitary tumor tissue was homogenized and the cytosols were prepared by ultracentrifugation, after which the cytosolic DNA polymerase activity was assessed as the ability of the cytosols to promote the uptake of tritiated thymidine into activated calf thymus DNA [3].

A further estimate of proliferation was obtained by immunostaining with the antibody Ki-67 using frozen sections. A total of 87 tumors was assessed. The method was first described by Gerdes et al. [5] from Kiel and this is the origin of the abbrevation. The antibody is directed against a nuclear antigen which is present in all phases of the cell cycle except in the G_0 and the early G_1 phase [6]. The results were expressed as the percentage of positively staining nuclei.

Results

In the 1121 operations we found an invasion rate of 23.3%. Among 1024 transsphenoidal operations, 205 tumors (this is about 20%) were found to be invasive. At transcranial surgery, however, the percentage was much higher: 57.7% (Fig. 1). Among the different endocrinological diseases, invasion was most commonly found in Nelson's syndrome and thyrotropinomas. It was slightly less frequent in acromegaly and in inactive adenomas. In Cushing's disease, invasion was exceedingly rare. All acromegalic patients who required operations by both approaches within short intervals had invasive tumors, and the same was true for half of the inactive adenomas.

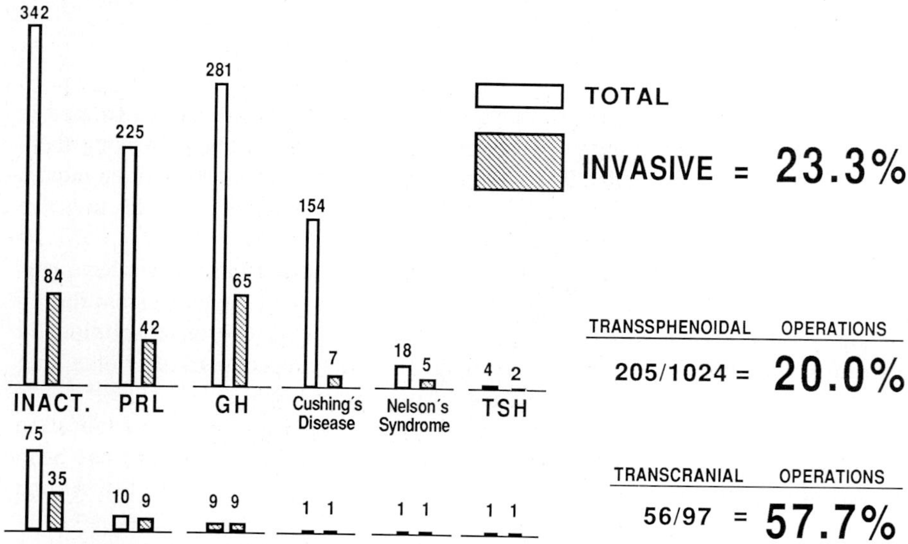

Fig. 1. Incidence of invasion in different types of pituitary adenomas operated upon via the transsphenoidal or transcranial route (1121 operations, 1 December 1982 – 31 December 1990)

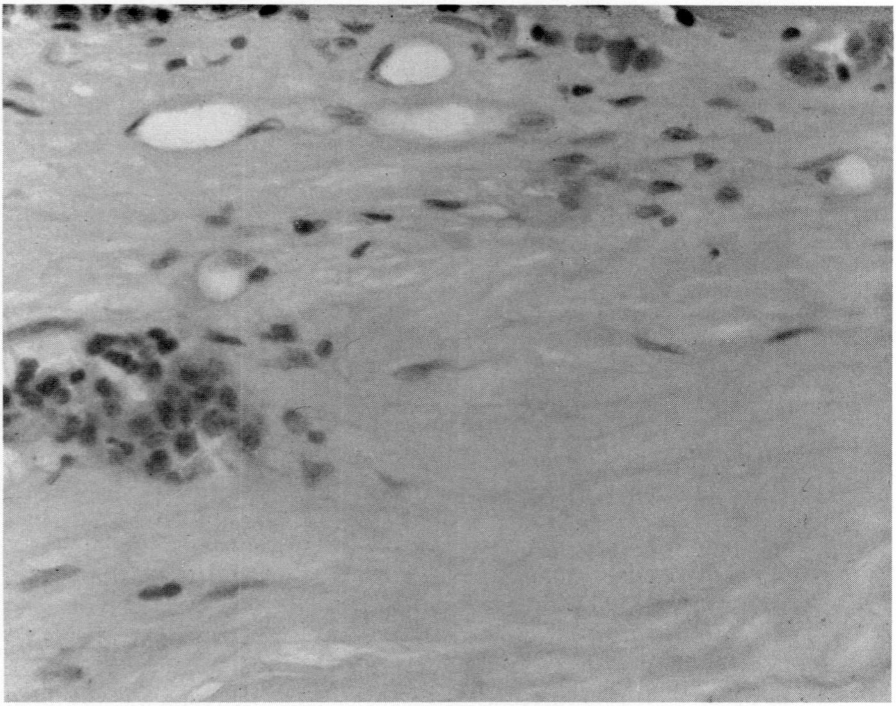

Fig. 2. Histological section of a dural biopsy revealing invasion by clumps of tumor cells within the fibrous layer of the endosteum

It is not surprising that the invasive character correlates very well to the tumor volume. Invasion was found in 2% of our microadenomas, 20% of the macroadenomas, and in 80% of the giant adenomas, when only cases undergoing primary surgery were considered.

Surgical invasion was found in 17% of the primary operations and in 28% of secondary operations, in which patients had had previous therapy for their pituitary adenoma. There was nearly no difference in the site of invasion, which was most commonly found into the cavernous sinus and rarely into the diaphragm only. Diffuse infiltration to all these structures was found in about one-third of the patients.

The histological examination of 310 basal dura specimens revealed that 199 were normal fibrous tissue and 111 showed some signs of invasion, e.g., clumps of cells within the fibrous layers of the basal dura (Fig. 2). The surgeon had recognized only 59 of these 111 tumors to be invasive.

By investigating the DNA polymerase activity in the adenoma tissue of 81 patients, it was shown that there is a significant difference of the replication enzyme activity when microadenomas and invasive pituitary macroadenomas were compared (Fig. 3). Enclosed macroadenomas and macroprolactinomas which were exposed to bromocriptine for some weeks or months before surgery showed a higher DNA polymerase activity as compared with noninvasive microadenomas. However, here the difference was not significant. Immunohistology for Ki-67 on frozen sections of adenoma tissue showed that there was a significant difference in Ki-67 positive cells when microadenomas and invasive macroadenomas were compared (Fig. 4). Enclosed macroadenomas were shown to have a somewhat higher Ki-67 positive cell rate but here the difference was not significant.

Discussion

Our figures on the incidence of invasion in a large surgical series of pituitary adenomas are basically compatible with findings in the literature [4, 9]. They represent the subjective impression of the surgeon during operation. It is, however, generally agreed that sometimes it is difficult to decide intraoperatively if the tumor is or is not invasive. Differences in patients who underwent different operative approaches simply reflect our selection criteria for transsphenoidal and transcranial surgery. There was an obvious correlation between the tumor size and the rate of invasion. Furthermore, irrespective of tumor size, invasion was found most frequently in adenomas with a defective feedback mechanism. The discrepancy found in evaluating endosteal biopsies suggests to us that in a considerable percentage of invasion is hidden to the surgeon [4, 10]. There has been considerable discussion whether these dura infiltrations represent ectopic pituitary tissue, but in functioning adenomas the

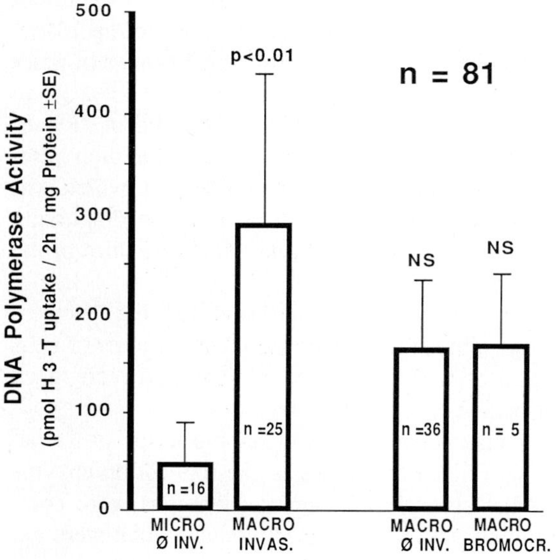

Fig. 3. DNA polymerase activity of noninvasive microadenomas (*MICRO ø INV.*, invasive (*MACRO INVAS.*) and noninvasive macroadenomas (*MACRO ø INV.*), and macroprolactinomas pretreated by bromocriptine (*MACRO BROMOCR.*). *NS*, not significant

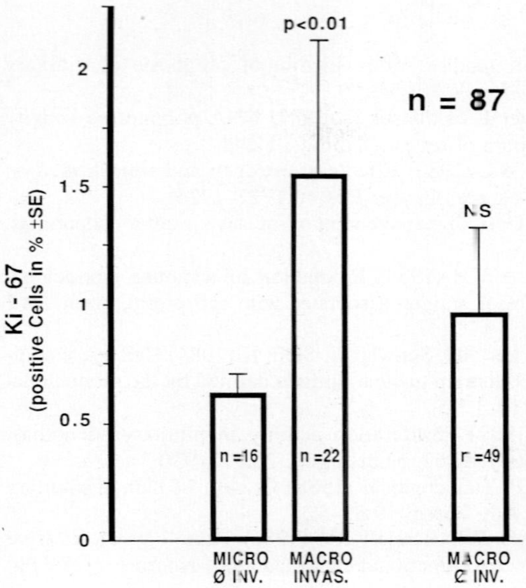

Fig. 4. Percentage of Ki-67 staining cells in noninvasive microadenomas (*MICRO ø INV.*) and invasive (*MACRO INVAS.*) and noninvasive macroadenomas (*MACRO ø INV.*). *NS*, not significant

histological impression that there is an unphysiological distribution of cells is confirmed by immunohistological findings [9]. Strongly positive immunostaining for the respective pituitary hormone in a secreting adenoma is good evidence that the dura infiltrations actually represent tumor infiltration into the endosteum. Assessing the DNA polymerase activity and immunostaining for Ki-67 are both widely accepted and sensitive methods to quantify proliferative activity. Assessing the rate of Ki-67 positive cells has already been applied to pituitary tumor by other authors [7, 8], while determining the DNA polymerase activity in human adenomas was introduced by our group [2], although it has been used to study estrogen-induced rat pituitary tumors [12]. Whereas others have shown that the determination of the mitosis rate is practically useless in these slowly growing tumors [1], our demonstration of two independent proliferation parameters basically documenting comparable results virtually rules out mere laboratory phenomena. Altogether these findings seem to support our concept that more aggressively growing tumors actually do have an increased growth potential. It is worth noting the potential practical and clinical use of laboratory assessment of proliferation in these benign tumors as described in this report. It may be possible to utilize DNA polymerase and Ki-67 measurement to predict the likelihood of regrowth or recurrence of pituitary adenomas, and thus which patients will require additional treatments and more careful postoperative observation.

References

1. Anniko M, Wersäll J (1988) DNA studies for prediction of prognosis of pituitary adenomas? Adv Biosci 69:45–52
2. Buchfelder M, Adams EF, Honegger J, Fahlbusch R (1989) DNA polymerase activity in human pituitary tumours. J Endocrinol Invest (Suppl 2) 12:44
3. Edwards DP, Methy SR, McGuire WL (1980) Effects of estrogen and antiestrogen on DNA polymerase in human breast cancer. Cancer Res 40:1722–1726
4. Fahlbusch R, Buchfelder M (1989) Current management of invasive pituitary adenomas. Contemp Neurosurg 11 (17):1–6
5. Gerdes J, Schwab U, Lemke H, Stein H (1983) Production of a mouse monoclonal antibody reactive with a human nuclear antigen associated with cell proliferation. Int J Cancer 31:13–20
6. Gerdes J, Lemke H, Baisch H, Wacker HH, Schwab U, Stein H (1984) Cell cycle analysis of a cell proliferation-associated human nuclear antigen defined by the monoclonal antibody Ki-67. J Immunol 133:1710–1715
7. Knosp E, Kitz K, Pernetzky A (1989) Proliferation activity in pituitary adenomas: Measurement by monoclonal antibody Ki-67. Neursurgery 25:927–930
8. Landolt AM, Shibata T, Kleihues P, Tuncdogan E (1988) Growth of human pituitary adenomas: Facts and speculations. Adv Biosci 69:53–62
9. Scheithauer BW, Kovasc KT, Laws ER, Randall RV (1986) Pathology of invasive pituitary tumors with special reference to functional classification. J Neurosurg 65:733–744
10. Selman WR, Laws ER, Scheithauer BW, Carpenter SM (1986) The occurrence of dural invasion in pituitary adenomas. J Neurosurg 64:402–407
11. Shaffi OM, Wrightson P (1975) Dural invasion by pituitary tumors. N Z Med J 81:386–390
12. Wiklund JA, Gorski J (1982) Genetic differences in estrogen-induced deoxyribonucleic acid synthesis in the rat pituitary: Correlations with pituitary tumor susceptibility. Endocrinology 111:1140–1149

Intraoperative Antibiotic Prophylaxis in Neurosurgery: A Prospective Randomized Trial in 840 Patients

J. Zentner[1], J. Gilsbach[2], and T. Gaillard[3]

Summary

The efficacy of a single dose of cefotiam as prophylaxis for postoperative infection was analyzed in a prospective randomized study of 840 patients undergoing either carniotomy (group I, $n=711$) or cerebrospinal fluid shunting (group II, $n=129$). The main interest was centered on the rate of bone flap infection and shunt sepsis requiring operative revision. Data were evaluated in the total groups and various subgroups formed for high risk patients. Our results show a highly significant difference for postoperative bone flap infection, with 0.3% in the cefotiam group versus 5.1% in the control group ($p < 0.001$). The overall rate of postoperative deep wound infections including meningitis and abscess (group I) was also significantly different (3.1% vs 9.0%, $p < 0.005$). This was also true for wound infections in high risk patients (3.1% vs 10.6%) as well as for postoperative sepsis and pneumonia. The overall rate of shunt infections (group II) was 7.5% in the cefotiam group and 12.9% in the control group, with the differences not being statistically significant either for the main group or for high risk subgroups. In summary, antibiotic prophylaxis has proven to be effective for prevention of postoperative infection in patients undergoing craniotomy. Although our results in shunt patients do not reach statistical significance, we also recommend single dose prophylaxis in these cases, since there is a clear difference of infection rate between patients receiving and not receiving the antibiotic.

Introduction

Postoperative infection rates in clean neurosurgical craniotomies range from 0.8% to 6.%, with 3%–4% being the expected average [2, 3, 7, 14, 17, 18, 24, 26, 28]. The occurrence of shunt infections usually varies between 10% and 15% [1, 10, 22, 27]. Nevertheless, antibiotic prophylaxis in neurosurgery has always been a controversial subject [12]. This controversy, however, mainly results from the lack of careful studies of its efficacy. Therefore, we have focused again on this issue with a prospective randomized trial in order to clarify the value of antibiotic

[1] Neurochirurgische Universitätsklinik, Sigmund-Freud-Str. 25, W–5300 Bonn 1, FRG.
[2] Neurochirurgische Klinik der RWTH, Pauwelstr. 30, W–5100 Aachen, FRG.
[3] Neurochirurgische Universitätsklinik, Hugstetter Str. 55, W–7800 Freiburg, FRG.

Advances in Neurosurgery, Vol. 20
K. Piscol, M. Klinger, M. Brock (Eds.)

prophylaxis in neurosurgery with respect to patients undergoing craniotomy and cerebrospinal fluid (CSF) shunting.

Patients and Methods

During 2- and 1-year periods, respectively, all patients undergoing either craniotomy ($n=918$, group I) or cerebrospinal fluid shunting ($n=134$, group II) in the Neurosurgical University Clinic Freiburg were enrolled in this prospective and randomized trial. Only clean or clean-contaminated cases were included. Randomization was achieved by computerized lists. Patients operated on more than once in this period were counted separately for each occasion, except for immediate reoperation due to complications. Cefotiam was administered intravenously in a single 2-g dose with induction of anesthesia. The surgical procedure was standardized. The patient's hair was totally shaved the day before the operation with an electrical razor and again immediately before surgery using a razor blade in the region of skin incision, which was prepared with a polyvidone-iodine solution. Data analyzed in particular were medical history, actual diagnoses, details on operation, intensive care and medical therapy, the postoperative course and infectious complications, including late results obtained 6 months after surgery. Infections were defined as deep wound infections and/or bacterial meningitis with clinical symptoms and bacterial contamination of CSF requiring surgical and/or antibiotic therapy. Data collection and evaluation was computerized (dBASE III+) using 118 singular items per case.

Final data were available in 711 patients of group I (craniotomy) and in 129 patients of group II (shunt).

Statistical analysis was based on the confirmation of structural equality and comparability of the cefotiam and control groups followed by χ^2-test with double-sided p.

Results

Group I: Craniotomy

The overall wound infection rate including meningitis and abscess formation was 11 out of 356 cases (3.1%) in the cefotiam group and 32 out of 355 cases (9.0%) in the control group. The difference is statistically significant ($p < 0.005$). Regarding bone flap infection alone, we found a 0.3% infection rate in the cefotiam group and 5.1% in the control group (Table 1).

Several subgroups were formed to evaluate the effect of cefotiam in high risk patients. The results are shown in Table 2. The total infection rate was 3.1% in the cefotiam group and 10.6% in the control group. The difference is statistically significant ($p < 0.005$).

We encountered 14 patients with postoperative sepsis. Five (1.4%) belonged to the cefotiam and nine (2.5%) to the control group. Postoperative pneumonia was

Table 1. Postoperative wound infections in 711 patients undergoing craniotomy (group I): the difference between the cefotiam and the control group is statistically significant ($p < 0.005$)

Postoperative wound infections	Patients Cefotiam ($n=356$)		Control ($n=355$)	
	n	%	*n*	%
No late results	28	7.9	22	6.2
Bone flap infection alone	1	0.3	18	5.1
Meningitis	5	1.4	9	2.5
Bone flap infection + meningitis	1	0.3	4	1.1
Shunt sepsis	3	0.8	–	–
Abscess	1	0.3	1	0.3
Total infections	11	3.1	32	9.0

Table 2. Postoperative wound infections in high risk patients of group I (craniotomy): the difference between the cefotiam and the control group is statistically significant ($p < 0.005$)

Risk factors	Patients Cefotiam		Control		Total
	n	%	*n*	%	
Malignant tumor	0	0	7	8.4	180
Preoperative steroids	3	3.8	13	17.6	152
Postoperative steroids	4	2.9	13	9.6	271
Severe internal disease	2	3.2	8	13.3	122
Reoperation	5	4.7	7	9.1	183
Total infections	14	3.1	28	10.6	

observed in 42 patients, 14 (3.9%) in the cefotiam group and 28 (7.9%) in the control group. The differences are statistically significant ($p < 0.01$ and $p < 0.05$, respectively).

Group II: Shunt

Among the 129 patients undergoing shunting procedures, 112 (86.8%) received va shunts, 13 (10.1%) vp shunts and 4 (3.1%) lp shunts. The total infection rate

Table 3. Postoperative infections in 129 patients undergoing cerebrospinal fluid shunting: the results for both normal risk and high risk patients are not statistically significant

Risk factors	Patients Cefotiam ($n=67$)		Control ($n=62$)		Total
	n	%	n	%	
Normal risk	1	4.3	3	14.3	44
High risk	4	9.1	5	12.2	85
Total	5	7.5	8	12.9	129

was 13 (10.1%), with five patients (7.5%) belonging to the cefotiam group and 8 (12.9%) to the control group. The difference is not statistically significant.

Evaluating the subgroups for high risk patients (internal disease, intensive care, steroid therapy) separately, we found infections in 4 of 44 patients (9.1%) in the cefotiam group and in 5 of 41 cases (12.2%) in the control group. The difference is not statistically significant (Table 3).

Discussion

There has been a great deal of interest and controversy regarding the value of routine perioperative antibiotic prophylaxis in clean neurosurgical procedures. Some uncontrolled studies have been reported which have not supported antibiotic prophylaxis [5, 19] or have reached indeterminate conclusions [1, 14, 23], while other studies have supported antibiotic prophylaxis [18, 20, 21, 25]. It was concluded at that time that existing information was inconclusive and supported the positions favoring and opposing antibiotic prophylaxis with equal weight [13].

Several controlled studies have focused on this issue again and suggested that perioperative antibiotic prophylaxis does indeed reduce the risk of postoperative wound infection in clean neurosurgical operations [4, 11, 16, 23]. Accordingly, our prospective randomized study shows a significant effect of a single dose of cefotiam administered with induction of anesthesia for prevention of postoperative wound infection in craniotomy both for the main group and for high risk subgroups. Moreover, postoperative sepsis and pneumonia were reduced significantly in the prophylaxis group. Although total infection rate was also reduced in shunt patients receiving prophylaxis (7.5% vs 12.9%), the difference is not statistically significant. Basically, infection rate can be expected to be higher in surgery involving implantation of a foreign body and connection of the ventricles to the atrium or peritoneum.

Therefore, only with a much higher number of patients might statistically significant results be expected.

The general principles of antibiotic prophylaxis are well established. The antibiotic must be specific for the organisms likely to cause postoperative infection, and administration should be started shortly before the operation so that maximal tissue levels are present at the time of skin incision [13]. The most studied regimen is that of Malis [15] using intramuscular gentamycin or tobramycin, intravenous vancomycin, and topical streptomycin. However, excellent results have also been reported with cephazolin, clindamycin, ampicillin, oxacillin and others [6, 8, 9, 20, 25]. As stated by Hains [13], no single regimen is likely to be the best in every hospital and a careful inspection of patterns of infection and types of organisms seen in the individual institution should lead to selection of an appropriate antibiotic for prophylaxis.

Cefotiam is a cephalosporin of the second generation which has a broad spectrum including staphylococci, beta-lactamase producing bacteria, and gram-negative bacteria. Cefotiam penetrates soft tissue and bone. On the basis of previously performed antibiograms cefotiam was considered to be an adequate antibiotic for prophylaxis in our hospital. No cases of allergy or serious side effects were observed in our 918 patients.

In conclusion, our results clearly demonstrate the efficacy of a single dose of cefotiam as a prophylaxis for postoperative infection in patients undergoing craniotomy. Although results in shunt patients do not reach statistical significance, the infection rate was lower in the prophylaxis group than in the control group. Therefore, single-dose antibiotic prophylaxis can also be recommended for patients undergoing CSF shunting.

References

1. Ajir F, Levin AB, Duff TA (1981) Effect of prophylactic methicillin on cerebrospinal fluid shunt infections in children. Neurosurgery 9:6–8
2. Balch E (1967) Wound infections complicating neurosurgical procedures. J Neurosurg 26:41–45
3. Blomstedt GC (1985) Infections in neurosurgery. Acta Neurochir (Wien) 78:81–90
4. Blomstedt GC, Kytta J (1988) Results of a randomized trial of vancomycin prophylaxis in craniotomy. J Neurosurg 69:216–220
5. Brandt RA, Feres H (1979) Antibioticos profilaticos em neurocirurgia. Arq Neuropsiquiatr 37:42–47
6. Bullock R, van Dellen JR, Kelebey W, Reinach SG (1988) A doubleblind placebo-controlled trial of perioperative prophylactic antibiotics for elective neurosurgery. J Neurosurg 69:687–691
7. Cruse PJE, Foord R (1973) A five-year prospective study of 23,649 surgical wounds. Arch Surg 107:206–210
8. Dempsey R, Rapp RP, Young B, Johnston S, Tibbs P (1988) Prophylactic parenteral antibiotics in clean neurosurgical procedures: a review. J Neurosurg 69:52–57
9. Djindjan M, Fevrier MJ, Otterbein G, Soussy JC (1986) Oxacillin prophylaxis in cerebrospinal fluid shunt procedures: results of a randomized open study in 60 hydrocephalic patients. Surg Neurol 25:178–180

10. Gardner BP, Gordon DS (1982) Postoperative infection in shunts for hydrocephalus: are prophylactic antibiotics necessary? Br Med J 284:1914–1915
11. Geraghty J, Feely M (1984) Antibiotic prophylaxis in neurosurgery. A randomized controlled trial. J Neurosurg 60:724–726
12. Haines SJ (1980) Systemic antibiotic prophylaxis in neurological surgery. Neurosurgery 6:355–361
13. Haines SJ (1989) Efficacy of antibiotic prophylaxis in clean neurosurgical operations. Neurosurgery 24:401–405
14. Haines SJ, Goodman ML (1982) Antibiotic prophylaxis of postoperative neurosurgical wound infection. J Neurosurg 56:103–105
15. Malis LI (1979) Prevention of neurosurgical infection by intraoperative antibiotics. Neurosurgery 5:339–343
16. Mollman HD, Haines SJ (1986) Risk factors for neurosurgical wound infection. A case control study. J Neurosurg 64:902–906
17. Quadery LA, Medlery AV, Miles J (1977) Factors affecting the incidence of wound infection in neurosurgery. Act Neurochir (Wien) 39:133–141
18. Quartey GRC, Polyzoidis K (1981) Intraoperative antibiotic prophylaxis in neurosurgery: a clinical study. Neurosurgery 8:669–671
19. Raggueneau JL, Cophiguon J, Kind A, Rey A, Goldstein A, Thurel C, Dematons C, George B, Roux FX (1983) Analyse des suites infectieuses de 1000 interventions neurochirurgicales incidence de l'antibiotherapie prophylactique. Neurochirurgie 29:229–233
20. Reale F, Biancotti R, De Falco D, Gambacorta D (1987) Antibiotic prophylaxis in neurosurgery. Acta Neurochir (Wien) 86:75–78
21. Savitz MH, Katz SS (1986) Prevention of primary wound infection in neurosurgical patients: a 10 year study. Neurosurgery 18:685–688
22. Schoenbaum SC, Gardner BP, Shillito J (1975) Infections of cerebrospinal fluid shunts: epidemiology, clinical manifestations, and their therapy. J Infect Dis 131:543–552
23. Shapiro M, Wald U, Simchen E, Pomeranz S, Zagzay N, Michowiz SD, Cahn SE, Wax Y, Shuval R, Kahane N, Sacks T, Shilit M (1986) Randomized clinical trial of intra-operative antimicrobial prophylaxis of infection after neurosurgical procedures. J Hosp Infect 8:283–295
24. Tenney JH, Vlahor D, Salcman M, Ducker T (1985) Wide variations in risk of wound infection following clean neurosurgery. J Neurosurg 62:243–247
25. Urciuoli R, Russo GL, Zeme S, Canotte M (1983) Traitment antibiotique prophylactique des complications infectieuses postoperatoires en neurochirurgie. Agressologie 24:237–238
26. Van EKG, Bakker FP, van Dulken H, Dijkmans BAC (1986) Infections after craniotomy: a retrospective study. J Infect 12:106–109
27. Venes JL (1976) Control of shunt infection: report of 150 consecutive cases. J Neurosurg 45:311–314
28. Wright RL (1966) A survey of possible etiologic agents in postoperative craniotomy infections. J Neurosurg 25:125–132

Subject Index

M. Samii, Hannover Medical School;
E. Knosp, University of Vienna

Approaches to the Clivus

Approaches to No Man's Land

1992. Approx. 180 pp. 122 figs. 4 tabs.
Hardcover ISBN 3-540-54015-6

A different kind of book! The clivus of the skull base is an area difficult to reach in neurosurgery, otorhinolaryngology, maxillo-facial surgery, plastic surgery, reconstructive surgery, and orthopedic surgery. It is for this reason that the various specialties have found different approaches for different operations.

This book shows the various approaches to the clivus. Each of the chapters shows a different approach; all of them follow the same format which includes a brief history, key aspects of anatomy, possible pathological processes, the surgical approach, and a summary with indications, limits, advantages and disadvantages.

Springer-Verlag
Berlin
Heidelberg
New York
London
Paris
Tokyo
Hong Kong
Barcelona
Budapest

Druck: Mercedesdruck, Berlin
Verarbeitung: Buchbinderei Lüderitz & Bauer, Berlin